BEST PRACTICES II
The Classroom As An Intervention Context

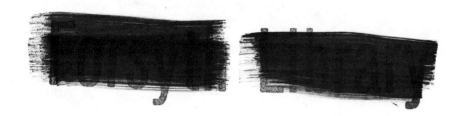

Katharine G. Butler, PhD
Editor, *Topics in Language Disorders*
Syracuse University
Syracuse, New York

TOPICS IN LANGUAGE DISORDERS SERIES

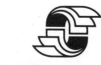

AN ASPEN PUBLICATION®
Aspen Publishers, Inc.
Gaithersburg, Maryland
1994

Library of Congress Cataloging-in-Publication Data

Best practices / Katharine G. Butler, editor.
p. cm.
Compilations from Topics in language disorders.
Includes bibliographical references and index.
Contents: 1. The classroom as an assessment arena—2. The
classroom as an intervention context.
ISBN: 0-8342-0586-6 (v. 1)—ISBN: 0-8342-0587-4 (v. 2)
1. Handicapped children—Education—Language arts. 2. Language
disorders in children—Treatment 3. Speech therapy for children.
4. Speech disorders in children—Diagnosis.
5. Learning disabled children—Education—Language arts.
I. Butler, Katharine G.
II. Topics in language disorders
LC4028.B47 1994
371.91'4—dc20
93-36264
CIP

Editorial Resources: Ruth Bloom

Library of Congress Catalog Card Number: 93-36264
ISBN: 0-8342-0587-4
Series ISBN: 0-8342-0590-4

Printed in the United States

1 2 3 4 5

Table of Contents

Best Practices II: The Classroom As an Intervention Context

Preface

Topics in Language Disorders is a transdisciplinary journal that is devoted to discussion of issues surrounding language acquisition and its disorders. *TLD* has the following major purposes: (1) providing relevant information to practicing professionals who provide services to those who are at-risk or have language disabilities; (2) clarifying the application of theory and research to practice; (3) bringing together professionals across disciplines, who are researchers and clinicians from the health and education arenas both as authors and as readers; (4) clarifying the application of theory to practice among professionals and students-in-training; and (5) contributing to the scientific literature while making each issue accessible and relevant to an interdisciplinary readership.

Typically, each *TLD* journal is devoted to a single topic, although the constellation of articles may vary. A few may be wholly clinical in nature, while most blend practice and research. In the *TLD* book series, each book provides a critical but highly sensitive evaluation of current research and translates that analysis into a framework for service delivery. Hence, in this *TLD* book, the reader will find a distillation of the best of the journal's current offerings as well as some seminal articles that may enhance the readers' conceptual knowledge. Offerings are provided by professionals in a variety of disciplines: speech-language pathologists; allied health professionals, including augmentative and alternative communication (AAC) and autism experts; special educators, such as those specializing in early childhood intervention and learning disabilities and regular educators, including reading, instruction and curriculum specialists.

The authors represented within the covers of *Best Practices II: The Classroom As an Intervention Context* bring to the readers their distilled wisdom and experience. They address multiple aspects of classroom interventions

designed for children from early preschool through adolescence whose language and learning disorders range from mild to severe. The classroom contexts were selected to reflect a continuum of services. Available permutations of special, regular, and inclusive classroom instruction and intervention provided by multidisciplinary and transdisciplinary teams are described.

Individual as well as group instruction are not neglected, nor are the changing needs of children with a variety of language difficulties as they move into, through, and out of the educational system. Finally, dyadic interaction between children and their parents, children and their teachers, and children and their intervention specialists in both clinical and classroom contexts is discussed.

PART I. CONTEMPORARY CLASSROOMS: YOUNGER CHILDREN IN SPECIAL AND INCLUSIVE SETTINGS

The theme for Part I reflects current research which indicates that "language," whether it be listening, speaking, reading, or writing, does not begin when children enter the educational system. Children comprehend spoken language within their first year of life, and learning about print begins in infancy (Dickenson & McCabe, 1991; van Kleeck, in press; Wallach & Butler, in press). While the jury is not in, and researchers continue to explore younger children's acquisition of speaking, reading, and writing, the evidence is piling up that spoken language skills are enhanced by early metalinguistic and cognitive development. Readers, sitting as members of the jury, will find themselves debating the probability of emergent literacy acquisition among younger children whose development is impeded by severe speech and physical impairments.

Part I also addresses the recurrent issue of how might language and learning disabled (LLD) children, when difficulties in phonological awareness are present, fare in classroom settings where reading instruction is based on a whole language philosophy (Blachman, in press; van Kleeck, this text). While it is sometimes difficult to tell the prosecution from the defense or the status of the evidence, there remain a number of researchers and practitioners who support the concept that reading and writing instruction simultaneously develop with oral language. They maintain that direct instruction in early reading and in spelling is helpful; however, some see this as occurring in the whole language context, while others reflect that direct instruction is more helpful (Blachman, in press; Butler & Wallach, in press; Chaney, 1990; Halliday, 1982; Jagger, 1985; Mason, 1986; Schickedanz, 1990).

Van Kleeck begins Part I by introducing the topic of "Emergent Literacy: Learning about Print before Learning To Read." She makes her case as she stresses the importance of the early years of life, noting that language delays in the preschool years "foreshadow difficulties in reading, writing, and spelling during the early school years. " She reflects upon the wealth of knowledge that many preschoolers absorb prior to learning to read through family literacy events that assist them in demonstrating understanding of form, use, and content. At some level, normal children begin to understand the conventions of print, letter naming and writing, and the formal relationship of print to speech before entering school. Van Kleeck provides a number of suggestions for assessment and concludes the review of the rapidly growing and diverse body of research with a balanced view of the effects of preschoolers' "nascent knowledge" of print on their later development of reading and writing. She states, "Attention to emergent print literacy concepts during the preschool years will in no way eradicate subsequent reading disabilities. It will, however, provide a solid foundation on which to continue to build."

Koppenhaver and Yoder follow with an analysis of research and practice as it relates to children with severe speech and motor impairments, such as the cerebral palsied youngster, in their contribution entitled "Classroom Literacy Instruction for Children with Severe Speech and Physical Impairments (SSPI): What Is and What Might Be." If the jury is out on classroom reading instruction paradigm shifts, the jury has not yet been paneled regarding the best methods for language and reading intervention for the SSPI population. Summarizing the small body of literature that informs classroom teachers and specialists, the authors provide a model of classroom instruction that readers will find helpful. Noting what "is," Kopenhaver and Yoder provide a case for improving literacy instruction to children with SSPI and postulate what "might be." Having explored the frontiers of knowledge in this area, the authors also propose four steps that teachers and speech-language pathologists (SLPs) can take to enhance literacy learning of children with SSPI.

Taking the middle ground, in terms of the level of language disability exemplified by early elementary school age children with special needs, Westby and Costlow provide their view of "Implementing a Whole Language Program in a Special Education Class." They support the view that "whole language methodology can provide LLD students with enriched language contexts, meaningful reasons for communication, and contextual cues to support learning." They warn that implementing a successful whole language program with LLD students "requires understanding of their linguistic skills and deficits in order to structure contexts in which they will learn." Given this proviso, they go on to describe such a program, providing readers with the critical information required to observe, assess, and provide instruction and intervention within a whole language framework. Readers will benefit from the exemplars provided by children in their dialogue journals to parents and teachers.

A supportive metaphor for the whole language approach continues with Norris' "From Frog to Prince: Using Written Language As a Context for Language Learning." She suggests that addressing the needs of students with language disabilities through written language intervention is helpful when it is carefully integrated with the school curriculum. She presents an intervention method identified as *communicative reading strategies* within the classroom or clinical context. Noting that children with LLD have difficulty with abstract vocabulary, complex syntactic structures, elements of discourse, and metalinguistic concepts, Norris provides suggestions for interactive and communicative exchanges between clinician and child. Her lucid presentation assists readers in recognizing how elementary and middle school children can benefit from classroom-related activities. Frogs can become princes (and probably princesses as well).

Continuing the notion of semantic organizers, Pehrsson and Denner focus upon the importance of such strategies in their "Semantic Organizers: Implications for Reading and Writing." They advocate that *all* children be taught how to understand the internal organization of written texts, including children with language disorders. They suggest that even young children may benefit from the semantic-organizer approach, as a preventive measure. Older children who require advanced organizational skills will find such instruction essential as well. This article is replete with examples of the basic organizational patterns recommended. Readers who are encountering the authors' work for the first time will find their discussion of a "realia cluster" (for preschoolers and early elementary school students) to be most helpful, while problem solution organizers offer assistance to older children and adolescents. Described by the authors as a metacognitive approach to instruction, readers will find Phrsson and Denner's application to classroom and clinical contexts informative.

PART II. FROM CLINIC TO CLASSROOM: INTERVENTION SCENARIOS AMONG AND BETWEEN

A closer look is now taken at the themes from Part I, specifically, how intervention for children with SSPI and those with phonological awareness difficulties may be most appropriately addressed. As a corollary, the importance of integrating computers into intervention scenarios for not only children with SSPI but also those with mild-to-moderate language disorders is presented.

Part II begins with Blachman's work "Early Intervention for Children's Reading Problems: Clinical Applications of the Research in Phonological Awareness." For more than a decade, Blachman's research agenda has included teaching early reading to young children from minority backgrounds in large urban "inner city" schools, where many, if not most, are at risk for early reading and language failure. Her work has led her to agree with Adams (1990) who states "the evidence is compelling: Toward the goal of efficient and effective reading instruction, explicit training of phonemic awareness is invaluable." (See Blachman, this text.) Blachman is convinced that professionals must continue to explore "exactly what it is that children must understand about the connections between print and speech to become literate." Fortunately for practitioners, she and her students have been engaged in reaching that understanding through school-based application of current research findings. Equally fortunate is that the intervention applications suggested are predominantly classroom-based, although they are also useful in clinical settings. She continues by describing interventions built around sound categorization, phonemic segmentation, and metalinguistic activities within play-based formats. In addition, she provides readers with assessment suggestions from experimental tasks as well as published tests. In conclusion, she emphasizes that research here and abroad has demonstrated a causal relationship between phonological awareness and reading success; thus, she urges supporters of traditional approaches to reading and advocates of whole language to integrate phonological awareness activities into rich oral language classroom environments.

Advocating that clinicians embed computerized activities within the context of a total language program, Steiner and Larson discuss "Integrating Microcomputers into Language Intervention with Children." They suggest that computers can be integrated into both individual and group therapy. They urge that the clinician maintain an interactive role with students, rather than permitting student-microcomputer interaction to be the focus of the intervention. Steiner and Larson provide a series of seven guidelines for enhancing clinician-student interaction. Noting that computers are currently underused, they provide guidance on software applications that may be helpful in school-based intervention settings. The authors close with the thought that the "most sophisticated tool" is the clinician's expertise, a thought to warm the hearts of all practitioners.

Returning to recurrent themes in Part I and II, Pierce and McWilliam address intervention possibilities in "Emerging Literacy and Children with Severe Speech and Physical Impairments (SSPI): Issues and Possible Intervention Strategies." Building upon Koppenhaver and Yoder's predictions of "what might be," Pierce and McWilliam discuss emerging literacy from the perspective of the child with SSPI, one who may not be physically capable of actively participating in play, in reading, in verbalizing thoughts and feelings, in acting out stories, or pretending to read and write. While it may seem simple for parents of children with SSPI to read *with* them, the lack of verbal responsiveness and the need to frequently reposition children so that they may be able to see the book and the text is extremely difficult. While recommending that

parents of such children make a concerted effort through the preschool years to provide their children with literacy experiences, the authors' comments reflect their understanding of the inherent difficulties encountered due to the child's motor problems and expressive language limitations. Readers are provided with suggestions for increasing literacy activities, particularly in connection with thematic play carried out with communication boards.

The last article in Part II, "Ethnography and the Clinical Setting: Communicative Expectancies in Clinical Discourse" by Kovarksy and Maxwell, reports on the outcomes of recent qualitative research that explored two clinical discourse styles—adult-centered and child-centered. The authors provide examples of the impact of adult discourse on the performance of children with language disorders. When children are presumed to be the "error makers," adults, in this case clinicians, tend to interpret responses as evidence of language incompetency. On the other hand, child-centered discourse does not assume that a child's utterances are right or wrong: "Instead, communicative appropriateness is established by the ability of participants to engage in and sustain a mutually intelligible conversation from the child's frame of reference." The authors urge that clinicians adopt a positive regard for children's communication intentions and try to reduce the client-as-error maker expectancy. Readers will find that the exemplars of adult-child interactions provide a pathway that, if followed, will positively modify their interactions with language-disordered children.

PART III OLDER CHILDREN: CHANGING NEEDS

Times change; children's needs change; even best practices change! Part III describes the changes that must be made if adolescents with language disorders are to be well served.

This final section begins with a seminal article by Wallach, "Magic Buries Celtics: Looking for Broader Interpretations of Language Learning and Literacy." The author's "sports" metaphor is anchored in her understanding of the research literature and her experience with children and adolescents with LLD. It is a certaintude, as she suggests, that language specialists are involved in a "complex business that requires constant reevaluation of interpretations about what it means to be literate and what it takes to help children acquire literacy." Just as "Magic Buries Celtics," a headline that can only be understood by the sports-literate, Wallach buries the notion that professionals who take an "either/or approach to reading, espousing either whole language or phonics approaches, ignore the reality that what they do with children has more to do with what the children are ready for rather than what a language or reading program promises." She recommends a broader framework, one that will emphasize the value of theory-driven intervention and the careful evaluation of all research. She states that one "consummate language intervention or reading program may never be identified as the best" but urges professionals to develop new practices based on the excellent research currently available. Her analysis of oral and written language differences, process differences, and form and style differences leads readers to their own conclusions about the importance of literate and syntactic modes to school success. Her intervention recommendations will help readers to reach a level playing field for and with their students, just as Magic found it on the basketball court.

In Part III's next offering, German presents a model for "Work-Finding Intervention for Children andAdolescents." German's research, assessment, and intervention efforts in the area of students' word-finding difficulties have been gathered over more than a decade. She, too, wishes to provide students with LLD assistance on the "memory" court. She discusses their retrieval difficulties, moving on with ease to an explanation of models for intervention. German's three-fold model for word-finding intervention reflects her interest in providing remediation, compensation, and self-advocacy. Readers who share that interest will appreciate her explanation of how limitations on lexical storage and/or word retrieval complicate the academic and personal lives of children who exhibit word-finding difficulties. Dividing such children and adolescents into three groups for intervention planning purposes, German provides five principles for intervention. She follows with a description of remediation components, with seven identifiable principles, and concludes with a discussion of self-advocacy instruction and compensatory programming. Her recommendations are based upon "child and adult psychological and neurological research and [her] own clinical work with children." She concludes the article with a cautionary statement, noting that as children become older, their control and flexibility in lexical accessing may go awry. She urges SLPs and other school personnel to provide appropriate intervention programming for students with word-finding and discourse problems.

Continuing with the theme of adolescents in trouble, Seidenberg recounts the emergence of the current view of the importance of strategic activities to support academic success. Much like Pehrsson and Denner in Part I, she notes that the LLD adolescent is viewed as an individual who does not spontaneously access or use task-appropriate cognitive strategies. Her review of learning disabilities and metacognition provides an integrated conceptual base for designing instructional intervention. Her suggestions for procedures for teaching cognitive strategies for complex academic tasks reflect her many years of experience in working with adolescents and young adults with learning disabilities. As does

German, Seidenberg emphasizes the importance of intervention programming rooted in scientific investigation. She describes a comprehensive program based on a metacognitive orientation. Such a program draws upon extant research and its finding that LLD students can be successfully taught in regular classroom settings.

Special educators Graham and Harris join Seidenberg in recommending strategy training for "Improving Composition Skills of Inefficient Learners with Self-Instructional Strategy Training." Their approach was developed based on the work of Meichenbaum; Brown, Campione and Day; Brown and Palinscar; and Deshler and his colleagues at the Kansas Institute for Research in Learning Disabilities. Having given credit where credit is due, Graham and Harris report on their own research "in developing and validating various composition strategies with both early adolescents and elementary school students." Based on a series of studies, they have found that self-instructional strategy-training procedures can be successfully applied in a flexible and individualized way to children. They stress that evaluation is to continue throughout the intervention process, and they provide guidelines and techniques to assure its successful conclusion. They emphasize that time-based intervention should give way to criterion or mastery-based completion and that training can be done individually or in small groups. These authors, as have others throughout this text, urge that strategy training must reflect both common sense and continuous monitoring of current research so that practitioners may adapt their approaches to the most recent findings.

Picking up on the general theme, but refocusing it to explore how conversational skills are necessary for adolescent success in academic settings, Hoskins calls attention to "Language and Literacy: Participating in the Conversation." She provides a framework for facilitating conversational interaction, using this interactive approach to first assist adolescents in developing "competence in nonverbal communication as a foundation skill for conversation." Conversation group sessions are triadic, providing for discussion, guided conversations, and verbal activities to build foundation skills. Teachers as well as clinicians can serve as facilitators to these groups. The author stresses that activities are selected that complement the curriculum and build linguistic-conceptual and social-cognitive skills. Hoskins provides facilitator guidelines, noting that facilitators act as "metalinguistic guides," thus reinforcing the cognitive processing approaches recommended by other authors in this text. She closes with the injunction that practitioners should continue to examine how an interactive view of language assists adolescents' willingness to participate "in a discourse through listening, speaking or writing."

In the final article, Lord joins Hoskins in her concern for conversational disabilities among adolescents in "Enhancing Communication in Adolescents with Autism." Lord summarizes the conversational and pragmatic difficulties observed in many adolescents with autism and the difficulties in securing adequate classroom placements, even for high-functioning autistic children. Noting that "there is still much about communication in autistic persons that is not well understood," Lord attempts to identify goals, resources, and strategies for communication by autistic adolescents. These goals include participating in age-appropriate social relationships and the ability to use language to independently participate in everyday experiences. She suggests, among other things, that functional objectives for communication in the community may be relatively easy to attain and maintain through planning structured teaching and guided practice.

This text's authors have provided a panoramic view of the ages and stages of children's and adolescents' language and learning disabilities. They have provided instructional frameworks and models for designing classroom and clinical interventions. They have addressed the cognitive, linguistic, and affective needs of these students and have established goals and objectives consonant with current views of language use in an interactive context. Through their interpretations of theory and research, they have sought to bring an interdisciplinary perspective to the language intervention in classrooms and clinics. While agreement is less than unanimous on some topics, the relevance of discourse in literacy, be it spoken or written, is held paramount. While authors have taken care to share with readers research at the cutting edge, there is a timeless quality about participating in the conversation, as Hoskins would have it. Indeed, Jonathon Swift (1667-1745), perhaps best known to

American readers for *Gulliver's Travels*, published in 1726, is less well known for this bit of comment about the "conversation," to wit:

> Conversation is but carving.
> Give no more to every guest
> Than he is able to digest.
> Give always of the prime,
> And but little at a time.
> Carve to all but just enough.
> Let them neither starve nor stuff
> And that you may have your due,
> Let your neighbor carve for you.
>   (Swift, J. (1738) *Conversation*)

Methinks that the carver is the facilitator, the guests are students, and the conversational intervention principles may have been established in the 17th century. I wonder.

REFERENCES

Adams, M.J. (1990). *Beginning to read: Thinking and learning about print.* Cambridge, MA: MIT Press.

Blachman, B. (In press). Early literacy acquisition: The role of phonological awareness. In G.F. Wallach & K.G. Butler's (Eds.), *Language learning disabilities in school-age children and adolescents, Second Edition.* Columbus, OH: Merrill/Macmillan.

Butler, K.G. & Wallach, G.F. (In press). Keeping on track to the 21st century: Queries, quandries and quibbles. In. G.F. Wallach & K.G. Butler (Eds.), *Language learning disabilities in school-age children and adolescents, Second Edition.* Columbus, OH: Merrill/Macmillan.

Chaney, C. (1990). Evaluating the whole language approach to language arts: The pros and cons, *Language, speech, and Hearing Services in Schools,* 21, 244–249.

Dickenson, D. & McCabe, A. (1991). The acquisition and development of language: A social interactionist account of language and literacy development. In J.G. Kavanagh (Ed.), *The language continuum: From infancy to literacy* (pp. 1–40). Parkton, MD: York Press.

Halliday, M.A.K. (1982). Three aspects of children's language development: Learning language, learning through language, and learning about language. In Y. Goodman, H. Haussler, & D. Strickland (Eds.), *Oral and written language development research: Impact on the schools.* Urbana, IL: National Council of Teachers of English.

Jagger, A.M. (1985). On observing the language learner: Introduction and overview. In A.M. Jaggar & M.T. Smith-Burke (Eds.), *Observing the language learner.* Newark, DE: International Reading Association.

Mason, J. (1986). Foundations for literacy: Pre-reading development and instruction. In S. De Castell, A. Luke, & K. Egan (Eds.), *Literacy, society, and schooling* (pp. 232–242). New York, NY: Cambrige University Press.

Schickedanz, J.A. (1990). The jury is still out on the effects of whole language and language experience approaches for beginning reading: A critique of Stahl and Miller's study. *Review of Educational Research, 60*(1), 127–131.

Swift, J. (1738). *Complete collection of genteel and ingenious conversation according to the most polite mode and method now used at court and in the best companies of England.* London: B. Motte & C. Bathurst.

van Kleeck, A. (In Press). Metalinguistic development. In G.F. Wallach & K.G. Butler (Eds.),

Lanuguage learning disabilities in school-age children and adolescents, Second Edition. Columbus, OH: Merrill/Macmillan.

Wallach, G.F. & Butler, K.G. (In press). Creating communication, literacy, and academic success: Concepts for consideration. In G.F. Wallach & K.G. Butler (Eds.), *Lanuguage learning disabilities in school-age children and adolescents, Second Edition.* Columbus, OH: Merrill/Macmillan.

—Katharine G. Butler, PhD
Editor, *Topics in Language Disorders*

Part I
Contemporary Classrooms: Younger Children in Special and Inclusive Settings

Emergent literacy: Learning about print before learning to read

Anne van Kleeck, PhD
Associate Professor
Program in Communication Sciences
and Disorders
Department of Speech Communication
University of Texas at Austin
Austin, Texas

RECENT RESEARCH from a variety of disciplines has begun to highlight the importance of the preschool years in laying the foundation for children's later development of print literacy. The critical importance of this information to professionals who work with language-delayed preschoolers lies in the fact that language delays very often foreshadow difficulties in reading, writing, and spelling during the early school years (Butler, 1988; Forrell & Hood, 1985; Lee & Shapero-Fine, 1984; Mattis, French, & Rapin, 1975; Padget, 1988; Stark, Bernstein, & Condino, 1984; Strominger & Bashir, 1977). However, the utility of this research clearly is not restricted to those who work with language-delayed preschoolers, since the foundations for print literacy are of great importance to the development of all children. The term "print literacy" is used

The author acknowledges Lynda Miller and Alice Richardson for their comments on an earlier draft of this article and C. Melanie Schuele for sharing new information on early print literacy with the author.

Top Lang Disord, 1990,10(2),25–45
© 1990 Aspen Publishers, Inc.

in this article to acknowledge that print is only one tool for accessing information and becoming literate.

For many years, educational practices in the United States have been based on what is typically referred to as a "reading readiness" approach. Implicit in the reading readiness approach, which is still prevalent in many school systems, is the notion that preparation for learning to read requires the structured, sequenced teaching of skills that lays foundations for the formal components of reading, such as the sounds and how they correspond to the visual characteristics of print. This approach has addressed reading almost exclusively while virtually ignoring writing.

More recent research calls into question numerous assumptions implicit in the reading readiness approach, including the notions that initial instruction should await formal schooling, follow a structured sequence, focus on formal aspects of reading to the exclusion of attention to the functions of print, and focus on reading only, while excluding writing. This current work focuses on the rudimentary knowledge about print literacy that is acquired during the years before formal schooling. Researchers in this newer tradition often use the term "emergent literacy" to refer to the wealth of knowledge many preschool children gain about print before they actually learn how to read (Clay, 1966; Hall, 1987; Mason & Allen, 1986; Teale & Sulzby, 1986).

Studies of emergent literacy have had numerous foci. Some have focused on the print literacy environment of the young child, noting artifacts related to print and print-related events in the home, thereby raising the conception of print literacy to the level of a social and cultural phenomenon (Cochran-Smith, 1984; Heath, 1983). Other investigators have been interested in the skills of children—their awareness of environmental print, their early writing behavior, their nascent metalinguistic abilities, and, in the cases of early readers, their self-taught ability to actually decode print (i.e., achieve the letter-sound correspondences and then blend the sounds to form meaningful words) (Downing & Valtin, 1984; Ferreiro, 1984, 1986; Lass, 1982). From the studies conducted to achieve these various goals, it is possible to gain insight into the role of the family environment in early literacy development and the kind of knowledge regarding the form, content, and use of print that is acquired during the preliterate years. This article reviews some of these findings and offers suggestions for assessment and facilitation of emergent literacy skills.

FAMILY ENVIRONMENT AND EMERGING LITERACY

Three types of research have focused on the early family environment for literacy. First, ethnographic observers studying homes in various communities have begun describing literacy objects (or artifacts, as the anthropologists call them) in the preschool child's home environment and literacy events to which they are exposed (Cochrane-Smith, 1984; Heath, 1983). These studies are helpful to the interventionist because they provide details regarding the literacy experiences of preschoolers from various cultures and backgrounds. Second, other descriptive studies have looked more specifically at the nature of the adult–child interactions that occur within literacy events (Snow, 1983). These studies illuminate possible ways that adults informally foster literacy development, and hence provide direction for the interventionist who wishes to facilitate such development. A third type of study has moved beyond description in an attempt to determine what aspects of preschool literacy experience actually affect later reading development (Share, Jorm, Mac-Lean, & Matthews, 1984). This type of study is intended to determine what specific aspects of preschool literacy experience best predict or correlate with later reading achievement. The following discussion draws from these three kinds of studies to describe literacy artifacts and events to which preschool children are exposed and to consider the specific nature of adult guidance within literacy events and the role such guidance plays in later reading development.

Ethnographic investigations

Descriptive ethnographic investigations have been conducted in families from various geographic areas with a wide variety of cultural, ethnic, and socioeconomic backgrounds. For example, Heath (1983) studied working-class African Americans, working-class white, and middle-class white communities in the Piedmont Carolinas. Cochran-Smith (1984) studied a community in Philadelphia consisting of Eastern and Western European, Jewish, Indian, Filipino, Egyptian, English, and African American families. Anderson and Stokes (1984) focused on low-income African American, Mexican-American, and Anglo-American families in San Diego, California.

These and other researchers have found literacy artifacts and print-related events to be pervasive in all kinds of homes in literate societies. However, the range and quantity of artifacts varies. For example, in studies in both Israel (Feitelson & Goldstein, 1986) and the United States (McCormick & Mason, 1986), the number of children's books purchased varied as a function of socioeconomic status, with lower-class families providing far fewer books for their children. However, this finding has not been consistent (see Chall et al., 1983; and Miller, 1982).

The importance of literacy artifacts in children's homes was pointed out in a study by Thorndike (1976), who examined reading comprehension in 15 countries. Results indicated that socioeconomic level and the availability of print in the home were the two factors that predicted reading achievement. A sample of the variety of these artifacts found in American homes is offered by Leichter's (1984) comprehensive, but by no means exhaustive, list:

Books; dictionaries; atlases and maps; encyclopedias; school workbooks, reports, and tests; letters to and from school; newspapers; magazines; television guides; comic books; junk mail; notes from one family member to another; captioned religious pictures; merit awards; personal letters; kitchen canisters; labels on food, jars, cans, and medicine and bathroom products; postcards; political fliers; coupons; laundry slips; cookbooks; wall plaques; games; name plates; shopping lists; postage stamps; coloring books; sport catalogs; diaries; Christmas cards; gift lists; record albums; sewing patterns; baseball cards; sweatshirts; photograph albums; identification cards; and tickets. (p. 41)

To Leichter's list, one can add Cochran-Smith's (1984) list of writing utensils and materials "such as pencils, markers, crayons, chalk, papers, pads, notebooks, chalkboards, and folders" (p. 49).

These literacy artifacts are embedded in various ways in the literacy events that take place in homes. As will be discussed later, it is in the context of these literacy events that much of the preschooler's knowledge about literacy is acquired. Children may either observe or actively participate in such events, which occur with varying frequency and duration in some homes and not at all in others. Indeed, the parents in the working-class African American community studied by Heath (1983) neither read to their children nor taught them reading and writing skills. Teale (1986) and Anderson and Stokes (1984) likewise found very little book reading to children in working-class families. In contrast, the highest frequency of print-related events in low-income homes falls into the "activities of daily living" category described below (Anderson & Stokes, 1984; Heath, 1983; Taylor, 1983; Teale, 1986).

The following sampling of potential literacy events is organized according to the broad functions they serve (some aspects of this list are expanded and revised from a listing provided by Anderson & Stokes, 1984):

- Activities of daily living include creating shopping lists (see a transcript of a mother discussing a shopping list with her child in Tizard & Hughes, 1984); searching newspapers, magazines, and leaflets for shopping coupons; reading the aisle signs, product labels, and sales notices in the supermarket; washing clothes; paying bills; getting welfare assistance and dealing with other bureaucratic processes (applying for permits, licenses, etc.); writing checks; signing credit card receipts; taking down telephone messages; reading instructions for household appliances and devices; reading street signs and building signs; preparing food (reading recipes; reading boxes, jars, and cans containing foods and spices); looking up information such as phone numbers and addresses; keeping the family budget; and dressing the children (reading slogans on clothing, sizes on clothing labels).

- Entertainment activities for older children include reading novels, reading stories to children, doing crossword puzzles, playing word games, reading instructions for parlor games, playing computer and video games involving print, reading a television guide, reading a local paper for movie listings, reading words occurring on television (such as on game shows); for young children, entertainment activities include pretending to read and write in symbolic play, drawing, "writing," and coloring.

- Practicing religion includes reading the Bible.

- Using print for interpersonal communication includes writing notes to family members, writing letters to out-of-town family and friends, and sending greeting and holiday cards.

- Using print for intrapersonal communication includes keeping lists of things to do, writing in a personal journal, and writing poetry or stories.

- Using print to gather information, which often overlaps with entertainment, includes reading newspapers, magazines, fliers received in the mail, nonfiction books, and encyclopedias.

- Using print at home that is related to one's livelihood includes keeping records related to work; billing clients; reading books, journals, and magazines (and for teachers, papers and tests) related to work; and writing reports, articles, and books by using typewriters or personal computers.

While lists such as the above attest to a print-rich environment in our literate culture, not all children are exposed to the same range of print-related experiences (Anderson & Stokes, 1984; Heath, 1983; McCormick & Mason, 1986; Teale, 1986). In addition, even in cases where middle-socioeconomic status mothers report a high degree of uniformity in print-related activities (Hiebert, 1981; Mason, 1980), children demonstrate great variation in their print-related knowledge. This variation leads to questions regarding the nature of children's print-related experiences, since exposure alone does not appear to be sufficient.

Adult–child interaction

One consistent finding about the nature of most literacy events occurring in the young child's home (with the exception of book-reading routines) is that they are

---

Using print for interpersonal communication includes writing notes to family members, writing letters to out-of-town family and friends, and sending greeting and holiday cards.

---

embedded very naturally in ongoing social interactions in order to accomplish real-life, practical goals (Anderson & Stokes, 1984; Cochran-Smith, 1984; Heath, 1983; Taylor, 1981). Indeed, in studying low-income families, Teale (1986) found that 90% of the time the focus or motive for activities involving print was not literacy itself. In a study by Taylor (1981), children in fact resisted parental attempts at formal didactic teaching of letter names.

Although informal in nature, parents' teaching attempts may often be very deliberate. In a study by Tobin and Pikulski (1983), 37% of the parents reported that they were in fact deliberately teaching their nursery school and kindergarten aged children to read. The informal nature of these early print experiences, whether used to deliberately teach print-related skills or not, stands in stark contrast to traditional, highly structured methods of teaching reading readiness and early reading.

In the past few years, programs that advocate extending methods of formal, didactic teaching almost to birth have become increasingly popular. Such programs purport to teach a variety of athletic and academic skills, include reading (Doman, 1963; Englemann & Englemann, 1986; Ledson, 1983; Ludington-Hoe, 1985). These "superkid" programs, as they are often called, have raised alarm among some child development experts because the programs ignore the natural, spontaneous, and informal approach to learning that best suits the cognitive abilities of the preschool child. Elkind (1987) states that "there is absolutely no evidence that such teaching gives children any lasting advantage in reading or that it has any effect on a child's brightness" (p. 13). On the contrary, Elkind notes that too much, too soon can in fact cause serious, permanent damage to a child's self-esteem, kill the child's natural desire to learn, and block the child's natural talent.

It appears that children benefit most from early literacy experiences that are informal rather than structured. Observing or participating in informal print literacy events is not, however, sufficient for developing literacy knowledge, as Hiebert (1986) points out:

While research supports the idea that print-related learning results from informal experiences rather than didactic or highly structured ones, the process is not one of children acquiring information about print via osmosis from a print-saturated environment. In one manner or another, children's attention needs to be directed to the print in these informal experiences. (p. 151)

The need for guidance and support by a literate person (in this culture, frequently a parent) has been documented in an array of studies looking at the impact of early literacy experiences on children's acquisition of various aspects of knowledge about print. The guiding roles of parents in book reading has been noted in several studies (Cochran-Smith, 1984; DeLoache & DeMendoza, 1986; Ninio & Bruner, 1978; Snow & Goldfield, 1981, 1983; Snow & Ninio, 1986). However, several researchers have found that parents who read to their children do not carry out book reading in the same fashion (Heath, 1982; Thomas, 1985; Wells, 1985). Parents of early readers (Thomas, 1985) and parents of children who achieve success in school (Heath, 1983; Wells, 1985) go beyond just reading books and eliciting labels for objects and details of events.

Such findings indicate that children need to be guided in relating information in books to events in the real world; in discussing reasons, motives, and evaluations; and in interpreting and making inferences.

The positive effects of parental direction and guidance in other literacy events have also been documented. Numerous researchers have shown that, left to their own devices to "read" the print, children will focus on contextual features of environmental print, such as the stylized representations of the logos, to "read" the print (Dewitz, Stammer, & Jenson, 1980; Hiebert, 1978; Masonheimer, Drum, & Ehri, 1984). Hence, a child may say "McDonald's" in response to the arches in the logo, even if a word other than "McDonald's" is substituted for the print. Children are capable of attending to the graphic features (i.e., the letters) of environmental print, however, if their attention is directed to it (Masonheimer et al., 1984).

In a study by Mason (1980), there were two home influences that correlated significantly with four-year-olds' word reading—children watching Sesame Street, and their parents engaging them in discussion about the program's content. Here again, adult guidance was a key factor. Teale (1978) noted that parental responsiveness to children's print-related questions was an important factor in the children's success as early readers.

Snow (1983) identified the specific nature of parental guidance in book reading as well as other literacy events in a case study involving her son Nathaniel. She argued that the specific parental behaviors known to facilitate language development are the same as those that support general literacy development. These include semantic contingency (staying on topics introduced by the child), scaffolding (structuring and constraining the linguistic and nonlinguistic context to facilitate the child's success), accountability procedures (requiring that a child contribute to and complete tasks at the level she or he is capable of), and routines (highly predictable, repetitive structure that recurs frequently, as in book reading).

Snow's claims were supported by Thomas's (1985) finding that family members of early readers used more instances of these devices than did families of non–early readers. Snow (1983) believes that these interactive strategies of families, and not differences in access to print, perhaps account for the later "large and reliable" (p. 165) social class differences in reading achievement that have been repeatedly documented. Teale (1986) tempers this conclusion, saying that it is how parents rear their children and not socioeconomic status per se that accounts for these differences. And indeed, White (1982), in a meta-analysis conducted on nearly 200 studies, concluded that it was not socioeconomic status that contributed most directly to early reading achievement, but rather other family characteristics related to academic guidance, attitude toward education, aspirations of the parent for the child, conversations in the home, reading materials in the home, and cultural activities.

The importance of the support and guidance of adults or any literate others in children's early literacy experiences has led many researchers to adopt the social-interaction–based Vygotskian theory to

explain the process of this early learning (Cochran-Smith, 1984; Heath, 1982; Ninio & Bruner, 1978; Scollon & Scollon, 1981; Teale, 1984; Wells, 1985). In Vygotskian theory, children learn all psychological functioning in social interaction with a more competent, experienced member of their culture. Initially, the adult (or a more competent child) provides a great deal of support to ensure the child's successful participation at whatever level she or he is capable of. Over time, the adult gradually relinquishes control of the interaction to the child, who can eventually perform the task independently. Vygotsky (1978) refers to this shift as movement from other-regulation to self-regulation, or from interpsychological to intrapsychological functioning.

Schieffelin and Cochran-Smith (1984) apply Vygotskian theory to literacy development, stating that,

Adults initially played all the parts in literacy events, completely producing and comprehending print for the children and behaving as if the children themselves intended for print to be used in particular ways and as if the children themselves were using the print. Little by little, however, the nursery school children took over the various roles in literacy events and needed less and less help from adult intermediaries. (p. 8)

While Vygotskian theory provides a powerful explanation of the nature of many family literacy events reported in this literature, it is most important to note that not all children are taught in such a manner. Heath (1983), reporting on the working-class African American community of Trackton in the Piedmont Carolinas, found that talk addressed to children was not simplified, nor was children's reading material available. So, Vygotskian principles do not provide a universal explanation of early literacy learning, even within American culture. Olson (1984) believes the style of deliberate guidance of oral language teaching may be a technique adopted by highly literate parents. In so doing, "the literate parent is teaching the child an orientation to language that has everything to do with literacy" (p. 189), even though it is not necessary for oral language learning.

Even if Vygotskian principles were universal, they would not be adequate for explaining the entirety of early literacy development. Particularly in the area of early writing behaviors, the role of the child in actively constructing knowledge regarding how writing works points to important ways that Piagetian theory can also shed light on early literacy development (examples will be provided in the next section). As Sulzby (1986) notes, "children construct ideas about reading and writing that are not taught to them, are not modeled for them, and are not yet conventional" (p. 52).

Olson (1984) views the contributions of Piagetian and Vygotskian theory as essentially providing explanations of children's literate capacities at two different levels of description—the psychological and the social. These levels are best summed up in the question he poses: "Do we look into the mental activities of children, an essentially piagetian undertaking, or do we look into the tutorial practices of parents, an essentially durkheimian, vygotskyan, or brunerian undertaking?" (p. 186). Whether child constructed, adult guided, or a combination of both, children's experiences with print before they reach formal schooling

lead to their developing knowledge regarding numerous aspects of the form, content, and use of print.

AREAS OF PRESCHOOLER LITERACY KNOWLEDGE

The three broad components of oral language development set forth by Bloom and Lahey (1978)—form, content, and use—also provide a useful way of categorizing the areas of knowledge about print developed by preliterate children.

Form

Children develop knowledge of the formal aspects of print in five areas: (a) mastery of the conventions of print, (b) phonological awareness, (c) letter naming and writing, (d) realization of the formal relationship of print to speech, and (e) comprehension of macrostructures for organizing written language text (such as story grammars).

Conventions of print

Conventions of print mastered by most preschoolers include how to handle books. At the most basic level, they learn how to hold a book upright. Even without being able to read, they are often aware that

---

Whether child-constructed, adult-guided, or a combination of both, children's experiences with print before they reach formal schooling lead to their developing knowledge of the form, content, and use of print.

print in English is organized from left to right on each line, from top to bottom on each page, from the left to the right page, and from the front page to the back page in a book. These types of awareness were universally demonstrated by English and bilingual 3-, 4-, and 5-year-olds from Tucson, by urban African American and rural lower- to lower-middle class white children in Alabama, and by 5- and 6-year-old Papago Indian children (Goodman, 1986). Children begin formal reading without full awareness of other conventions, such as the use of spaces to separate words in print and the function of punctuation marks (Goodman, 1986).

Children's early writing attempts also reveal some emerging concepts of print conventions. As young as 1½ years, scribbling can hold fascination for children (Gibson & Levin, 1975). At this point, scribbling is uncontrolled and bears little resemblance to print (Fields, 1989). A bit later, however, scribbling begins to take on the linear, repetitive qualities of print and is sometimes called "scribble writing." This activity reflects at least rudimentary attention to conventions of written language.

Scribbling may reveal some surprisingly advanced knowledge of conventions of print. Heath (1983), for example, reported on a 4-year-old child named Mel whose scribble writing demonstrated an understanding of the locations of the date, salutation, body, closing, and signature used in letter writing.

Phonological awareness

Of all the foundations for print literacy laid during the preschool years, none has been as extensively studied nor as directly tied to a most important role in early reading as phonological awareness (see Wagner & Torgesen, 1987, for a review of the causal role of phonological processing in reading acquisition). The exact nature of the relationship between phonological awareness and reading remains a debated issue (e.g., is it a precursor to or a result of learning to read, or is the relationship a reciprocal one?); however, few would disagree that becoming aware of words as consisting of discrete phonemic segments is eventually of crucial importance to reading ability in an alphabetic writing system such as English. Exemplary of such findings is one recent study (Share, Jorm, MacLean, & Matthews, 1984) that found phoneme segmentation ability on entry to school was the best predictor of 39 measures of reading achievement 2 years later.

The culminating skill of phonological awareness, the ability to segment words into their component phonemes, is mastered rather late in comparison to other foundations for print literacy discussed in previous sections. Furthermore, mastering phoneme segmentation may require explicit instruction for most children, unlike the informal context of other emerging literacy skills. And indeed, phoneme segmentation has been successfully taught to prereaders in a formal, didactic manner with a positive impact on subsequent reading achievement (Lundberg, 1988; Rosner, 1974; Sawyer, 1988; Treiman & Baron, 1983). The very well documented and incontrovertible role of phoneme segmentation ability in reading acquisition warrants consideration of underlying precursory skills, including earlier segmentation abilities and rudimentary phonological awareness skills (such as rhyming and alliteration). Both of these skills can and often do emerge in informal contexts during the years before formal schooling.

Prior to being able to segment words into component phonemes, children demonstrate the ability to segment other units of language. The very earliest manifestation of segmentation ability occurs when children divide sentences into semantic propositions. Karpova (1966) gives an example of a child who indicated that "Galya and Vova went walking" had two words, "Galya went walking and Vova went walking." According to Fox and Routh (1975), the ability to segment sentences into words emerges next (one half of sentences were segmented into words by age 3 years), followed by the more clearly phonologically based skill of segmenting words into syllables (one third of words were segmented into syllables by age 3 years). The ability to segment words into phonemes emerges last (one quarter of words were segmented into phonemes by age 3 years). Other researchers have supported the general order of emergence of these skills, although the children in these studies have typically been somewhat older due to the greater difficulty of tasks used to assess segmentation skills (Ehri, 1975; Holden & MacGinitie, 1972; Huttenlocher, 1964; Liberman, 1973; Liberman, Shankweiler, Fisher, & Carter, 1974).

Producing rhymes and alliteration requires attention to the sounds in words and is a skill that is clearly within the purview of many preschool children (Chukovsky, 1963; Dowker, 1989; Rogers, 1979; Weir, 1962). Chukovsky (1963) discussed the fascination of Russian children with rhymes from the very onset of oral language development. Weir (1962) has many charming examples of the spontaneous play with the sound of language that was produced in the bedtime soliloquies of her son Anthony. One example is Anthony's nonsense poem:

> Bink
> Let Bobo bink
> Bink ben bink
> Blue kink. (p. 105)

Recently, McLean, Bryant, and Bradley (1987) demonstrated that knowledge of nursery rhymes as well as the ability to detect and produce rhymes and alliteration at 3 years of age was related to early reading at approximately 4½ years of age. One can conclude from the work of McLean and his colleagues and subsequent training studies conducted by Bradley (1988) that "word play, singing games, and nursery rhymes need to be a part of the everyday experience of our preschool children" (Bradley, 1988, p. 160) because of the positive impact on later reading and spelling achievement.

In addition to rhyming and alliteration, nascent phonological segmentation abilities are occasionally spontaneously produced by young children. Van Kleeck and Schuele (1987) document several such examples, including a child just shy of 3 years old who commented, "/w/ starts *witch, watch, water*" (p. 27).

Letter naming and writing

Letter naming has traditionally been a very important ingredient in reading readiness programs. However, one study has demonstrated that training in letter naming alone has no effect on learning to read in English (Samuels, 1971).

The ability to write alphabet letters may emerge gradually from scribbling, to mock letters, to recognizable letters that may often vary from conventional shapes and orientations. The basic configuration of writing may be presaged in the child's early scribbles. Differences have been noted between the scribbling of Hebrew- and Bengali-speaking 4-year-olds (Goodman, 1986), and between Arabic- and English-speaking 4-year-olds (Harste, Woodward, & Burke, 1984). Indeed, the 4-year-old Saudi Arabian child in the Harste, Woodward, and Burke study even commented on her scribbling, "Here, but you can't read it, cause I wrote it in Arabic and in Arabic we use more dots than you do in English" (Row & Harste, 1986, p. 240).

Formal relationship of print to speech

Both letter detection and phonological awareness are component skills in children's ability to realize the formal relationship between speech and print. The relationship between print and speech in English (and other alphabetic writing systems) relies on a rough correspondence between the phonemes (or sounds) in speech and the graphemes (or letters) in writing. Prior to arriving at the idea that graphemes correspond to phonemes, however, children may come up with other notions regarding the relationship of speech to print.

A very young child may believe that it is pictures rather than print that correspond to speech. Such a child might point to a picture when asked to show what we read, or, conversely, draw a picture when asked to write something. However, across a variety of languages and cultures, between the ages of 3 and 5 years, nearly all children know that it is print and not pictures that one reads (Goodman, 1986).

Once children become aware that print conveys meaning, they might adopt any of a variety of strategies for participating in the act of writing, although their attempts will show no specific relationship between speech and print. Five such strategies are (a) scribble writing; (b) scribbling plus some letters or letter-like characters (Henderson, 1986), which Goodman (1986) claims is used by 50% of 3-year-olds; (c) producing a combination of letters and numbers (Ferreiro, 1986); (d) copying environmental print (Sulzby, 1986); and (e) writing by repeating well-learned units, such as letters from one's name or from the alphabet (Clay, 1975; Genishi & Dyson, 1984; Sulzby, 1986). Sulzby (1986) gives an example of the "copying environmental print" strategy that was produced by a 5-year-old subject, Chad. He was asked to write about a race with silly, wind-up toys that had just been conducted and discussed. Chad's story, which was to be written for "someone who wasn't there," relied on print from a nearby crayon box and a tape recorder. He wrote:

> SONY CRAYOLA
> BINNEY & SMITH
> END
> ONN

Some children may believe that their inventions actually carry meaning and

---

Once children become aware that print conveys meaning, they might adopt any of a variety of strategies for participating in the act of writing, although their attempts will show no specific relationship between speech and print.

"read" them to adults or, alternatively, insist that only an adult who knows how to read can decipher them. Others will realize that their invention does not carry meaning, and make comments such as, "I didn't write anything" (Sulzby, 1986, p. 73).

Some children may display somewhat more advanced strategies that attempt to make a correspondence between units of speech and units of print, although the nature of the correspondence remains child-invented and completely arbitrary. Children may construct a rule of one grapheme per word, as Ferreiro's 4-year 11-month-old subject who labeled each of three cats with a "P-like" grapheme and a butterfly with an "A" (1984, p. 166). Note that the particular letters he chose had no logical connection to the words they were used to represent. This rule may be embellished by adding graphemes for bigger, heavier, or older objects (Ferreiro, 1986; Goodman, 1984). Other children may believe that the correspondence is between graphemes and syllables. Ferreiro's Spanish-speaking subject, Abraham, who was 4 years 7 months, was asked to prepare cards for a toy shop. With a repertoire of only five different graphemes, he used four of them to represent each of the four syllables in "muñeca" (doll), three to represent each of the syllables in "barquitos" (little boats), and so forth. Some children will develop a "minimum number" principle and believe that a word must have a minimum of three graphemes in order to be a word (Ferreiro & Teberosky, 1982).

The most sophisticated level of matching speech to print occurs when children begin to realize the correspondence that actually adheres in English orthography—that of letters to sounds. Initially, children may adopt a strategy in which they use one grapheme to represent just one sound in an entire syllable or word. Ferriero's (1986) subject Santiago displayed the syllable strategy when, at age 3 years 9 months, he wrote his name, "SiO." Santiago's choice of the "S" and the "O" correspond to findings noted earlier that children first begin to distinguish only initial, and sometimes final, sounds of words (Ehri, 1985; Mason, 1980; Morris, 1981).

The code is finally "cracked" with the realization that each sound in speech is represented, more or less, by one phoneme (one of the child's subsequent tasks will be to realize how truly rough this correspondence is). At this juncture, children may produce spelling that is not yet conventional but does adhere to the sound–letter correspondence principle. This phenomenom is called invented spelling, and it has been very widely studied. Sulzby's (1986) subject Betsy wrote of the wind-up toy race mentioned earlier, "WELL WATE HAPPEND FRST WAS I PICKT A RASRE AND STATD IT UP . . ." (Well, what happened first was I picked a racer and started it up . . .). She demonstrates a combination of invented and conventional spelling.

Whether there is an invariant developmental sequence in children's approaches to early writing remains inconclusive. Several studies have claimed that there is no developmental sequence (Clay, 1975; Graves, 1983; Harste, Woodward, & Burke, 1984; Sulzby, 1986), while several others report finding a developmental sequence (Ferreiro & Teberosky, 1982; Henderson & Beers, 1980; Temple, Nathan, & Burris, 1982). Sulzby (1986) suggests that the developmental level of writing exhibited by a child may be more task than age related, indicating that children may harbor several conceptions regarding the nature of print simultaneously. The same child might spell her or his name, family members' names, and some common words conventionally, but revert to scribble writing when asked to write a story. The print to speech correspondence, then, emerges gradually over time and is manifested earlier in some tasks than others.

Macrostructures for organizing written language

Parents who read to their children may begin doing so when the children are as young as 3 to 6 months of age (Cochran-Smith, 1984; Heath, 1983). The critical importance of being read to in the early years for later literacy development has been underscored by numerous researchers (see especially Wells, 1985 and, for a review, Teale, 1984).

Children learn about print from a wide variety of print-related experiences, but it is in the context of being read to that they gradually abstract the global framework for the organization of stories that are often called story grammars. The major constituents of a story grammar designated in the seminal work of Stein and Glenn (1979) include the setting, the initiating event, the internal response, the attempt, the consequence, and the reaction or the ending.

Applebee's (1978) work shows that children begin to be sensitive to the schematic structure of stories from a very young age. For instance, he found that children recognize such features as formal opening phrases (e.g., "Once upon a time"), formal closings, and consistent use of the past tense beginning as early as 2 years of age, when 70% used at least one of these three devices in stories they produced. Applebee further demonstrated how the form of the child's story concept changes with age throughout the preschool years. This knowledge of story grammar is important in that it can facilitate children's comprehension of both spoken and written language (Just & Carpenter, 1987; Perfetti, 1985).

Use

Functions of print

As a consequence of their many and varied print-related experiences, children come to realize that print may serve a wide variety of functions, including such things as a primary way of acquiring knowledge, a memory support, a way of entering a world of fantasy, a means of self expression, a form of entertainment, a way to initiate problem solving, a tool for financial negotiations, a means of maintaining relationships, a way of dealing with emotions, a way to convey instructions, and a way to make announcements (Anderson & Stokes, 1984; Schieffelin & Cochran-Smith, 1984).

Researchers have noted a surprising array of more specific functions in young children's symbolic play. Some specific examples include taking meeting notes, making calendars, writing shopping lists, and keeping a diary (Schickedanz, 1984); taking restaurant orders (Baghban, 1984); writing traffic tickets (Kammler, 1984); sending letters, taking messages (Harste et al., 1984); and buying goods with food stamps and getting prescriptions from doctors (Jacob, 1984).

Hall (1987) discusses a study in which he and his colleagues (Hall, May, Moores, Shearer, & Williams, 1986) provided literacy materials (writing utensils and materials for writing on) for the "home corner" of a nursery classroom. For example, the telephone had directories, notepads, pens, and pencils placed near it. The effects of providing literacy artifacts were dramatic. "Children filled hundreds of sheets of paper with writing. They sent letters, and filled notebooks, diaries and calendars. They took messages, created restaurants and took orders. They also engaged in a lot of reading behaviors" (p. 44). In two other studies (Baghban, 1984; Harste et al., 1984), the types of literacy instruments provided for children were shown to be important. Children would not write telephone messages with crayons, for example, since this is not what adults do.

Rules for interaction with print

Snow and Ninio (1986) elucidate a variety of rules for interacting with print that mothers convey, either implicity or explicitly, during the book reading routine. These include learning that books are for reading, not manipulating; in book reading, the book controls the topic; pictures are not things but representations of things; pictures are for naming (especially when children are in the single and two-word utterance stage); pictures, though static, can represent events; book events occur outside real time; and books represent an autonomous fictional world. In their study, these researchers provide numerous segments of transcripts in which these rules are being taught.

Answering questions about information in books

In the course of the book-reading routine engaged in with parents, children are socialized in "patterns of language use related to books" (Heath, 1982, p. 50). Snow and Goldfield (1981) discuss the ways in which parents gradually increase the level of their demands in the questions they ask and comments they make during the book-reading routine. Questions and comments progress from simple ones about the labels of objects, to ones that ask for more detailed information about objects, to ones about names of events, to ones requiring that the child elaborate on aspects of events, to ones about motives and causes, to evaluations or reactions to information in books, and finally to comments and questions that relate the events in books to events in the real world. The last three types of comments and questions require that the child think beyond the actual words in the text in order to respond. Heath (1982) proposes that a hierarchy similar to that proposed by Snow and Goldfield is typical of the kinds of language usage children will encounter throughout their academic careers.

An important aspect of print literacy socialization that is occurring as children learn to answer questions from books is related to the social dominance issue of "display" and how it operates in American culture. In American culture (unlike, for example, British culture), the dominant member of an asymmetrical pair often functions as a spectator while the subordinate member exhibits skills (Bateson, 1972; Mead, 1977). As subordinate members, children are expected to exhibit their knowledge to adults (Scollon & Scollon, 1981). The book-reading routine is a prime example of a context in which children learn to answer questions that are not true requests for information, since they clearly know the adult already possesses the answer. These questions function instead as requests for the child to display his or her knowledge.

Content

Print is meaningful

A most basic realization regarding the content of print is that it represents meaningful ideas. While this may appear to be so simple as to be completely obvious, consider the utter confusion of a child who would enter formal reading instruction devoid of this fundamental insight.

Language about language

Children begin to develop a specialized vocabulary for dealing with print during the preschool years. They come to understand words such as *read, write, draw, page, story,* and *book,* although they cannot yet define them as an adult would. They may begin formal reading instruction without being able to demonstrate an understanding of words such as *letter,*

The book-reading routine is a prime example of a context in which children learn to answer questions that are not true requests for information, since they clearly know the adult already possesses the answer.

---

number, capital, and *word* (Goodman, 1986). A child who lacks the vocabulary to talk about print-related phenomena will be at risk for failure in early reading instruction not because of a lack of conceptual knowledge, but because of deficits in the basic vocabulary used in such instructional contexts.

Decontextualized nature of print

In the process of being read to and engaging in other print-related activities, young children gain insight into a basic characteristic of written text—the meaning resides in the printed words alone and is independent of the immediate social context. Learning to disembed language from the concrete, social context in which children first learn to speak is a crucial task for being able to gradually make the transition into the instructional uses of language that prevail in classrooms. It should be noted that using the term *decontextualization* to discuss the nature of written prose is debatable, since interpreting all discourse, including that which is written, relies on prior knowledge of many kinds of contexts (Nystrand, 1982; Rader, 1982; Tannen, 1985). Thus, it might be more accurate to say that a child is learning to embed print into contexts that are increasingly complex and removed from the here and now.

ASSESSMENT

Not surprisingly, the wealth of research findings that has accumulated in the last few years on foundations for print literacy prior to formal schooling has led to the development of several standardized tests for assessing this knowledge in preschool and kindergarten children. These tests include the following: *Analysis of the Language of Learning* (ALL) by Blodgett and Cooper, ages 4:0 to 9:11; *Concepts about Print* (CAP), *Sand* (1972) and *Stones* (1979b) by Clay, ages 5:0 to 7:3; *Early School Inventory* (ESI)-*Preliteracy* by Nurss and McGauvran, ages 5:0 to 7:0; *Linguistic Awareness in Reading Readiness* (LARR) by Downing, Ayers, and Schaefer, ages 4:0 to 6:0; *Sawyer's Test of Awareness of Language Segments* (TALS) by Sawyer, ages 4:6 to older; *Test of Early Reading Ability* (TERA/2) by Reid, Hresko, and Hammill, ages 3:0 to 9:11; *Written Language Awareness Test* (WLAT) (Experimental Edition) by Taylor and Blum, ages 4:0 to 7:0.

Of these tests, the *Concepts about Print* (Clay, 1972, 1979a, 1979b) is the least adequately standardized. The *Early School Inventory—Preliteracy* (Nurss and McGauvran, 1986) provides the best norms in terms of sample size, having been standardized on 2,500 5- to 7-year-olds.

While the norms provided in these tests are helpful for situations where standardized test scores are necessary, it is quite apparent from reviewing the procedures of these tests that all of the information they provide could as easily be obtained informally. In fact, considering the savings in administration time, it is undoubtedly easier to assess emerging literacy knowledge informally. Indeed, Hall (1987) reports that a group of teachers he worked with found the *Linguistic Awareness in Reading Readiness Test* (Downing, Ayers, & Schaefer, 1982) more useful for providing the basis for a general discussion with the children than it was as a formal

test. Some suggested that the areas listed on the test score sheet formed a useful checklist. Goodman (1981) has made similar observations regarding the *Concepts about Print* test.

Many of the tests have items designed to ascertain whether a child knows about print conventions such as how to hold a book upright; what one reads (print, not pictures); where the print begins on a page and where it proceeds from there (left to right and top to bottom);what constitutes a word in print, a letter, a number, a capital letter; and how stories are organized. One could easily observe a child's command of such concepts by informally asking questions in a book-reading context. Informal questioning could likewise shed light on a child's segmenting abilities, ability to name and write letters and associate them with sounds, writing skills, and information regarding various functions of print. In fact, many children might even be better able to exhibit such knowledge in an informal context than in a structured, formal test context.

FACILITATING FOUNDATIONS FOR LITERACY: A SUMMARY

From the research reviewed above, four general approaches for promoting the development of foundations for print literacy in normal or language delayed preschoolers can be gleaned.

1. Interaction should be guided in informal, everyday activities involving print. Given the guiding role that must be played by an adult or literate person, the clinician or teacher may wish to foster the development of parental behaviors believed to facilitate children's learning from early

literacy experiences. This might be done by modeling facilitating behaviors for the parents or by recommending books written for parents based on new emerging literacy research (Bettleheim & Zelan, 1981; Fields, 1989; Graves & Stuart, 1985; Time-Life Editors, 1987).

2. Literacy-related episodes should be promoted in pretend play. Much of children's learning takes place in play, where trying new behaviors can flourish in a risk-free context. As noted earlier, some research has demonstrated the dramatic impact of supplying print-related materials for children's play. Clinicians might share the value of providing "literacy artifacts" for young children's play with parents, teachers, and day care providers.

3. Game-like activities should be encouraged. Rhyming and alliteration skills have been found to greatly facilitate a child's ability to focus on sounds in language, hence enhancing later reading and spelling achievement (Bradley, 1988). Furthermore, all kinds of language games are more prevalent in the homes of early readers (Tobin, 1981). Teachers or clinicians might strongly encourage parents to read nursery rhymes to infants and toddlers. Ideas for many other language games that could effectively be embedded in therapy activities or encouraged in families are provided in a book written for a parent audience by McCabe entitled, *Language games to play with your child* (1987).

4. Direct instruction may be necessary for phoneme segmentation skills. Researchers believe that direct instruction may be necessary for most children to develop phoneme segmentation abilities. For children of kindergarten age or older, teachers

and clinicians might consider formal training in segmentation skills similar to that employed in training studies by Sawyer (1988) and Lundberg (1988).

• • •

From this rapidly growing and diverse body of research, four general conclusions can be drawn regarding the role of the preschool years in literacy development.

1. Almost from birth, children gradually begin learning a great deal about print, even though they may not learn how to actually decode print until they are formally taught to do so in school.

2. Children's knowledge of print stems from learning about both reading and writing, both of which develop simultaneously and are closely related processes.

3. Children learn about print by encountering it in meaningful, real-life social interactions where it is used to get real things done.

4. While some very general stages can be noted in early literacy development, ages at which children pass through these stages vary markedly. In addition, there is also a great deal of variability in the strategies that children employ in dealing with print.

The development of reading is an extremely complex process. Facilitating preschool children's nascent knowledge of what print is, how it works, and why it is used is clearly only a first step in introducing children to print literacy. Attention to emergent print literacy concepts during the preschool years will in no way eradicate subsequent reading disabilities. It will, however, provide a solid foundation on which to continue to build.

REFERENCES

Anderson, A., & Stokes, S. (1984). Social and institutional influences on the development and practice of literacy. In H. Goelman, A. Oberg, & F. Smith (Eds.), *Awakening to literacy*. Exeter, NH: Heinemann Educational Books.

Applebee, A. (1978). *The child's concept of story*. Chicago: The University of Chicago Press.

Baghban, M. (1984). *Our daughter learns to read and write: A case study from birth to three*. Newark, DE: International Reading Association.

Bateson, G. (1972). *Steps to an ecology of mind*. New York: Ballantine.

Bettelheim, B., & Zelan, K. (1981). *On learning to read*. New York: Random House.

Blodgett, E., & Cooper, E. (1987). *Analysis of the language of learning*. Moline, IL: LinguiSystems.

Bloom, L. (1974). Talking, understanding, and thinking: Developmental relationship between receptive and expressive language. In R. Schiefelbusch & L. Lloyd (Eds.), *Language perspectives: Acquisition, retention, and intervention*. Baltimore: University Park Press.

Bloom, L., & Lahey, M. (1978). *Language development and language disorders*. New York: Wiley.

Bradley, L. (1988). Rhyme recognition and reading and spelling in young children. In R. Masland & M. Masland (Eds.), *Pre-school prevention of reading failure*. Parkton, MD: York Press.

Butler, K. (1988). Preschool language processing performance and later reading achievement. In R. Masland & M. Masland (Eds.), *Preschool prevention of reading failure*. Parkton, MD: York Press.

Chall, J., Snow, C., Barnes, W., Chandler, J., Hempill, L., Goodman, I., & Jacobs, V. (1983). *Families and literacy* (Final Report). Cambridge, MA: National Institute of Education, Harvard Graduate School of Education.

Chukovsky, K. (1963). *From two to five* (M. Morton, Trans.). Berkeley: University of California Press. (Original work published 1925)

Clay, M. (1966). *Emergent reading behavior*. Unpublished doctoral dissertation, University of Auckland, New Zealand.

Clay, M. (1972). *Sand—The Concepts About Print Test*. Portsmouth, NH: Heinemann Educational Books.

Clay, M. (1975). *What did I write? Beginning writing behavior*. Portsmouth, NH: Heinemann Educational Books.

Clay, M. (1979a). *The early detection of reading difficulties: A diagnostic survey with recovery procedures* (2nd ed.). Portsmouth, NH: Heinemann Educational Books.

Clay, M. (1979b). *Stones—The Concepts About Print Test*. Portsmouth, NH: Heinemann Educational Books.

Cochran-Smith, M. (1984). *The making of a reader*. Norwood, NJ: Ablex.

DeLoache, J., & DeMendoza, O. (1986). *Joint picturebook reading of children*. Champaign, IL: University of Illinois.

Dewitz, P., Stammer, J., & Jenson, J. (1980, December). *The development of linguistic awareness in young children from label reading to word recognition*. Paper presented at the annual meeting of the National Reading Conference, San Diego, CA.

Doman, G. (1963). *Teach your baby to read*. London: Jonathan Cape.

Dowker, A. (1989). Rhyme and alliteration in poems elicited from young children. *Journal of Child Language, 16*, 181–202.

Downing, J., Ayers, D., & Schaefer, B. (1982). *Linguistic Awareness in Reading Readiness (LARR)*. Slough, England: The NFER-Nelson Publishing Co.

Downing, J. & Valtin, R. (Eds.). (1984). *Language awareness and learning to read*. New York: Springer-Verlag.

Ehri, L. (1975). Word consciousness in readers and prereaders. *Journal of Educational Psychology, 67*, 204–212.

Ehri, L. (1985). Effects of printed language acquisition on speech. In D. Olson, N. Torrance, & A. Hildyard (Eds.), *Literacy, language, and learning: The nature and consequences of reading and writing*. Cambridge, MA: Cambridge University Press.

Elkind, D. (1987). *Miseducation: Preschoolers at risk*. New York: Knopf.

Englemann, S., & Englemann, T. (1986). *Give your child a superior mind*. New York: Cornerstone.

Feitelson, D., & Goldstein, Z. (1986). *Effects of reading series-stories to first graders on their comprehension and use of language*. Haifa, Israel: University of Haifa, School of Education.

Ferreiro, E. (1984). The underlying logic of literacy development. In H. Goelman, A. Oberg, & F. Smith (Eds.), *Awakening to literacy*. Exeter, NH: Heinemann Educational Books.

Ferreiro, E. (1986). The interplay between information and assimilation in beginning literacy. In W. Teale & E. Sulzby (Eds.), *Emergent literacy*. Norwood, NJ: Ablex.

Ferreiro, E., & Teberosky, A. (1982). *Literacy before schooling*. Exeter, NH: Heinemann Educational Books.

Fields, M. (1989). *Literacy begins at birth*. Tucson, AZ: Fisher Books.

Forrell, E., & Hood, J. (1985). A longitudinal study of two groups of children with early reading problems. *Annals of Dyslexia, 35*, 97–116.

Fox, B., & Routh, D. (1975). Analyzing spoken language into words, syllables, and phonemes: A developmental study. *Journal of Psycholinguistic Research, 4,* 331–342.

Genishi, C., & Dyson, A. (1984). *Language assessment in the early years.* Norwood, NJ: Ablex.

Gibson, E., & Levin, H. (1975). *The psychology of reading.* Cambridge, MA: MIT Press.

Goodman, Y. (1981). Test review: Concepts about print tests. *The Reading Teacher, 34,* 445–448.

Goodman, Y. (1984). The development of initial literacy. In H. Goelman, A. Oberg, & F. Smith (Eds.), *Awakening to literacy.* Exeter, NH: Heinemann Educational Books.

Goodman, Y. (1986). Children coming to know literacy. In W. Teale & E. Sulzby (Eds.), *Emergent literacy.* Norwood, NJ: Ablex.

Graves, D. (1983). *Writing: Teachers and children at work.* Exeter, NH: Heinemann Educational Books.

Graves, D., & Stuart, V. (1985). *Write from the start: Tapping your child's natural writing ability.* New York: New American Library.

Hall, N. (1987). *The emergence of literacy.* Portsmouth, NH: Heinemann.

Hall, N., May, L., Moores, J., Shearer, J., & Williams, S. (1986, August). *Literacy events in the "home" corner of a nursery school.* Paper presented at the World Congress on Reading, London.

Harste, J., Woodward, V., & Burke, C. (1984). *Language stories and literacy lessons.* Portsmouth, NH: Heinemann Educational Books.

Heath, S. (1982). What no bedtime story means. *Language and Society, 2,* 49–76.

Heath, S. (1983). *Ways with words: Language, life, and work in communities and classrooms.* New York: Cambridge University Press.

Henderson, E. (1986). Understanding children's knowledge of written language. In D. Yaden & S. Templeton (Eds.), *Metalinguistic awareness and beginning literacy.* Portsmouth, NH: Heinemann Educational Books.

Henderson, E., & Beers, J. (1980). *Developmental and cognitive aspects of learning to spell.* Newark, DE: International Reading Association.

Hiebert, E. (1978). Preschool children's understanding of written language. *Child Development, 49,* 1231–1234.

Hiebert, E. (1981). Developmental patterns and interrelationships of preschool children's print awareness. *Reading Research Quarterly, 16,* 236–260.

Hiebert, E. (1986). Issues related to home influences on young children's print-related development. In D. Yaden & S. Templeton (Eds.), *Metalinguistic awareness and beginning literacy.* Portsmouth, NH: Heinemann Educational Books.

Holden, M., & MacGinitie, W. (1972). Children's conceptions of word boundaries in speech and print. *Journal of Educational Psychology, 63,* 551–557.

Huttenlocher, J. (1964). Children's language: Word–phrase relationships. *Science, 143,* 264–265.

Jacob, E. (1984). Learning literacy through play: Puerto Rican kindergarten children. In H. Goelman, A. Oberg, & F. Smith (Eds.), *Awakening to literacy.* Exeter, NH: Heinemann Educational Books.

Just, M., & Carpenter, P. (1987). *The psychology of reading and language comprehension.* Boston: Allyn and Bacon.

Kammler, B. (1984). Ponch writes again: A child at play. *Australian Journal of Reading, 7,* 61–70.

Karpova, S. (1966). The preschooler's realization of the lexical structure of speech. In F. Smith & G. Miller (Eds.), *The genesis of language: A psycholinguistic approach.* Cambridge, MA: The MIT Press.

Lass, B. (1982). "Portrait of my son as an early reader." *The Reading Teacher, 36*(1), 20–28.

Ledson, S. (1983). *Raising brighter children.* Toronto: McClelland and Stewart.

Lee, A., & Shapero-Fine, J. (1984). When a language problem is primary: Secondary school strategies. In G. Wallach & K. Butler (Eds.), *Language learning disabilities in school-age children.* Baltimore: Williams & Wilkins.

Leichter, H. (1984). Families as environments for literacy. In H. Goelman, A. Oberg, & F. Smith (Eds.), *Awakening to literacy.* Exeter, NH: Heinemann Educational Books.

Liberman, I. (1973). Segmentation and the spoken word. *Bulletin of the Orton Society, 23,* 65–77.

Liberman, I., Shankweiler, D., Fisher, F., & Carter, B. (1974). Explicit syllable and phoneme segmentation in the young child. *Journal of Experimental Child Psychology, 18,* 201–212.

Ludington-Hoe, S. (1985). *How to have a smarter baby.* New York: Rawson Associates.

Lundberg, I. (1988). Preschool prevention in reading failure: Does training in phonological awareness work? In R. Masland & M. Masland (Eds.), *Preschool prevention of reading failure.* Parkton, MD: York Press.

Mason, J. (1980). When do children begin to read: An exploration of four-year-old children's letter and word reading competencies. *Reading Research Quarterly, 15,* 203–227.

Mason, J., & Allen, J. (1986). A review of emergent literacy with implications for research and practice in reading. In C. Rothkopf (Ed.), *Review of research in education* (Vol. 13). Washington, DC: American Educational Research Association.

Masonheimer, P., Drum, P., & Ehri, L. (1984). Does environmental print lead children into word reading? *Journal of Reading Behavior, 12,* 257–272.

Mattis, S., French, J., & Rapin, I. (1975). Dyslexia in children and young adults: Three independent neuropsychological syndromes. *Developmental Medicine and Child Neurology, 17,* 150–163.

McCabe, A. (1987). *Language games to play with your child.* New York: Fawcett Columbine.

McCormick, C., & Mason, J. (1986). Intervention procedures for increasing preschool children's interest in and knowledge about reading. In W. Teale & E. Sulzby (Eds.), *Emergent literacy.* Norwood, NJ: Ablex.

McLean, M., Bryant P., & Bradley, L. (1987). Rhymes, nursery rhymes and reading in early childhood. *Merrill-Palmer Quarterly, 33,* 255–282.

Mead, M. (1977). End linkage: A tool for cross-cultural analysis. In J. Brockman (Ed.), *About Bateson.* New York: E. P. Dutton.

Miller, P. (1982). *Amy, Wendy and Beth: Learning language in South Baltimore.* Austin: University of Texas Press.

Morris, D. (1981). Concept of word: A developmental phenomenon in the beginning reading and writing process. *Language Arts, 58,* 659–668.

Ninio, A., & Bruner, J. (1978). The achievements and antecedents of labelling. *Journal of Child Language, 5,* 1–15.

Nurss, J.R., & McGauvran, M. (1986). *Early School Inventory-Preliteracy.* New York: Harcourt, Brace, Jovanovich, Inc.

Nystrand, M. (1982). Rhetoric's "audience" and linguistics' "speech community": Implications for understanding writing and text. In M. Nystrand (Ed.), *What writers know: The language, process, and structure of written discourse.* New York: Academic Press.

Olson, D. (1984). "See! Jumping!" Some oral antecedents of literacy. In H. Goelman, A. Oberg, & F. Smith (Eds.), *Awakening to literacy.* Exeter, NH: Heinemann Educational Books.

Padget, S.Y. (1988). Speech- and language-impaired three and four year olds: A five year follow-up study. In R. Masland & M. Masland (Eds.), *Preschool prevention of reading failure.* Parkton, MD: York Press.

Perfetti, C. (1985). *Reading ability.* New York: Oxford University Press.

Rader, M. (1982). Context in written language: The case of imaginative fiction. In D. Tannen (Ed.), *Spoken and written language: Exploring orality and literacy.* Norwood, NJ: Ablex.

Reid, D., Hresko, W., & Hammill, D. (1989). *Test of Early Reading Ability (TERA-2).* Austin, TX: PRO-ED.

Rogers, T. (1979). *Those first affections: An anthology of poems composed between the ages of two and eight.* London: Routledge & Kegan Paul.

Rosner, J. (1974). Auditory analysis training with prereaders. *The Reading Teacher, 27*(4), 379–384.

Row, D., & Harste, J. (1986). Metalinguistic awareness in writing and reading: The young child as circular

informant. In D. Yaden & S. Templeton (Eds.), *Metalinguistic awareness and beginning literacy.* Portsmouth, NH: Heinemann Educational Books.

Samuels, S. (1971). Letter name versus letter sound knowledge in learning to read. *Reading Teacher, 24,* 604–608.

Sawyer, D. (1987). *Test of Awareness of Language Segments.* Austin, TX: PRO-ED.

Sawyer, D. (1988). Studies of the effects of teaching auditory segmenting skills within the reading program. In R. Masland & M. Masland (Eds.), *Preschool prevention of reading failure.* Parkton, MD: York Press.

Schickedanz, J. (1984, December). *A study of literacy events in the homes of six preschoolers.* Paper presented at the National Reading Conference, St. Petersburg, FL.

Schieffelin, B., & Cochran-Smith, M. (1984). Learning to read culturally: Literacy before schooling. In H. Goelman, A. Oberg, & F. Smith (Eds.), *Awakening to literacy.* Exeter, NH: Heinemann Educational Books.

Scollon, R., & Scollon, S. (1981). *Narrative, literacy, and face in interethnic communication.* Norwood, NJ: Ablex.

Share, D., Jorm, A., MacLean, R., & Matthews, R. (1984). Sources of individual differences in reading acquisition. *Journal of Educational Psychology, 76*(6), 1309–1324.

Snow, C. (1983). Literacy and language: Relationships during the preschool years. *Harvard Educational Review, 53*(2), 165–189.

Snow, C., & Goldfield, B. (1981). Building stories: The emergence of information structures from conversation. In D. Tannen (Ed.), *Analyzing discourse: Text and talk.* Washington, DC: Georgetown University Round Table on Language and Linguistics, Georgetown University Press.

Snow, C., & Goldfield, B. (1983). Turn the page please: Situation-specific language acquisition. *Journal of Child Language, 10,* 551–569.

Snow, C., & Ninio, A. (1986). The contracts of literacy: What children learn from learning to read books. In W. Teale & E. Sulzby (Eds.), *Emergent literacy.* Norwood, NJ: Ablex.

Stark, R., Bernstein, L., & Condino, R. (1984). Four-year follow-up study of language-impaired children. *Annals of Dyslexia, 34,* 29–48.

Stein, N., & Glenn, C. (1979). An analysis of story comprehension in elementary school children. In R. Freedle (Ed.), *New directions in discourse processing, vol. 2.* Norwood, NJ: Ablex.

Strominger, A., & Bashir, A. (1977, November). *A nine-year follow-up of language-delayed children.* Paper presented at the annual convention of the American Speech-Language-Hearing Association, Chicago.

Sulzby, E. (1986). Writing and reading: Signs of oral and written language organization in the young child. In W.

Teale & E. Sulzby (Eds.), *Emergent literacy: Writing and reading*. Norwood, NJ: Ablex.

Tannen, D. (1985). Relative focus on involvement in oral and written discourse. In D. Olson, N. Torrance, & A. Hildyard (Eds.), *Literacy, language, and learning: The nature and consequences of reading and writing*. Cambridge, MA: Cambridge University Press.

Taylor, D. (1981). *Family literacy: The social context of learning to read and write*. Unpublished doctoral dissertation, Teachers College, Columbia University, New York.

Taylor, D. (1983). *Family literacy: Young children learning to read and write*. Portsmouth, NH: Heinemann Educational Books.

Taylor, N., & Blum, I. (1980). *Written Language Awareness Test* (Experimental Edition). Washington, DC: The Catholic University.

Teale, W. (1978). Positive environments for learning to read: What studies of early readers tell us. *Language Arts, 55*, 922–945.

Teale, W. (1984). Reading to young children: Its significance for literacy development. In H. Goelman, A. Oberg, & F. Smith (Eds.), *Awakening to literacy*. Exeter, NH: Heinemann Educational Books.

Teale, W. (1986). Home background and young children's literacy development. In W. Teale & E. Sulzby (Eds.), *Emergent literacy: Writing and reading*. Norwood, NJ: Ablex.

Teale, W., & Sulzby, E. (1986). Introduction: Emergent literacy as a perspective for examining how young children become writers and readers. In W. Teale & E. Sulzby (Eds.), *Emergent literacy: Writing and reading*. Norwood, NJ: Ablex.

Temple, C., Nathan, R., & Burris, N. (1982). *The beginnings of writing*. Boston: Allyn and Bacon.

Thomas, K. (1985). Early reading as a social interaction process. *Language Arts, 62*(5), 469–475.

Thorndike, R. (1976). Reading comprehension in 15 countries. In J. Merritt (Ed.), *New horizons in reading*. Newark, DE: International Reading Association.

Time-Life Editors. (1987). *First steps toward reading*. Alexandria, VA: Time-Life Books.

Tizard, B., & Hughes, M. (1984). *Young children learning: Talking and thinking at home and school*. London: Fontana.

Tobin, A. (1981). *A multiple discriminant cross-validation of the factors associated with the development of precocious reading achievement*. Unpublished doctoral dissertation, University of Delaware, Newark.

Tobin, A., & Pikulski, J. (1983, April). *Parent and teacher attitudes toward early reading instruction*. Paper presented at the annual meeting of the American Educational Research Association, Montreal.

Treiman, R., & Baron, J. (1983). Phonemic analysis training helps children benefit from spelling-sound rules. *Memory and Cognition, 2*, 382–389.

van Kleeck, A., & Schuele, M. (1987). Precursors to literacy: Normal development. *Topics in Language Disorders, 7*(2), 13–31.

Vygotsky, L. (1978). *Mind in society: The development of higher psychological processes*. In M. Cole, V. John-Steiner, S. Scribner, & E. Souberman (Eds.), Cambridge, MA: Harvard University Press.

Wagner, R., & Torgesen, J. (1987). The nature of phonological processing and its causal role in the acquisition of reading skills. *Psychological Bulletin, 101*(2), 192–212.

Weir, R. (1962). *Language in the Crib*. The Hague, Netherlands: Mouton.

Wells, G. (1985). Preschool literacy-related activities and success in school. In D. Olson, N. Torrance, & A. Hildyard (Eds.), *Literacy, language, and learning: The nature and consequences of reading and writing*. Cambridge, MA: Cambridge University Press.

White, K. (1982). The relation between socioeconomic status and academic achievement. *Psychological Bulletin, 91*, 461–481.

Classroom literacy instruction for children with severe speech and physical impairments (SSPI): What is and what might be

David A. Koppenhaver, PhD
Associate Director, The Carolina Literacy Center
Department of Medical Allied Health Professions
The University of North Carolina at Chapel Hill

David E. Yoder, PhD, CCC-SLP
Chair, Department of Medical Allied Health Professions
Director, The Carolina Literacy Center
The University of North Carolina at Chapel Hill
Chapel Hill, North Carolina

IN THIS ARTICLE, we have chosen to focus on instruction in conventional literacy (i.e., learning to read and write traditional orthography) for children with severe speech and physical impairments (SSPI). In this article, SSPI refers to persons with cerebral palsy, although our early experiences at the Carolina Literacy Center with individuals who have SSPI associated with other developmental disabilities suggest that there are many similar concerns (e.g., low expectations, limited learning opportunities). Literacy is no less relevant to individuals who may never become conventionally literate (see Koppenhaver, Coleman, Kalman, & Yoder, 1991), but there is little research to inform practice.

There is no question about whether literacy is important to persons with SSPI, but there are relevant questions related to the causes of the observed literacy-learning difficulties and the potential solutions. The state of our knowledge base regarding effective literacy intervention approaches

Top Lang Disord, 1993,13(2),1–15
© 1993 Aspen Publishers, Inc.

with persons with SSPI is that we know very little that will help us argue with certainty that one is more effective than another. An absence of certainty should not impede our efforts to improve literacy services for children and adults with SSPI, but educators should be seeking a balance of teaching strategies in the instructional programs they design for children with SSPI.

We begin our discussion by presenting a model to assist in understanding classroom instruction. We then review research conducted in classrooms of children with SSPI and present descriptions and explanations of some effective instructional strategies. We conclude with suggestions for implementing more effective literacy instruction in the classrooms of children with SSPI.

A MODEL OF CLASSROOM INSTRUCTION

If we are to make sense of the research to be reviewed in this article, it is important to understand some of the factors influencing classroom instruction. Dunkin and Biddle's (1974) model for the study of classroom teaching provides a useful organizing framework. Dunkin and Biddle contend that there are four major categories of variables of interest to instructional research: (1) presage, (2) context, (3) process, and (4) product. Hoffman (1991) provides the following definitions, which we will elaborate on, utilizing specific augmentative and alternative communication (AAC) examples:

- Presage variables are the personal characteristics, experiences, or qualities that teachers bring to the instructional setting (e.g., training in special

education, prior experience with persons with SSPI, motivation).
- Context variables refer to conditions within and surrounding classroom instruction (e.g., nature of the students' disabilities, AAC systems in use, classroom support services).
- Process variables are what teachers and students actually do in the classroom (e.g., answering yes/no or open-ended questions, composing text using word processors with synthetic speech feedback).
- Product variables refer to what is learned by students as a function of participating in classroom processes (e.g., literacy achievement, attitudes toward learning).

In essence, presage and context variables influence the kinds of processes teachers and students engage in and consequently the kinds of educational outcomes or products that result. For example, one teacher we know holds high expectations for all of her first graders (i.e., presage). While she typically teaches children with severe disabilities, she has excellent support staff, materials, and equipment (i.e., context). She engages all of her students in literacy activities and structures opportunities for them to interact with staff and each other about those activities (i.e., process). For the past three years, 30% to 50% of her students have moved on to full-inclusion settings because their literacy skills have progressed to grade-level performance (i.e., product).

CLASSROOM STUDIES OF CHILDREN WITH SSPI

Repeated searches of the literature (Koppenhaver & Yoder, 1992) reveal five studies to date that directly pertain to a description of the actions and interactions of teachers and students with severe disabilities during classroom literacy instruction. The first is an unpublished ethnographic report of the nature of literacy instruction provided to five children, ages 10 to 14 years, with cerebral palsy (Mike, 1987). The second is an unpublished observational study of the daily instruction provided to a set of six-year-old twins, one with SSPI and the other typically developing (Wasson & Keeler, 1984). The third is a descriptive study of the nature of teacher–student interaction in three school contexts involving a trio of children, ages 6 years and 6 months to 7 years and 11 months, with SSPI (Harris, 1982). The fourth is a recently completed, year-long, descriptive and qualitative study of literacy instruction provided to three boys in three self-contained classrooms for children with severe physical disabilities (Koppenhaver, 1991). A fifth study (Koppenhaver, Evans, & Yoder, 1991) provides descriptive data of classroom instruction through interviews.

Mike (1987) conducted 63.5 two-hour observations in a single self-contained classroom for five children with cerebral palsy. The observations were conducted over a 17-week period in the fall of the school year. The five subjects had a variety of types and degrees of disability: four had severe physical impairments and relied on wheelchairs for mobility, one was ambulatory, three had mild mental retardation, and one had a severe speech impairment. Mike's preliminary data analysis revealed that students received direct instruction in reading for an average of just 15 minutes per day, and they seldom interacted with each other (181 instances across 127 hours

of observation). When they did interact, it was largely unrelated to instruction. Details of the study are sketchy since it was never written as a paper.

Wasson and Keeler (1984) observed in the classrooms of a set of twins; one had severe disabilities, and the other was nondisabled. Both children had intelligence within normal limits and had been provided similar experiences to the extent possible prior to entering school. Very soon after starting first grade, however, the child who had no disabilities began excelling in literacy learning, while the child with disabilities made little progress. This occurred despite the fact that the former was in a classroom of 25 children with 1 teacher and no aides, while the latter was in a classroom of nine children with disabilities, one teacher, and two aides. Classroom observations revealed that the child with disabilities received 30 minutes of instruction for every 60 provided to her sister. Instructional time became secondary to transitions and toileting, technology repairs, therapies, and other management concerns. Further, despite the difference in adult–child ratio, the child with disabilities received one fifth the opportunities to communicate in the classroom (i.e., to answer or ask questions, to make comments).

Harris (1982) studied the nature of communication interaction between school-aged children who rely on AAC systems and their teachers in three school contexts: (1) free time, (2) individualized instruction, and (3) small group instruction. The individualized instructional activity consisted primarily of language experience story construction. The teachers would ask questions and write a story on the chalkboard based on the students' responses.

The small group instruction context consisted primarily of reading lessons in which the teacher would either read a story or discuss a topic and then ask the group questions. Speaking peers occasionally would be called on to read aloud.

Harris videotaped the communication interactions of students and their teachers in these contexts and then coded conversational turns, unit types within turns, communicative functions, and turn forms. Harris observed that while the frequency of teacher and child participation was similar, the teachers contributed much more information within turns and primarily initiated topics, while the children most often provided one-word responses to requests for information. Students seldom communicated via their AAC devices. Teachers also contributed a high number of initiations to fill the silence gap between the phrasing of a teacher question and the response of the student. Subjects rarely interacted with anyone except the teacher in any of the three contexts.

Koppenhaver (1991) observed and videotaped three boys, ages 10 to 14, with SSPI and their teachers during literacy instruction in three different self-contained classrooms. All teacher and student activities were analyzed using separate categorical coding frameworks. The teacher framework facilitated analysis of type of teacher activity performed, function of the instruction engaged in, and instructional grouping employed. Teachers devoted between 55% and 63% of the time they allocated for instruction to actual teaching activity. Remaining time was devoted to classroom management activities, work with other students, or activities unrelated to instruction. Much of the instruction

(68%–100% across teachers) was provided one-to-one or in small groups and consisted largely of assessment activities such as asking questions or providing feedback as to the correctness of response (58%–66%). The average daily instructional time devoted to each of these activities may be found in Table 1. Across teachers, less than 2% of instructional time was devoted to teaching students how to accomplish literacy tasks (e.g., how to determine the main idea of a paragraph or how to write an outline).

The student framework permitted analysis of the type of activity students engaged in, the mode of student participation in that activity, the level of text engaged in during instructional activities, and in the case of writing, the nature of the writing task. Students engaged in more nonliteracy activities (34%–38%; e.g., waiting, management, being off-task or out of the room during instructional time) than any single literacy activity. In descending frequency, students engaged in reading (23%–29% of allocated instructional time across students), listening (15%–22%), writing (10%–16%), and AAC (6%–9%). The

Table 1. Range of teacher use of time allocated for literacy instruction

Teacher activity	Average daily time (hours: minutes: seconds)	Percent of time allocated for literacy instruction (%)
Literacy instruction	47:07–1:01:12	55–63
Small group or one-to-one instruction	35:50–41:56	37–56
Assessment or feedback	27:06–40:35	33–40

vast majority of literacy instruction focused on words and sentences in isolation, fill-in-the-blank exercises, and spelling practice (47%–100% of reading, writing, listening, and AAC activity across students). The average daily instructional time devoted to these various student activities may be found in Table 2. Further microanalysis of reading comprehension lessons suggested they were largely teacher-directed, text-based exercises in assessment of student comprehension of factual details. Similar analysis of written composition lessons suggested that they were teacher-directed, collaborative exercises in text production. Students supplied specific content while teachers maintained control of topic, organization, syntax, and cohesion.

While it is not observational research, a fifth study is included here because it examines the school-based literacy instruction and experiences of individuals with SSPI through interviews. Koppenhaver et al. (1991) surveyed 22 highly literate adults with SSPI in the United States and Canada, asking them to reflect on literacy-learning experiences from their childhood. Respondents recalled having been regularly read to as well as engaging in regular reading themselves for pleasure and to complete assignments in school settings. Respondents also reported engaging in a great many activities that research suggests are linked to literacy gains (see, e.g., Anderson, Hiebert, Scott, & Wilkinson, 1984): reading and listening to taped stories; listening to adults read aloud; reading widely in self-selected materials; reading texts in order to answer questions posed by teachers beforehand; reading the same text repeatedly; and learning new vocabulary prior to reading a new assignment. Interestingly, although they were highly literate young adults and adults, the respondents reported few opportunities to write as school-aged children.

In summary, the five studies suggest that school-aged children with severe disabilities appear to receive less literacy instruction than do their nondisabled peers, participate in that instruction in fairly passive ways, seldom interact with peers during instruction, and experience frequent and regular interruptions despite receiving that instruction most often one-to-one or in small groups. On the other hand, while causality cannot be inferred, literate adults with severe impairments reported having regular and wide access to many literacy experiences supported by research. Whether such findings are representative of the nature of instruction provided to other children with severe disabilities has not yet been determined empirically.

We do know, however, that such findings are in concert with much of the

Table 2. Range of student use of time allocated for literacy instruction

Student activity	Average daily time (minutes: seconds)	Percent of time allocated for literacy instruction (%)
Nonliteracy	28:31–35:02	34–38
Literacy		
Reading	17:10–29:33	23–29
Listening	15:16–16:20	15–22
Writing	7:32–15:17	10–16
AAC	5:35–8:59	6–9
Words and sentences in isolation	34:55–56:31	47–100

previous descriptive research examining the nature of literacy instruction provided to children with learning disabilities, mild mental retardation, and reading disabilities. Students in these special education settings

- engage in many noninstructional activities during the time allocated for instruction (e.g., Allington, Stuetzel, Shake, & Lamarche, 1986; Haynes & Jenkins, 1986);
- seldom read or write texts of a paragraph or longer (e.g., Leinhardt, Zigmond, & Cooley, 1981; Ysseldyke, Christenson, Thurlow, & Bakewell, 1989); and
- spend substantial amounts of time completing worksheets (e.g., Baker & Zigmond, 1990) and focusing on the surface features of writing such as spelling and punctuation (e.g., Ysseldyke et al., 1989).

Each of these practices is negatively correlated with literacy achievement. In essence, the research suggests that often in the best of circumstances (i.e., experienced teachers who believe their students are capable of learning), students with mild to severe disabilities are engaged in activities that should not be expected to improve their reading and writing.

INTERVENTION STUDIES OF CHILDREN WITH SSPI

There are likewise very few intervention studies of school-aged children with SSPI, each of which might be characterized as pilot or exploratory in nature, and none of which has led to an ongoing line of research to date. The studies have essentially examined ways of increasing the rate

and accuracy of student response, primarily in classroom settings.

Increasing rate of response

Wasson and Keeler (1984) replaced previous modes of response with eye-pointing in multiple-choice drill and practice activities to more than triple the response opportunities of a six-year-old girl with SSPI. McNaughton and Drynan (1990) reported a case study of an 11-year-old boy with SSPI, whose typing speed increased from three to eight words-per-minute with a keyboard overlay that permitted single keystroke selection of high-frequency known words. Harris's (1982) study of the classroom interactions of three 6- to 7-year-olds with SSPI showed that longer wait times (i.e., the length of time between the teacher asking a question and then calling on a student to answer) were associated with more frequent and lengthier student contributions.

Increasing accuracy of response

Accuracy of student response has been improved by means of auditory feedback from speech synthesizers, cassette tapes, and the human voice. In the most carefully controlled study, Koke and Neilson (1987) employed a single-subject design to examine spelling accuracy in natural writing samples. Two of three young adults with SSPI committed fewer errors in their final drafts and made more self-corrections in the process while using a word processing program with synthesized speech feedback than without speech feedback. The third subject showed no clear pattern. Koppenhaver and Yoder (1989) taught two young adolescents with SSPI a spelling study strategy in which the students looked at each new word as the teacher spoke it aloud, were told to see and hear the words in their heads, then practiced spelling each word and self-correcting. Both children consistently improved, but the child with the stronger phonemic discrimination skills was able to retain the newly learned words longer.

Repeated listening to texts has improved listening comprehension and word recognition in reading passages in two studies. De Hoop (1965) examined the effects of compressed speech and normal speech on listening comprehension in three groups of individuals with cerebral palsy (ages 7–27 years) with a wide range of cognitive skills. Pre/post improvement on a 20-question test averaged 5.6 items with a range of 18 items. Koppenhaver and Yoder (1988) created slide-tapes of interesting, easy-to-read books for two young adolescents with SSPI. The students repeatedly read the texts (on slides) while listening to the stories read aloud. Progress was measured using a multiple-choice cloze version of the text (Guthrie, Seifert, Burnham, & Caplan, 1974) and was most rapid on the easiest-to-read texts.

None of these intervention studies is without flaws, many of them serious (for a more in-depth review and discussion, see Koppenhaver & Yoder, 1992). However, each has demonstrated that children with SSPI can and do improve their participation in and learning from literacy activities if given appropriate strategies and assistance.

SOME EXPLANATIONS FOR THE FINDINGS

In essence, a review of these two small bodies of observational and intervention research presents a disheartening picture of classroom instruction for children with SSPI. These children, because of the importance of literacy to their basic communication and the often severe difficulties they encounter in learning to read and write, should receive the best instruction possible. Nevertheless, much of their classroom time is lost to noninstructional activities; the instruction they do receive is grossly imbalanced toward word-level exercises; and the students are passively involved in that instruction, responding briefly when directed to do so. Finally, the instruction is costly since it is delivered one-to-one or in small groups. The following discussion relates research findings with reference to the model of classroom instruction introduced earlier.

Presage variables

Personal characteristics or qualities of teachers of children with SSPI seem unlikely reasons to explain the kinds of instruction observed. A more obvious explanation lies in the area of teacher training experiences. The teachers in Koppenhaver's (1991) study reported they had received little education in literacy teaching methods and no training in methods for promoting literacy in children with SSPI. These teachers are not unique. Eighty percent of the literacy instructors surveyed by Light, Koppenhaver, Lee, and Riffle (1992) reported they had received no education and training in teaching children who use AAC systems to read and write. There are only a handful of universities nationwide that provide more than a single course in AAC. Only one currently offers specific and intensive training in literacy teaching methods and AAC: the University of North Carolina at Chapel Hill.

Context variables

Context variables might be conceptualized as those within the student (e.g., abilities, attitudes) and those within the learning context (e.g., class size, instructional materials). The most obvious examples related to students would be assistive technology broadly, and AAC systems specifically. Children with SSPI live in technology-rich classroom environments, employing light technology such as book holders and rubber-tipped headsticks and high technology systems such as voice output communication aids and electronic page turners. There are no computer programs that enable children with SSPI to closely approximate the early and exploratory literacy experiences of their nondisabled peers. With the exception of microcomputers, most of these devices are above and beyond those used by nondisabled students, and each complicates the delivery of instruction to a certain degree and requires additional technical expertise in educators who work with children with SSPI. AAC systems create contextual differences in and of themselves, providing slow rates of transmission (Yoder & Kraat, 1983) and limited vocabulary access (Higginbotham, 1985) while requiring co-construction of message by AAC users and their communication partners (Colquhoun, 1982; Culp, 1982). While technology provides access to speech, text production, and supported learning activities, it also frequently can interfere with the central learner task of constructing meaning in texts.

The absence of any curriculum or body of instructional strategies for teaching children with SSPI is a less obvious contextual variable. Teachers who currently provide written language instruction for children with SSPI do so on their own initiative by searching out and adapting materials and strategies from texts written for nondisabled children, by inquiring of fellow teachers, and by creating what they cannot locate elsewhere. Creating a curriculum can be exhausting in the face of competing demands in the workplace and home, particularly if no additional school resources (e.g., time, personnel, materials, or training) are allocated for that purpose.

The nature of the child with SSPI is a further complicating contextual variable. SSPI is a low-incidence disorder regardless of etiology. Often teachers have not previously taught such a child, or have not taught a child with such severe impairments. In our experience at the Carolina Literacy Center in providing technical assistance, we find that support services are typically unable to address specifically the literacy needs of such children, and the teacher is left feeling isolated.

Process variables

The two studies that have examined the face-to-face interactions of school children with SSPI and their teachers (Harris, 1982; Koppenhaver, 1991) are consistent with studies of AAC users in other natural environments. AAC users often forego many conversational opportunities (Light, Collier, & Parnes, 1985a), provide yes/no and one- or two-word informational responses (Calculator & Luchko, 1983; Colquhoun, 1982), and typically choose efficiency of message delivery over effectiveness in message construction or conversational control (Farrier, Yorkston, Marriner, & Beukelman, 1985).

Explanations of these findings sort themselves into three categories: (1) the nature of the AAC user, (2) the nature of the AAC system (discussed above), and (3) the nature of the speaking partner. AAC users often lack proficiency with their communication systems (Kraat, 1987) due to infrequent opportunities to practice conversational skills (Smith-Lewis & Ford, 1987) and limited access to paralinguistic, kinesic, and proxemic cues that augment speech in nondisabled persons (Higginbotham & Yoder, 1982). Speaking partners typically initiate many more conversational topics, contribute both longer and more frequent comments and questions, and respond more readily to AAC users' responses than initiations (Calculator & Dollaghan, 1982; Light et al., 1985a, 1985b).

Instead of being able to focus solely on constructing meaning in and from texts, children with SSPI and their teachers may be distracted by continually needing to repair message breakdowns; include the AAC user more fully in the classroom interaction; and find tasks that the child can do within the restrictions of available vocabulary, time constraints, and physical access to materials. In essence, teachers of children with SSPI must juggle more instructional variables more quickly than teachers of nondisabled children.

Product variables

Accurate assessment of student literacy achievement is hindered by the absence of any research-tested instruments or methods. Timed assessments penalize children for their physical impairments. Oral reading, such as that required for miscue analysis or informal reading inventories, penalizes children for their speech impairments. Children with scanning devices are at a disadvantage because they have to hold more information in memory longer than nondisabled children. New methods in other fields such as the preferential-looking paradigm (Cauley, Golinkoff, Hirsh-Pasek, & Gordon, 1989) show some promise in this area. In this paradigm, children are presented with two silent videotapes playing simultaneously on adjacent monitors. Language comprehension is indicated by the child's preference to view the monitor that matches a stimulus. It would seem that written vocabulary knowledge and reading comprehension could be measured in like fashion with a visual print prompt.

In summary, the poor quality of literacy instruction provided to children with SSPI can be traced to many different, and overlapping, sources, including lack of teacher training programs, contextual complications introduced by assistive technology and the absence of a specific curriculum, the difficulties in communication that AAC users and speaking partners encounter across contexts, and the absence of valid and reliable literacy assessments to monitor student progress.

WHAT MIGHT BE

Anderson and colleagues (1984) wrote in the introduction to their review of reading instruction practices in the United States, "If the practices seen in the classrooms of the best teachers in the best schools could be introduced everywhere, the improvements would be dramatic" (p.

3). We believe a similar case could be built for improving literacy instruction for children with SSPI. Toward that end, we would like to present two brief descriptions of literacy instruction from two teachers achieving somewhat better outcomes than we typically observe.

Robbie

Robbie is an 11-year-old with congenital cerebral palsy, normal intelligence, and reading skills at a mid-first grade level. Robbie has profound hearing loss in one ear and uses American Sign Language, vocalizations, and gestures to communicate in the classroom. He received reading instruction in a class of second graders using a basal reading series.

In this lesson, the class is going to read a story about two boys who were good friends. Key vocabulary has been taught the previous day, and the teacher introduces the story by telling the class, "Today we're going to read a story about a boy named Jacob. Look at the picture on the first page, and tell me what you think the story is going to be about." The class makes various predictions, defending them with evidence from the picture. The teacher then directs the class, "Read to the bottom of the first page to find out what Jacob and Sam do together." As the class begins reading, she notices Robbie having difficulty getting started. She stands near him and begins quietly reading aloud to him as he points to the words. After the class finishes the first page, she repeats the question and the students respond. She then directs the students, "Read the next page to find out where they had to go and what they did together." The lesson continues.

In examining this simple lesson, we find a rich combination of practices supported by the research literature as beneficial to developing readers. First, central vocabulary has been taught, students predict story events, and a purpose for reading is set prior to the reading assignment (Stauffer, 1959; Tierney & Cunningham, 1984). Second, students spend much of the lesson reading text, not focusing on words in isolation (Leinhardt et al., 1981). Third, students follow up on the purpose set immediately following reading (Tierney & Cunningham, 1984), and, finally, the teacher reads the text aloud while the student follows along after he indicates difficulty (Koppenhaver et al., 1991; Smith, 1979).

Option 4 classroom

In the state of New York, children with disabilities are categorized into four educational placements, Option 4 being classrooms for children with the most severe disabilities. In fact, in the home school of this classroom, these students are referred to as "the wheelchair kids." Of the eight students, six of the children have congenital cerebral palsy, one has a degenerative neuromotor disorder, and one has spina bifida. Seven rely on wheelchairs for mobility, and one requires no assistive technology for mobility. Three of the students are anarthric, three severely dysarthric, one has a severe communication disorder, and one speaks without difficulty.

The children are taught by a full-time team of five educators: a special educator, a speech-language clinician, two teacher assistants (who carry out teacher lesson plans), and one teacher's aide (who assists but does not engage in instruction). Lessons are planned collaboratively by the special educator and speech-language clinician, and carried out in an integrated team approach by the five educators and other therapists (e.g., physical therapist, occupational therapist) in the classroom. The classroom is equipped with five Apple IIGS computers and a range of assistive technology that allows every child in the classroom to independently use a computer.

Literacy instruction includes a wide range of activities, including journal writing, skills instruction, interactive storybook reading, and integrated language and literacy activities. Journal writing is carried out for 30 minutes daily at the computers—their "pencils." Topics and tasks are self-selected and occasionally teacher-guided but range from copying spelling words to reflecting on a dispute on the bus. The children write as little as a few words to as much as several paragraphs. Skills instruction, too, is conducted largely at the computers. Instruction is fairly traditional and includes phonics activities, completion of fill-in-the-blank activities, and spelling practice using a program that provides auditory and visual feedback.

Storybook reading is made interactive by the inclusion of communication overlays allowing each child voice output for every book. For example, a repeated line story such as *Brown Bear, Brown Bear, What Do You See?* (Martin, 1967) will include the repeated lines and the names of the animals, which allows children to contribute specific lines, answer questions, or retell the story independently. Integrated language and literacy activities vary widely but always engage all of the children in real uses of oral and written

language to communicate, to entertain, to inform. For example, one activity included rehearsing and performing a play as well as gathering and making costumes and props.

In examining the range of activities in this classroom, again we find a rich combination of practices supported by the research literature as beneficial to developing readers. Computers are used as means to ends, to facilitate independent written or oral communication (Reinking & Bridwell-Bowles, 1991). Students engage in regular reading and writing of texts (Leinhardt et al., 1981). Students have opportunities to participate in their own learning, and to comment and ask questions (Lindfors, 1987). Teachers have high expectations for the students, and activities are structured to allow the students to experience success (Harris & Sipay, 1985). Research support aside, the most important thing about this classroom is that it works. The children clearly enjoy their lessons and delight in demonstrating their competence. For three consecutive years, between 30% and 50% of the students in this class have entered full-inclusion settings because of their literacy progress.

IMPLICATIONS FOR SCHOOL-BASED PROGRAMS

"There is so much we do not know, and so much we need to know, and the knowledge is of such pressing import for individuals with SSPI who wish to compete in mainstream educational and employment environments or engage in the sheer pleasure of recreational reading or writing" (Koppenhaver & Yoder, 1992, p. 189). While researchers continue to explore these frontiers, there are many steps that teachers and speech-language pathologists can take to further the literacy learning of children with SSPI.

First, practitioners should carefully examine exactly how time gets used by children with SSPI in their classrooms. Instructional time is lost almost imperceptibly a few minutes at a time as children wait during set-up, device repair, or transition between activities or classrooms. None of the children in the Koppenhaver (1991) or Wasson and Keeler (1984) studies engaged in literacy activities for more than 66% of the time allocated for instruction. In essence, one third of the available time for instruction (60 possible literacy instruction days over the course of a 180-day school year) was lost. Some time loss is inevitable (e.g., computer malfunction), but better management can circumvent many other time losses (e.g., booting up the computer and loading software programs before students arrive in the morning).

Teachers and clinicians must be meticulous in providing independent literacy activities to engage students when instruction or therapy is unavoidably interrupted. The three adolescent students in the Koppenhaver (1991) study seldom were provided with something to do while teachers engaged in management activities. Each of the three lost the equivalent of at least 16 full literacy instructional periods (projected over a full school year) to sitting and waiting with no productive task to occupy them. Instead, students might read independently from slide-taped books, study spelling words, try to solve a word puzzle, or interact with peers to accomplish a brief task.

Second, teachers should seek greater balance across their instructional activities and use of materials. The optimal mix of oral language versus written language activity or skills practice versus reading and writing for meaning is not known. However, students in the Koppenhaver (1991) study had more than twice the opportunity to read as to write and two to three times the opportunity to listen as to communicate. Words and sentences in isolation were the focus of more than 95% of all writing, 64% of all reading, 72% of all communication, and 47% of all listening. The implicit assumption in such an imbalanced instructional program is that by studying the components of literacy, children will be able to synthesize and employ this knowledge in meaningful literacy activities. However, with so few opportunities to practice skills in the context of reading and writing texts, children are unlikely to make these connections on their own (Leinhardt et al., 1981).

Third, teachers should examine just how much control students have over their own learning. Students in the observational studies described above seldom volunteered information, asked questions, or read or wrote for their own purposes, and activities were not designed to allow them to do so. Students should have opportunities to construct meaningful texts, to manipulate oral and written language for different purposes and in different texts, and to talk with other students and teachers before, during, and after those activities. Initial ideas for beginning such a program may be found in Koppenhaver, Coleman, Steelman, and Yoder (in press). In addition, many of the innovative AAC communication interaction strategies that speech-language clinicians have developed may be easily adapted to literacy activities (e.g., Goossens' & Crain, 1986).

Fourth, teachers should use the resources at their disposal. These are not numerous, but they are growing. For example, the Carolina Literacy Center (CLC) at the University of North Carolina at Chapel Hill annually offers a two-week intensive summer seminar on literacy and AAC as well as a two-day symposium each spring on literacy and individuals with SSPI. The CLC also has published a wide array of reports that are available to educators, parents, and others interested in literacy and SSPI. The University of Nebraska at Lincoln incorporates literacy into many of their AAC course offerings as well as research and development projects (e.g., Beukelman, Garrett, Lange, & Tice, 1988). The International Society for Augmentative and Alternative Communication (ISAAC) operates the CONFER bulletin board through which teachers and clinicians can communicate worldwide with others who work with children with SSPI.

FUTURE DIRECTIONS

Technological developments over the next few years are likely to provide the tools needed to overcome many of the barriers to effective literacy instruction described above, particularly in the area of training. For example, fiber optics and interactive video technology will soon make distance learning a real and affordable medium for inservice education. A pilot project currently is under way in North Carolina that will link universities, community colleges, and public schools in direct communication with one another across distances of several hundred miles. Such a system could encourage wider use of limited resources through distance education and consultation.

Policy changes under way at the federal level are likely to affect research efforts and service delivery. For example, former President Bush, in his State of the Union address and other public speeches, has stated that *all children* will enter school prepared to learn and *all adults* will be literate by the year 2000. The National Institute on Disability Research and Rehabilitation has taken the lead in the area of literacy and persons with disabilities in three progressive measures:

1. calling for a regional information exchange including literacy and persons with disabilities in its 1992–1993 funding priorities,
2. holding a national consensus conference on AAC in which literacy was 1 of 10 solicited background issue papers, and
3. issuing an invitational priority for research on the impact of AAC systems on literacy learning.

The greatest progress in providing appropriate, timely, and efficient literacy services will occur as intervention research and assessment tool development come to be the focus of research and development efforts. Interdisciplinary collaboration is essential as we begin to explore what works with whom, for how long, and why. There is a great deal to be gained by studying what has already been learned in much more developed fields of study such as psycho- and sociolinguistics, cognitive psychology, educational anthropology, and reading and writing instructional research.

REFERENCES

Allington, R., Stuetzel, H., Shake, M., & Lamarche, S. (1986). What is remedial reading? A descriptive study. *Reading Research and Instruction, 26*(1), 15–30.

Anderson, R.C., Hiebert, E.H., Scott, J.A., & Wilkinson, I.A.G. (1984). *Becoming a nation of readers: The report of the Commission on Reading.* Washington, DC: National Institute of Education.

Baker, J., & Zigmond, N. (1990). Are regular education classes equipped to accommodate students with learning disabilities? *Exceptional Children, 56,* 515–527.

Beukelman, D.R., Garrett, K., Lange, U., & Tice, R. (1988). *Cue-write: Word processing with spelling assistance and practice* [Computer program]. Tucson, AZ: Communication Skill Builders.

Calculator, S., & Dollaghan, C. (1982). The use of communication boards in a residential setting. An evaluation. *Journal of Speech and Hearing Disorders, 47,* 281–287.

Calculator, S. & Luchko, C. (1983). Evaluating the effectiveness of a communication board training program. *Journal of Speech and Hearing Disorders, 48,* 185–191.

Cauley, K.M., Golinkoff, R.M., Hirsch-Pasek, K., & Gordon, L. (1989). Revealing hidden competencies: A new method for studying language comprehension in children with motor impairments. *American Journal on Mental Retardation, 94,* 53–63.

Colquhoun, A. (1982). *Augmentative communication systems: The interaction process.* Paper presented at the meeting of the American Speech-Language-Hearing Association, Toronto, Canada.

Culp, D.M. (1982). *Communication interactions—Nonspeaking children using augmentative systems.* Unpublished manuscript, Callier Center for Communication Disorders, Dallas, TX.

De Hoop, W. (1965). Listening comprehension of cerebral palsied and other crippled children as a function of two speaking rates. *Exceptional Children, 31,* 233–240.

Dunkin, M., & Biddle, B. (1974). *The study of teaching.* New York, NY: Holt, Rinehart & Winston.

Farrier, L.D., Yorkston, K.M., Marriner, N.A., & Beukelman, D.R. (1985). Conversational control in nonimpaired speakers using an augmentative communication system. *Augmentative and Alternative Communication, 1,* 65–73.

Goossens', C., & Crain, S. (1986). *Augmentative communication intervention resource.* Birmingham, AL: Sparks Center for Developmental and Learning Disorders.

Guthrie, J., Seifert, M., Burnham, N., & Caplan, R. (1974). The maze technique to assess, monitor reading comprehension. *Reading Teacher, 28,* 161–168.

Harris, A.J., & Sipay, E.R. (1985). *How to increase reading ability* (8th ed.). New York, NY: Longman.

Harris, D. (1982). Communicative interaction processes involving nonvocal physically handicapped children. *Topics in Language Disorders, 2*(2), 21–37.

Haynes, M.C., & Jenkins, J.R. (1986). Reading instruction in special education resource rooms. *American Educational Research Journal, 23,* 161–190.

Higginbotham, D.J. (1985). *Message formulation using augmentative communication systems: Studies in social communication and interaction.* Unpublished doctoral dissertation, University of Wisconsin, Madison.

Higginbotham, D.J., & Yoder, D.E. (1982). Communication with natural conversational interaction: Implications for severe communicatively impaired persons. *Topics in Language Disorders, 2*(2), 1–19.

Hoffman, J.V. (1991). Teacher and school effects in learning to read. In R. Barr, M.L. Kamil, P.B. Mosenthal, & P.D. Pearson (Eds.), *Handbook of reading research* (Vol. 2). New York, NY: Longman.

Koke, S., & Neilson, J. (1987). *The effect of auditory feedback on the spelling of nonspeaking physically disabled individuals.* Unpublished master's thesis, University of Toronto, Toronto, Ontario.

Koppenhaver, D.A. (1991). *A descriptive analysis of classroom literacy instruction provided to children with severe speech and physical impairments.* Unpublished doctoral dissertation, University of North Carolina at Chapel Hill.

Koppenhaver, D.A., Coleman, P.P., Kalman, S.L., & Yoder, D.E. (1991). The implications of emergent literacy research for children with developmental disabilities. *American Journal of Speech-Language Pathology, 1*(1), 38–44.

Koppenhaver, D.A., Coleman, P.P., Steelman, J.D., & Yoder, D.E. (in press). Enhancing literacy learning in children and adults. In D.E. Pressman (Ed.), *Handbook of augmentative communication.* Stoneham, MA: Andover Medical Publishers.

Koppenhaver, D.A., Evans, D.A., & Yoder, D.E. (1991). Childhood reading and writing experiences of literate adults with severe speech and motor impairments. *Augmentative and Alternative Communication, 7,* 20–33.

Koppenhaver, D.A., & Yoder, D.E. (1988). Independent reading practice. *Aug-Communique, 6*(3), 9–11.

Koppenhaver, D.A., & Yoder, D.E. (1989). Study of a spelling strategy for physically disabled augmentative communication users. *Communication Outlook, 10*(3), 10–12.

Koppenhaver, D.A., & Yoder, D.E. (1992). Literacy issues in persons with severe speech and physical impairments. In R. Gaylord-Ross (Ed.), *Issues and research in special education* (Vol. 2). New York, NY: Columbia University, Teachers College Press.

Kraat, A.W. (1987). *Communication interaction between aided and natural speakers: A state of the art report* (2nd ed.). Madison, WI: Trace R & D Center.

Leinhardt, G., Zigmond, N., & Cooley, W.W. (1981). Reading instruction and its effects. *American Educational Research Journal, 18,* 343–361.

Light, J., Collier, B., & Parnes, P. (1985a). Communicative interaction between young nonspeaking physically disabled children and their primary caregivers: Part I—Discourse patterns. *Augmentative and Alternative Communication, 1,* 98–107.

Light, J., Collier, B., & Parnes, P. (1985b). Communicative interaction between young nonspeaking physically disabled children and their primary caregivers: Part II—Communicative functions. *Augmentative and Alternative Communication, 1,* 98–107.

Light, J., Koppenhaver, D., Lee, E., & Riffle, L. (1992). *The home and school literacy experiences of students who use AAC systems.* Manuscript in preparation.

Lindfors, J.W. (1987). *Children's language and learning.* Englewood Cliffs, NJ: Prentice-Hall.

Martin, B. (1967). *Brown bear, brown bear, what do you see?* New York, NY: Holt, Rinehart & Winston.

McNaughton, D., & Drynan, D. (1990, August). *Assessment and intervention issues for written communication: A case study.* Paper presented at the biennial meeting of the International Society for Augmentative and Alternative Communication, Stockholm, Sweden.

Mike, D.G. (1987, December). *Literacy, technology, and the multiply disabled: An ethnography of classroom interaction.* Paper presented at the meeting of the National Reading Conference, St. Petersburg Beach, FL.

Reinking, D., & Bridwell-Bowles, L. (1991). Computers in reading and writing. In R. Barr, M.L. Kamil, P.B. Mosenthal, & P.D. Pearson (Eds.), *Handbook of reading research* (Vol. 2). New York, NY: Longman.

Smith, D.D. (1979). The improvement of children's oral reading through the use of teacher modeling. *Journal of Learning Disabilities, 12,* 172–175.

Smith-Lewis, M., & Ford, A. (1987). A user's perspective on augmentative communication. *Augmentative and Alternative Communication, 3,* 12–17.

Stauffer, R.G. (1959). A directed reading-thinking plan. *Education, 79,* 527–532.

Tierney, R.J., & Cunningham, J.W. (1984). Research on teaching reading comprehension. In P.D. Pearson (Ed.), *Handbook of reading research.* New York, NY: Longman.

Wasson, P., & Keeler, J. (1984). *Changing response ratios of normal and handicapped children.* Unpublished raw data.

Yoder, D.E., & Kraat, A.W. (1983). Intervention issues in nonspeech communication. In J. Miller, D. Yoder, & R.L. Schiefelbusch (Eds.), *Contemporary issues in language intervention* (ASHA Report No. 12). Rockville, MD: American Speech-Language-Hearing Association.

Ysseldyke, J.E., Christenson, S.L., Thurlow, M.L., & Bakewell, E. (1989). Are different kinds of instructional tasks used by mentally retarded, learning disabled, emotionally disturbed and nonhandicapped elementary students. *School Psychology Review, 18,* 98–111.

Implementing a whole language program in a special education class

Carol E. Westby, PhD
Research Associate
University of New Mexico
Albuquerque, New Mexico

Linda Costlow, MS
Early Childhood Intervention Specialist
Albuquerque Public Schools
Albuquerque, New Mexico

THE WHOLE IS MORE than the sum of its parts. Three-year-olds can draw horizontal and vertical lines—the parts of a square—but they cannot draw squares. Squares have more than horizonatal and vertical lines; squares also have corners. Corners appear only in the whole square, not in its parts. Like a square, language is more than the sum of its parts. Language may be composed of phonemes, syntax, semantics, and pragmatics, but as Halliday (1978) stated, "Language comes to life only when functioning in some environment. We do not experience language in isolation—if we did, we would not recognize it as language—but always in relation to a scenario, some background of persons and actions and events from which the things are said to derive their meaning" (p. 28). Meaningful language exists only in a context.

Whole language methodology is part of the holism movement in many fields. Holism is a philosophy, a way of viewing the world, that suggests that we can under-

Top Lang Disord, 1991,11(3),69–84
© 1991 Aspen Publishers, Inc.

stand our world only by looking at the whole context (Rhodes & Dudley-Marling, 1988). Educators are considering not only children's cognitive and language development in school, but also their social and emotional development in their families and communities and are emphasizing teaching of reading and writing across the curriculum (Fulwiler & Young, 1982). Educators are also growing increasingly aware that knowledge and learning cannot be fragmented. Teaching language, reading, writing, or any other form of learning as isolated skills strips away meaning and makes learning more difficult (Rhodes & Dudley-Marling, 1988; Smith, 1973). Whole language is not a language arts curriculum, but a philosophy for all education; it is not a particular methodology, but a philosophical stance that puts learning in meaningful contexts (Goodman, 1986; Newman, 1985). Whole language philosophy seeks to have all children take an active role in all modes of communication: listening, speaking, reading, and writing. Fillion and Brause (1987) maintain that "In a culture where written language is prominent and readily available, basic literacy is a natural extension of an individual's linguistic development, given adequate environmental conditions" (p. 216).

Knowledge of how normal children acquire oral and written language provides support and direction for the whole language movement. (For further discussion and a somewhat differing viewpoint, see Sawyer, "Whole Language in Context: Insights into the Current Great Debate," this issue.) Normal children not only learn to listen and speak during the preschool years, but many also learn to read and write. Normal language learners acquire language by using language and by negotiating the meaning of the messages (Wells, 1987). They are immersed in a rich language environment that provides both language models and motivation to stay involved. Despite differences in oral and written language (written language requires knowledge of a print code and in many situations is more decontextualized, and hence requires more explicit vocabulary and complex structure), both develop when there are reasons to communicate to someone who will assist in negotiating the meaning of the message. Normal children learn to listen and speak in natural contexts. The information they acquire is part of a schema, or cognitive context, that often involves who did what, with what or whom, where, when, and how in spatial and causal relationships (Nelson, 1985).

Normal children also acquire reading and writing in real contexts as they become aware that one can communicate in print like one can communicate in speech (Bissex, 1980; Clay, 1975; Goodman, 1986). They learn to recognize print in context (Stop, McDonald's, Crest, Tide), and they learn to put their oral messages into print (NO GRLZ ALOUD [no girls allowed]). Mosenthal (1984) explained the importance of contexts to normal readers' comprehension of texts. He proposed multiple contexts that impinge on readers and affect their reading abilities:

- the organizer's (or adult's) context, which determines the type of interaction or negotiation between the adult and child during the reading activity;
- the text context, which refers to the

content and structure of the material to be read;

- the reader context, which is represented by the readers and their experiential background, intelligence, skills, and maturation;
- the task context, which represents what the reader will have to do to demonstrate comprehension; and
- the setting context, which is the location in which the reading activity occurs.

Readers' decoding skills, vocabulary knowledge, or syntactic skills cannot alone account for their success or lack of success in comprehending what they read. Evaluators must also consider the effects of the contexts of the reading activity on the reading process.

Holistic approaches to language and reading instruction may be especially valuable to learning-disabled students. If contexts are critical to the learning of normal children, they may be even more critical for language learning-disabled students who experience particular difficulty in learning through language alone. Whole language methodology can provide language learning-disabled students with enriched language contexts, meaningful reasons for communicating, and contextual cues to support learning. Whole language philosophy, however, does not provide a simple answer to meeting the developmental needs of learning-handicapped children. If language learning-disabled children learned language by the usual interactions in their environment, they would not be learning disabled. Teachers and speech-language pathologists who attempt to implement whole language methodology with language learning-disabled

Teachers and speech-language pathologists who attempt to implement whole language methodology with language learning-disabled children must be alert to what makes whole language whole.

children must be alert to what makes whole language whole. They must be aware of the framework of cognitive and linguistic knowledge that must underlie whole language activities (Vail, 1989) and the cognitive and linguistic skills that the learning-disabled students possess.

Language learning-disabled students have difficulty in listening, speaking, reading, and writing. Some students have difficulty in only one mode, whereas others have difficulty in two, three, or all four modes of language. Harste, Woodward, and Burke (1984) maintain that listening, speaking, reading, and writing all require the same language components:

- a *pragmatic reason* for communicating,
- a message with *semantic meaning,*
- a *syntactic form* to convey the meaning, and
- a *phonemic or graphemic code* for the message.

Deficits in these pragmatic, semantic, syntactic, and graphophonemic language components have been documented in language learning-disabled students (Butler, 1986). Some students exhibit deficits in only one component, whereas others may exhibit deficits in all components. Implementing a successful whole language program with learning-disabled students requires understanding of their linguistic skills and deficits in order to structure contexts in which they will learn.

This article describes a program for language learning-disabled students that used whole language philosophy to structure contexts that developed students' pragmatic, semantic, syntactic, graphophonemic, and metacognitive abilities that underlie speaking, listening, reading, and writing language competencies. The program considered

- the context of the setting—a pleasant, literacy-rich environment;
- the context of the children—their abilities, disabilities, and needs;
- the context of the teachers—the nature of the communicative interactions between adults and children;
- the context of the texts—discourse and texts matched to children's oral interactive, narrative, and expository language levels; and
- the context of the task—tasks sequenced so that they began with maximal support from all of the other contexts.

Particular attention in this article is given to the contexts for development of the children's writing.

THE PROGRAM

The environment

The program exemplified the characteristics of many whole language programs. The program provided a rich language environment. In the large classroom, books were prominently displayed in a comfortable area with a carpet, large easy chair, and beanbag. A centrally located writing area offered paper of assorted colors, sizes, and textures; stickers; rubber stamps; and assorted crayons, markers, pencils, and pens. A tiled portion of the room was devoted to hands-on activities for art, cooking, science, and social studies. A smaller, separate playroom down the hall, used by the speech-language pathologist, was organized for play and creative dramatics. The playroom had areas for a home, store, small toys (blocks, puppets, Fisher-Price and other action sets), and changeable dramatic play (doctor's office, campground, airport, etc.).

The entire morning was devoted to whole language activities. During the first half of the morning, all children in the class participated in cooking, art, science, and building projects related to the current topic or theme being studied. After morning recess, the class was divided. Half went with the speech-language pathologist for pretend-play and creative-dramatics activities, and the other half of the class remained with the classroom teacher for story reading, group storytelling, and book report time. In the afternoons, children's programs were individualized. Some children attended occupational therapy sessions or adaptive physical education, or were mainstreamed into a regular class for music, art, or math. Others remained in the classroom for individual or small-group math, fine motor, or visual–spatial activities.

The whole language program involved the children in meaningful listening, talking, reading, and writing about the activities in which they were engaged. The meaning of the language activities was negotiated among the children and adults in the program, and for the activities to be successful, the participants had to monitor their communication. There were numerous adults available to negotiate the activities with the children. A teacher and aide were always in the room. A speech-language pathologist was available to the room for half of each day, a *grandparent* from the city's senior citizens program came several half-days a week, and parents were always welcome.

The children

Initial characteristics

Eight to 10 students per year, ages 5 to 9 years, were enrolled in this self-contained classroom for children having severe communication disorders. All children entered the program with significant deficits in listening and speaking and without being able to read or write. Although the children exhibited differing patterns of speech and language skills, they all exhibited delayed and disordered oral language and listening skills. Several children had moderate to severe articulation disorders. All the children had syntactic skills that were delayed to varying degrees, and all the children exhibited a limited range of pragmatic communicative functions. They used language primarily for need-meeting purposes, and rarely, if ever, for reporting past experiences, predicting, reasoning, or projecting into thoughts and feelings of others.

Several children did not engage in extended conversations. They would answer a specific question with a single word or phrase, but did not spontaneously provide additional information, and they rarely initiated conversation. Those children who did engage in extended conversations generally used nonspecific vocabulary, did not provide the listener with sufficient information, and were poor at maintaining their topics.

The majority of the children exhibited listening (or auditory processing) problems. Some children responded impulsively before they had listened to the entire message; other children exhibited marked delays before they responded. All children required frequent repetition and rephrasing of instructions.

None of the children were able to produce a personal narrative about a past experience, even when the teacher provided leading questions, and none of them were able to produce a true story in response to a wordless picture book or poster picture. The best speakers provided descriptions of discrete actions in the pictures.

Previous to the implementation of the program, none of the children leaving the classroom at age 9 were able to read and write. However, after 3 years of the whole language program, it was extremely rare for a child to leave the program without some functional reading and writing skills, and many children were able to be mainstreamed into regular classes.

Observation and assessment

The staff used knowledge of normal oral language, reading, and writing development to provide language input that was comprehensible to the students. Adults followed Krashen's (1982) concept of providing children with language input slightly above their present level (Input + 1 or I + 1). To do this, staff had to be sensitive to students' current levels of language development in all aspects of language.

This required assessment of children's pragmatic, semantic, syntactic, and graphophonemic language abilities and their metacognitive, metalinguistic, and text schema and text structure knowledge.

Program staff evaluated children's phonological, syntactic, and semantic language abilities from language samples collected in play settings and from stories told by the children from wordless picture books and poster pictures. Pragmatic language functions were evaluated using Tough's (1979) listing of language functions (self-maintaining, directing self and others, reporting, predicting, projecting into thoughts and feelings of others, and reasoning). Pragmatic discourse skills were evaluated using Damico and Oller's *Spotting Language Problems* (1985). Children were observed conversing with an adult or another child and were rated, using a 1 to 5 scale, on their linguistic nonfluency, revisions, poor topic maintenance, inappropriate responses, delays before responding, failure to provide sufficient information, need for repetition of information from the discourse partner, and use of nonspecific vocabulary. Syntactic skills were monitored by noting T-unit length, use of clause modification (prepositional phrases), and for linguistically more advanced children, subordinate clauses (Scott, 1988). Metalinguistic awareness was evaluated and monitored through the children's development of reading and writing. Metacognitive abilities were evaluated by activities requiring the children to think aloud as they performed activities and to comprehend and use words such as *know, remember, forget,* and *guess* (Wellman, 1985). Content schema and text structure knowledges were assessed through children's production of stories and expos-

itory passages (see Westby, 1989, for a description of the levels). The classroom teacher, classroom aide, speech-language pathologist, and speech-language consultant met weekly to discuss children's current language levels and needs and to plan the activities for the following week.

Language learning through thematic contexts

With this information about the students' language abilities, adults were able to provide the students with "I + 1" comprehensible input: input that would be understandable but would, at the same time, facilitate development to higher levels. In listening and speaking, particular attention was devoted to assisting the children in conversing with adults and other children by increasing the variety of reasons for communicating, the informativeness of their communication, and their ability to maintain the topic (Brinton & Fujiki, 1989).

Throughout the day, the students, teacher, aide, *grandparent,* and speech-language pathologist engaged in meaningful communication around thematic topics, for example, the state fair, geology of New Mexico, ballooning, animals that come from eggs, and so forth. Organizing activities around themes provided a means of developing semantic networks and facilitating expansion of children's schema knowledge. Words and concepts were taught in relationship to other words and concepts, not in isolation. An experience approach helps children to organize information and recognize relationships, which then facilitates their ability to engage in inductive and deductive thought needed to plan and problem-solve (Clarke, 1990). A theme might last a week or several months. Children engaged in art, cooking, science, and building activities related to the themes, took field trips, listened to and read books about the themes, wrote stories about the themes, and responded to messages written in their journals about what they were seeing and doing. All activities involved negotiation of meaning among the children, their peers, and adults in the program.

Children began a unit on life in New Mexico by walking around their neighborhood, talking to community members, and noting the adobe homes and stucco buildings. They looked at an issue of *New Mexico Magazine* with pictures displaying how to make adobe bricks. Then the children and adults dug clay from the playground, mixed it with water and straw, and poured it into molds to make adobe brick. They spent a day with a Native American graduate student at her home pueblo a few miles from the school. They constructed ornos (bread ovens) and a pueblo from adobe clay and bricks using photographs as a guide. They made handlooms and wove small rugs to place in the pueblo, and they made coils of clay, formed the coils into pots, and fired the pots in the school kiln.

During all of these activities, adults were alert to facilitating all aspects of children's language in meaningful contexts. They modeled communication for a variety of functions (Tough, 1979):

- Self-maintaining: "I need more mud." "Those are my bricks."
- Directing self and others: "I'm finishing molding my pot and then I'll put it in the kiln." "Show John how to cut the straw."
- Reporting: "Julia's grandmother put

> *During all of these activities, adults were alert to facilitating all aspects of children's language in meaningful contexts.*

the bread in the orno to bake." "First we soften the clay in our hands. Then we roll it to make long snakes. Then we form the snakes into a pot."
- Predicting: "Tomorrow we'll see how tortillas are made."
- Reasoning: "We'll use clay because it will get harder than sand."
- Projecting: "Justin's proud of the rug he made." "Maria gets mad when you take her crayons."

Syntactic complexity was adjusted to the children's levels.

Adults used strategies to involve children in using Tough's (1979) language functions. They modeled metacognitive think aloud procedures as they carried out activities; as children became more verbal, they were required to think aloud. The adults used metacognitive words as they discussed their activities:

- "I *think* this is how Jennifer's aunt kneaded the bread."
- "I *forgot* what Ms. Garcia did after she added the flour. Go ask her."
- "I *remember* how good the bread smelled when it came out of the oven."
- "I *know* how to make adobe bricks from clay, straw, and water."

Adults oriented children to the various language functions by the comments and questions they asked (Tough, 1979):
- Directing self and others: "Tell Kim

to work with Peter." "Tell yourself what you're doing as you're weaving."

- Reporting: "How did you make your pot?"
- Predicting: "What will happen if you mix all that water in the clay?"
- Reasoning: "Why do we fire our pots in the kiln?"
- Projecting: "How does Michael feel when you share your popcorn with him?"

Contexts for literacy

Books were provided that had narrative content or structures at or slightly above the students' current narrative levels (Westby, 1989). Narrative and expository texts were integrated into all activities. In preparation for the annual Balloon Fiesta, the teachers provided the children with a wide variety of literature on balloons. They looked at wordless picture books about balloon flights and generated stories to go with the pictures. They looked at informational books about balloons and talked about the parts of and operation of hot air balloons. They watched the Reading Rainbow videotape of LeVar Burton reading *Hot Air Henry* (Calhoun, 1981) and going to a balloon fiesta, and they listened to and read fiction and nonfiction books about balloons. They followed procedural texts to make a hot air balloon out of garbage bags, heated the air in it over a camp stove, and watched how high it floated over the school grounds. They also made papier-mâché balloon mobiles in the classroom. Schema knowledge about ballooning gained from texts was expanded by a field trip to the Balloon Fiesta.

Children were exposed to print and were expected to communicate in print from the time they entered the program. Journal writing was selected over other possible beginning writing activities because of its greater similarities to oral conversation than the literate style of texts. Entries in the journals were directed to a specific child and referred to his or her own experiences, rather than to unfamiliar content. As in oral conversation, these interactive journal messages required a response. A major goal of the journal was to enable children to realize that writing carried a message. One did not read simply to say the words, but to gain the message that was in the text. (Johns & Ellis, 1976, reported that many children think that sounding out the words, rather than getting the meaning, is the main task in reading.)

All children received a spiral-bound notebook for their journals. The teacher explained that she or someone else in the school would be writing messages to them each day and that they were to read the messages and return an answer. Initially, many children told the teacher that they could not read. The teacher informed the children that the writer of the message was not the person who would read the message to the child. If children could not read the messages in their books, they were encouraged to find someone who could read the messages to them.

Daily, the classroom teacher, aide, or speech-language pathologist wrote a personal message in each child's journal. Generally, questions were asked about recent experiences the child had, such as, "Did you see that big elephant at the zoo yesterday? What was he eating?" "I'm glad your mom brought ice cream for your birthday. What's your favorite ice cream?"

Journal dialogue

During the 2 to 3 years the children were in the classroom, they exhibited the following developmental stages of metalinguistic knowledge in their journal writing:

Recurrent writing. Early responses often represented prewriting stages with the children producing recurring lines or figures (Clay, 1975; Temple, Nathan, Burris, & Temple, 1988). From the beginning, all of the children recognized that writing was not drawing pictures, and their journals reflected this. This does not mean that they wrote letters or words, but rather that the pencil marks were not pictures. Even the youngest and most limited children exhibited awareness that writing was recurrent; that is, they repeated similar-looking marks (Figure 1).

Copying. Gradually, children developed awareness that writing had a distinctive look; it was not simply repetitions of curves and marks. They began to copy portions of the message written by the teacher. Initially, they copied directly under the teacher's printing (Figure 2), but then they moved the copied letters to the end of the teacher's message. Shortly thereafter, the children initiated a modified copying, selecting words and letters from the message and placing them below the teacher's comments.

Simple message awareness. At this level, children indicated an understanding that the teacher's writing was a message to them and, like an oral comment or message, required a response. Initial responses were often "yes" or "no" or single words, often in invented spelling that was not always readable to others (Figure 3).

Extended response. Once children were

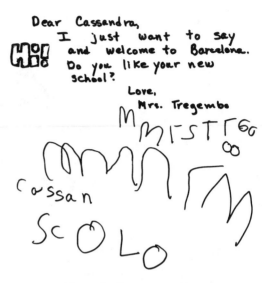

Figure 1. Recurrent writing.

able to give single-word responses to written messages, they began to produce extended responses that they generated themselves. The children responded to the message with print that represented several words, usually using invented spelling. In early forms of this level, an initial consonant might stand for an entire word. In Figure 4 Ron responds "NOID DUSW," meaning "No I didn't, did you see one?"

Sentence-length readable response. Finally, the students' responses became easily readable, although the students continued to rely heavily on invented spelling (Figure 5).

Evaluating messages. After students realized that the teacher's printing was a message to be responded to, and they were able to give a direct response, they began to attend to the specifics of the message. The teacher took advantage of this awareness by writing messages that required the children to judge the truth value of the message. For example, Figure

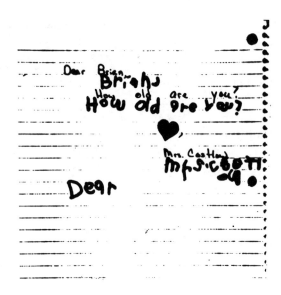

Figure 2. Copying.

6 shows what the teacher wrote in Ernestine's book and Ernestine's reply. Although Ernestine did not comment on the incorrect name in her journal, she did know that she had not played with anyone named Lucy yesterday.

Commenting and beginning initiation. Once children began to monitor their reading for truth value, they began to comment on the message received and to initiate a message in return. Children initially originated messages when they had a strong emotional response. For example, the children had read the book, *Miss Nelson is Missing,* the story of a pleasant teacher with a classroom of misbehaving students. One day Miss Nelson is not at school. Substituting for her is Miss Swamp, a strict teacher who brought the unruly children under control. On Halloween,

the classroom teacher, Mrs. Costlow, was missing, and the substitute teacher was none other than Miss Swamp (Mrs. Costlow wearing a black wig and dressed in a large black dress padded with a pillow). Later in the week, Miss Swamp wrote in the children's books. She signed her name using a rubber stamp with a picture of Miss Swamp. Ernestine had a strong response to this message, as seen in Figure 7.

The children did not know that Miss Swamp was Mrs. Costlow. It took them

Children initially originated messages when they had a strong emotional response.

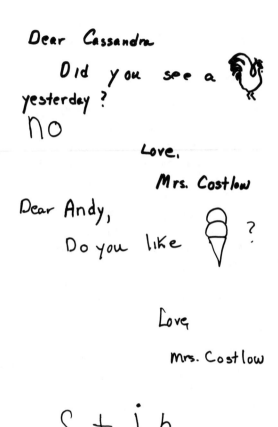

Dear Cassandra

Did you see a 🐓 yesterday?

no

Love,

Mrs. Costlow

Dear Andy,

Do you like 🍦?

Love

Mrs. Costlow

S t i b e

Figure 3. Simple message awareness.

Dear Ron,

Did you see a ⛄ this summer? Are you 🙂 to be back at school?

NOiD   DUSW

Love,

Mrs. Costlow

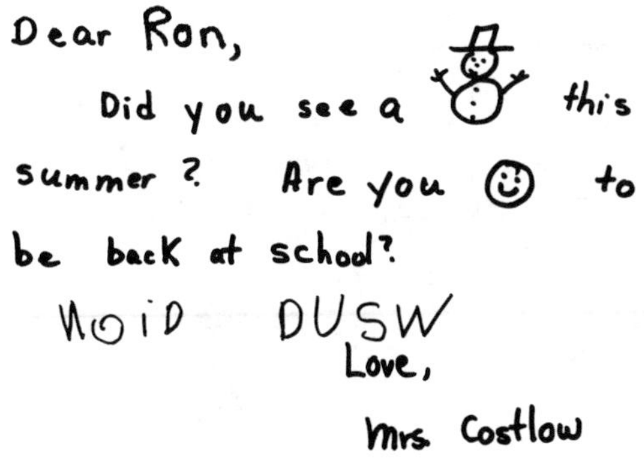

Figure 4. Extended response.

moved the costume and other related activities (journal writing, writing to Detective McSmogg to try to discover where Miss Swamp lived, story writing) would not have been done. The children treated the experience as a mystery to be solved. This represented Ernestine's first message that went beyond the response demands of the teacher's message.

Student-initiated questions and teacher's messages. Once students became comfortable with their ability to respond to a message written to them, they began to direct messages to people writing in their journals, and they began to leave notes for people (Figure 8).

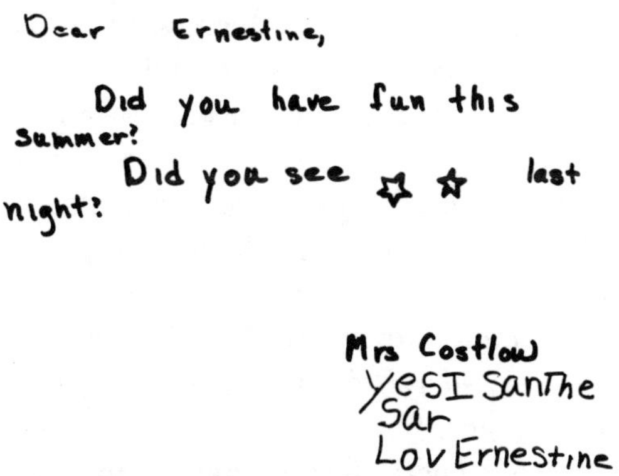

Dear Ernestine,

Did you have fun this summer? Did you see ✩ ✩ last night?

Mrs Costlow
YeSI SanThe
Sar
Lov Ernestine

Figure 5. Sentence-length readable response.

several months to figure this out. Ernestine was the first one to put the pieces together. Mrs. Costlow had intentionally left Miss Swamp's wig and dress in places where the children eventually found them. They never showed any fear about Miss Swamp—more surprise at the choice of the substitute teacher and excitement to tell others who their substitute teacher was. They spent time planning how they might deal with Miss Swamp. They delighted in reading other Miss Nelson stories and eventually wrote their own Miss Swamp stories. If the children had shown any fear, Mrs. Costlow would have re-

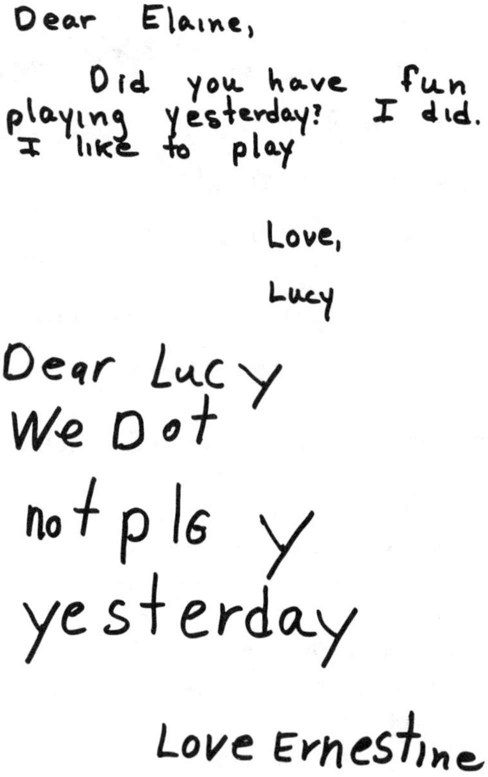

Dear Elaine,

    Did you have fun playing yesterday? I did. I like to play

        Love,

        Lucy

Dear Lucy
We Do t
not p l6 y
yesterday

      Love Ernestine

Figure 6. Evaluating messages.

Monologue

Once children were able to give extended responses to dialogue initiated by another and were able to initiate a dialogue, they began to produce writing that was not directed to a specific audience and that required them to sustain a monologue. When the teacher observed this development, she provided the children with bound diaries in which they could write.

Beginning narratives. Initially, entries were very short, reflecting on only a single event (Figure 9).

Extended narratives. Gradually, the narratives became longer: reflections on past experiences and evaluation of the experi-

ences, such as a trip to the airport and a hamburger restaurant (Figure 10).

Spontaneous letters. By the time students were producing extended narrative texts, many of them were reading and writing as well as or better than children in the regular classes. (Writing had not been emphasized in the regular classroom.) At this point, several students were mainstreamed into regular second- and third-grade classes for as much as half the day. Ernestine now had less frequent contact with her special education teacher, but she clearly had a close attachment to that teacher. Notes occasionally appeared on the teacher's desk (Figure 11).

Parent involvement

Wells (1986) reported that the two best predictors of children's success in school were related to their (a) having been read to by their parents during the preschool

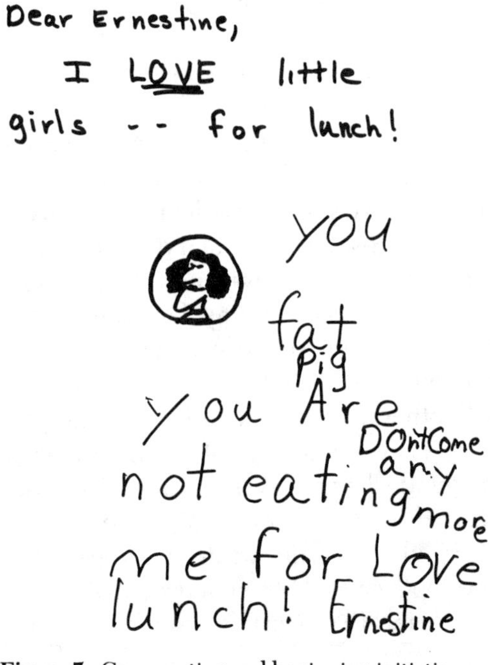

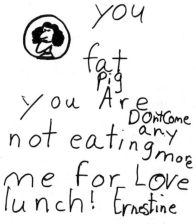

Dear Ernestine,
    I LOVE little girls -- for lunch!

      you
      fat pig
you Are DOntCome
not eating any moe
me for Love
lunch! Ernestine

Figure 7. Commenting and beginning initiation.

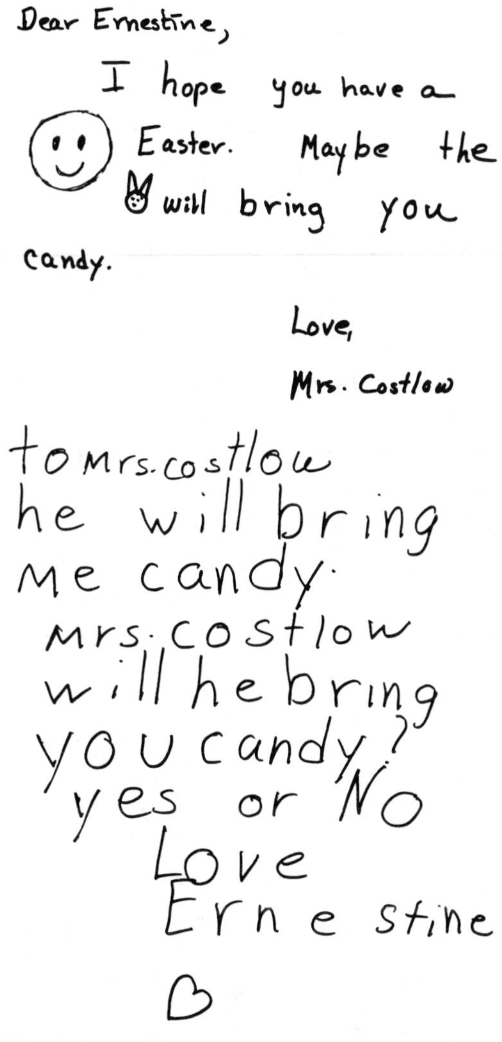

Dear Ernestine,

I hope you have a 😊 Easter. Maybe the 🐰 will bring you candy.

Love,

Mrs. Costlow

to mrs. costlow
he will bring
me candy.
mrs. costlow
will he bring
you candy?
yes or No
Love
Ernestine
♡

Figure 8. Student-initiated question and message.

years and (b) seeing their parents write. Whole language philosophy maintains that children should be surrounded by language- and literacy-enriched environments in all contexts, not just in school (Taylor, 1983).

Many of the parents of children in the program had themselves experienced academic difficulties or, for a variety of reasons, had not completed high school. All of them were concerned that their children might not learn to read, and reading was their primary goal for their children. To extend children's experiences with literate language outside the school environment, parents were invited on field trips and were always welcome in the classroom. A home book-reading program was established. Children checked books out of the classroom library, and parents read to them. Book report forms developed by the classroom staff provided parents with guidelines on how to talk with their children about books.

Parents were also encouraged to write. The teacher provided parents with a notebook that could serve as a diary. They were asked to write down any observations they had regarding their child's developing language and literacy. Ramon was a very quiet child who seldom spoke. His mother was pleased to report in her notebook: "When eating peanuts he asked if they grew in the garden. Saw a program on Benji and asked questions. 'Why the big dog chasing the little dog?'" Miguel's grandmother observed the following: "Miguel liked the Popcorn story. He recognized the letters m and c, for munch and crunch. He also learned another *at* word, eat and ate."

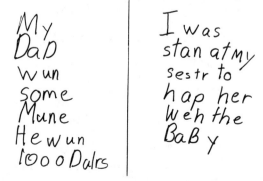

My
DaD
wun
some
Mune
Hewun
1000 Dulrs

I was
stan atmy
sestr to
hap her
weh the
BaBy

Figure 9. Beginning narrative.

The TiMe ToThe air port
We wen to go see the
air p lanes we had fun
and we went to go See the lady who
Call
we wen togosee a m ach ine
that you have to but your
purs in the ma ch ine
if it beeps that means
If you have Some
Sharp things they well
not let you go in the
plane and we wen to
Hardy's they gave
us a free dollar
we got a hamberger
and a cok and fries and
mr. mc. Don sand toke
us around we say them
make hamberger and
we say them got a milk
Shake and I got a m.lk
Shake and Eloy got a big
Cookie we where goin to
help the man
load up the truck
we where going to but
boxs on top of the truck
The End   ERnestine m ontoya

Figure 10. Extended narrative.

Once children demonstrated awareness of the message nature of journal writing in school, journals were also established between parents and children. The children brought the home journals to school once a week, and the teacher or speech-language pathologist would make comments to the parents about the journal. Only positive comments and suggestions were given. Comments were never made about the parent's writing or spelling. The teacher or speech-language pathologist commented about an event the parent had mentioned, noted that the child had talked about something in school that the parent had written in the journal, or praised the parents for creative ideas (as when some parents began to make rebus messages by

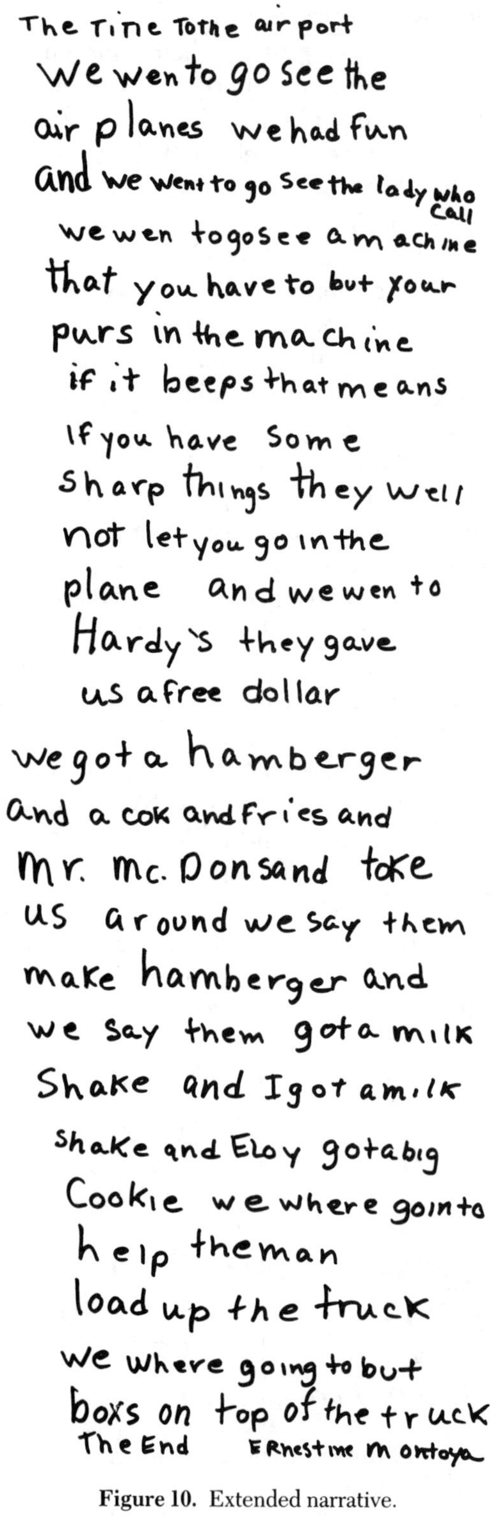

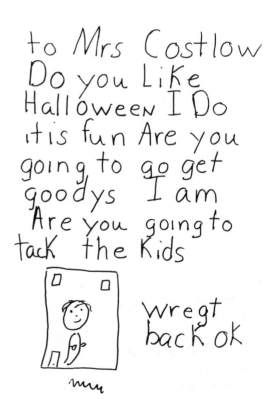

to Mrs Costlow
Do you Like
Halloween I Do
it is fun Are you
going to go get
goodys I am
Are you going to
tack the Kids

wregt
back ok

Figure 11. Spontaneous letter.

cutting pictures out of magazines). The goal was to develop parents' comfort with writing and to encourage them to write frequently. Some parents used the journals as a personal diary to discuss their own worries or joys:

Dear Ben,
I wanted to share some happy news with you. i finally got to buy my own bible this mourning, and guess what. the people i bought it from are going to engrave my own name on it for free. Isn't that nice! DO you think that as soon as you get to learn how to read real good, you'll want your own little Bible??
?Let me Gnow!?

P.S.   Love
I love you   mom

Some used the format they had observed in the classroom journals (Figure 12): The extension of the language program to the children's homes had a benefit beyond increasing the children's literacy levels. A number of parents reported that they became more confident of their own literacy skills, and they returned to school to obtain their graduation equivalency diplomas (GEDs).

• • •

Smith (1973) presented a tongue-in-cheek list of 12 ways to make learning to read difficult, including aiming for mastery of rules, teaching letters and words one at a time, encouraging avoidance of errors, discouraging guessing, providing immediate feedback, and identifying and giving attention to students experiencing difficulty as soon as possible. He proposed one rule for making learning to read easy: make learning easy. Making learning to read easy requires an understanding of the

reading process and what the child is trying to do. Making learning of anything easy can be accomplished by responding to what the child is trying to do. This requires that adults understand what children are trying to do and that they know ways to facilitate children's accomplishment. A successful whole language pro-

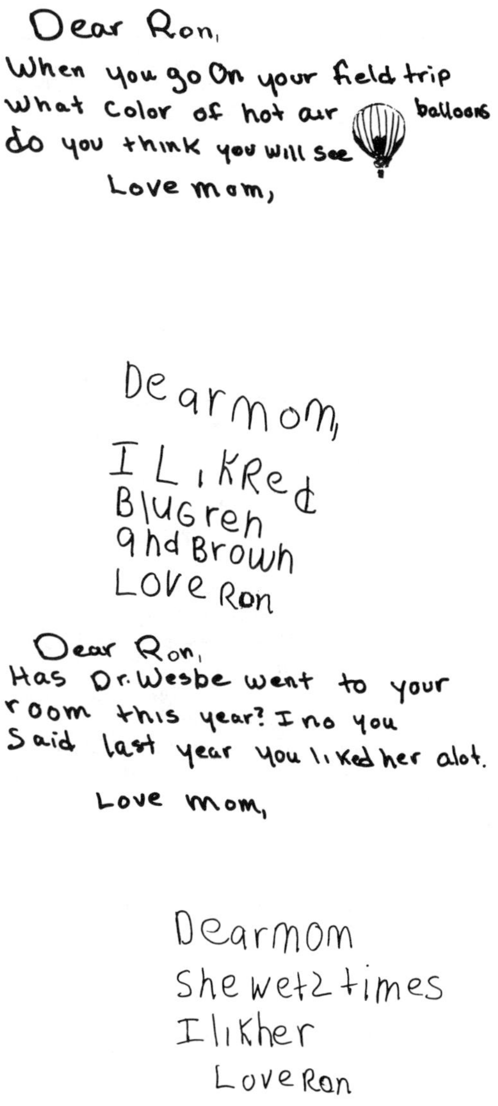

Figure 12. Parent journals.

gram for special education students requires that teachers:

- create contexts that will motivate children to communicate through speech and print;
- understand what the students are attempting to do; and
- understand the students' language

abilities and the normal developmental characteristics of language so that they can provide comprehensible language models. Whole language philosophy provides a basis for developing whole children—children who are able to participate effectively in the world around them.

REFERENCES

Bissex, G.L. (1980). *GNYS AT WRK: A child learns to write and read.* Cambridge, Mass.: Harvard University Press.

Brinton, B., & Fujiki, M. (1989). *Conversational management with language-impaired children.* Rockville, Md.: Aspen Publishers.

Butler, K.G. (1986). *Language disorders in children.* Austin, Tex.: PRO-ED.

Calhoun, M. (1981). *Hot air Henry.* New York, N.Y.: William Morrow.

Clarke, J.H. (1990). *Patterns of thinking.* Needham Heights, Mass.: Allyn & Bacon.

Clay, M.M. (1975). *What did I write?* Portsmouth, N.H.: Heinemann.

Damico, J., & Oller, J. (1985). *Spotting language problems.* San Diego, Calif.: Los Amigos Research Associates.

Fillion, B. & Brause, R. (1987). Research into classroom practice: What have we learned and where are we going? In J. Squire (Ed.), *The dynamics of language learning.* Urbana, Ill.: ERIC. (pp. 201–225)

Fulwiler, T., & Young, A. (Eds.). (1982). *Language connections: Reading and writing across the curriculum.* Urbana, Ill.: National Council of Teachers of English.

Goodman, K. (1986). *What's whole in whole language.* Portsmouth, N.H.: Heinemann.

Halliday, M.A.K. (1978). *Language as social semiotic.* Baltimore, Md.: University Park Press.

Harste, J.C., Woodward, V.A., & Burke, C.L. (1984). *Language stories and literacy lessons.* Portsmouth, N.H.: Heinemann.

Johns, J., & Ellis, D. (1976). Reading: Children tell it like it is. *Reading World, 16,* 115–128.

Krashen, S. (1982). *Principles and practice in second language acquisition.* New York, N.Y.: Pergamon.

Marshall, J. (1977). *Miss Nelson is missing!* New York, N.Y.: Scholastic.

Mosenthal, P. (1984). Reading comprehension research from a classroom perspective. In J. Flood (Ed.), *Promoting reading comprehension.* Newark, Del.: International Reading Association.

Nelson, K. (1985). *Making sense: The acquisition of shared meaning.* Orlando, Fla.: Academic Press.

Newman, J.M. (Ed.). (1985). *Whole language: Theory in use.* Portsmouth, N.H.: Heinemann.

Rhodes, L.K., & Dudley-Marling, C. (1988). *Readers and writers with a difference: A holistic approach to teaching learning disabled and remedial students.* Portsmouth, N.H.: Heinemann.

Scott, C. (1988). Spoken and written syntax. In M. Nippold (Ed.), *Later language development.* Boston, Mass.: College-Hill.

Smith, F. (1973). Twelve easy ways to make learning to read difficult. In F. Smith (Ed.), *Psycholinguistics and reading.* New York, N.Y.: Holt, Rinehart & Winston.

Taylor, D. (1983). *Family literacy.* Exeter, N.H.: Heinemann.

Temple, C., Nathan, R., Burris, N., & Temple, F. (1988). *The beginnings of writing.* Needham Heights, Mass.: Allyn & Bacon.

Tough, J. (1979). *Talk for teaching and learning.* Portsmouth, N.H.: Heinemann.

Vail, P.L. (1989). Watch out for the hole in whole language: Keep the wonder, the work, and the welcome. *The New York Branch of the Orton Dyslexia Society Newsletter, 13*(1), 1.

Wellman, H. (1985). The origins of metacognition. In D. Forrest-Pressley, G. Mackinnon, & T. Waller (Eds.), *Metacognition, cognition and human performance.* Orlando, Fla.: Academic Press.

Wells, G. (1986). *The meaning makers.* Portsmouth, N.H.: Heinemann.

Wells, G. (1987). The negotiation of meaning: Talking and learning at home and school. In B. Fillion, C. Hedley, & E. DiMartino (Eds.), *Home and school: Early language and reading.* Norwood, N.J.: Ablex.

Westby, C. (1989). Assessing and facilitating text comprehension. In A. Kamhi & H. Catts (Eds.), *Reading disabilities: A developmental language perspective.* Boston, Mass.: College-Hill.

From frog to prince: Using written language as a context for language learning

Janet A. Norris, PhD
Associate Professor
Division of Communication Disorders
Louisiana State University
Baton Rouge, Louisiana

A S RESEARCHERS explore the language abilities of children with language and learning disorders, an increasing range of problematic areas is revealed. These problems include difficulty with abstract vocabulary and figurative language, discourse structure, properties of cohesion and coherence, complex syntactic structures, and metalinguistic concepts (Crais & Chapman, 1987; Ripich & Griffith, 1988; Roth & Spekman, 1986, 1989). The scope and complexity of the problems exhibited can be overwhelming for the speech-language pathologist, whose role it is to provide meaningful and comprehensive intervention for these children. Each problematic aspect of language is important to include in an intervention program, but the time available to address these many areas is extremely limited. Even with adequate time, separate activities designed to teach specific semantic, syntactic, and pragmatic skills results in intervention that is fragmented and lacks overall continuity (Damico, 1989).

Top Lang Disord, 1991,12(1),66–81
© 1991 Aspen Publishers, Inc.

Furthermore, the language that is taught may not be directly relevant to the child's school and classroom environment, resulting in language intervention that places additional learning demands upon the child who is already failing to keep up with curriculum demands (Allington, 1989). Generalization to other uses of language, such as reading, may be poor because the child may fail to recognize that the language associated with picture cards and word games is the same as that found in the reading book or used in classroom activities.

One method of simultaneously addressing many aspects of language in an integrated manner that is relevant to the school curriculum is to use written language as the basis for language intervention. Written language presents a single context in which difficult vocabulary, syntax, discourse structure, and figurative and metalinguistic uses of language all are an inherent part of the text. With adult assistance, children can become aware of these elements of language as they are encountered in text and learn how they function to communicate meaning. Written language provides a context for learning in which elements of language remain integrated and communicative, consistent with principles of whole language learning (Goodman, 1986). This article presents strategies, including those used in an intervention method referred to as communicative reading strategies (Norris, 1988, 1989), that can be used in the written language context to facilitate holistic language learning. An example of narrative discourse is presented to demonstrate how the adult can mediate learning, but the strategies represent general principles that can be adapted to expository text or other forms of written discourse.

IDENTIFYING ELEMENTS OF LINGUISTIC STRUCTURE AND KNOWLEDGE

All the aspects of language that have been shown to be problematic for children with language and learning disorders, including abstract vocabulary, complex syntactic structures, elements of discourse, and metalinguistic concepts, can be found in written text. These elements of language interact in written text, as they do in oral discourse, to express complex relationships of meaning and to accomplish goals or pragmatic functions (Harste, Woodward, & Burke, 1984). Analysis of the following excerpt from *The Strange Story of the Frog Who Became a Prince* (Horwitz, 1971) serves as a representative example of the types of vocabulary, syntax, and discourse structures that can be addressed when written language is used as a context for language intervention. The estimated readability level of the story is third grade (Fry, 1977).

The story begins by establishing elements of story structure (Applebee, 1978), including the time, the character, and the setting, in the first sentence. This is followed by nine additional sentences that clearly depict the ordinary existence, or the "status quo," of this setting.

(1) Many years ago there was a handsome frog who lived by a rather nice pond.

(2) He had fun all day and at night he had happy dreams.

(3) Every day was exactly the same as every other day.

(4) He liked to swim in the pond and hop in the grass.

(5) He hopped high and he hopped low.

(6) When he was feeling silly he hopped from side to side.

(7) In the grass and in the pond the handsome frog found caterpillars, grasshoppers, and many other good things to eat.

(8) His skin was green like the grass and brown like the pond and gold like the sun.

(9) He had black eyes which poked out on either side of his head.

(10) He was a very handsome frog indeed. (Horwitz, 1971*)

Each sentence provides numerous opportunities for language learning. Examples of the elements of language that can be addressed in intervention, including abstract and metaphoric uses of words, the syntactic structures that organize these ideas in temporal and logical relationships, and the cohesive ties and elements of discourse structure that unify these ideas, are delineated below.

Syntax

The passage contains many complex sentences that are used to express a variety of meaningful relationships among characters, ideas, actions, locations, and so forth. For example, sentence 1 begins with an adverbial clause and contains a relative clause, prepositional phrase, and several noun modifiers. The 10-sentence passage contains 3 relative clause constructions, 11 coordinating or subordinating conjunctions, 8 prepositional phrases, and 3 infinitive verb constructions in addition to nu-

merous adverbs and adjectives (Akmajian, Demers, & Harnish, 1984).

Morphology

Several inflectional morphological forms are used to specify meaning, including plurals and verb tense endings. Irregular past tense forms are present, such as the word *found* (sentence 7). Instances of derivational forms also occur in the passage, as in the adverb *exactly* (sentence 3; Akmajian et al., 1984).

Cohesion

The passage uses cohesive ties extensively. The pronouns *he* and *his* are used 11 times to refer to the frog, and the demonstrative form *the* is used to refer to previously given information on 7 occasions. The deletion of understood information, or ellipsis, occurs 6 times (sentences 4 and 8). Substitution of nonspecific words, such as *things* (sentence 7), are used to refer to background information that must be inferred by the child. Many lexical ties unify the passage through theme or topic, including the repeated use of thematic words (i.e., *frog, pond, hopped,* and *handsome*) and the use of related words to expand upon the topic (hop: *grass, high, low,* and *side to side;* Halliday & Hasan, 1976).

The coherence of the passage must be understood for the story to make sense. There is little reason for the elaborated description of the frog's playing and eating

---

The coherence of the passage must be understood for the story to make sense.

---

habits (sentences 4 to 7) except in reference to the earlier information that his
days were always the same (sentence 3).
His activities and personal appearance are
only significant when embedded in the
context of events that occur later in the
story. Ideas within and across sentences,
paragraphs, and pages must be interpreted
in a unified and coherent manner for the
information to exist as anything greater
than lists of facts (Halliday & Hasan, 1976,
1985).

Implicature

The passage relies on the listener/
reader's ability to use contextual cues and
general knowledge to infer much of the
intended meaning. For example, phrases
such as "Many years ago" and "rather nice
pond" (sentence 1) require the child to
infer an appropriate temporal and environmental context. Similarly, from the given
information that the frog liked caterpillars
and grasshoppers, other edibles must be
inferred from the phrase "many other
good things" (sentence 7; Grice, 1975).

Abstraction

Many phrases and sentences must be
interpreted at figurative, metaphorical levels of meaning (Grice, 1975). For example,
the story is confusing if the child cannot
assume the perspective of the frog. Without this shift in perspective, caterpillars
and grasshoppers would not be classified
as "good things to eat," and green skin and
eyes poking out of one's head would not be
considered "handsome." A literal interpretation will fail to capture the humor and
irony that makes the passage entertaining
(Halliday & Hasan, 1985).

The passage also contains metaphors,
such as comparing the frog's skin to grass,
the pond, and the sun (sentence 8). This
use of the word *like* requires comparison
of abstract properties. On a concrete level,
skin is not like grass, a pond, or the sun in
any manner. The interpretation of metaphors requires a primary focus upon some
feature or property common to these objects rather than the objects themselves. A
literal interpretation would conjure up a
curious picture of a frog with grass, water,
and a sun attached to his skin (Blank, Rose,
& Berlin, 1978; Halliday & Hasan, 1985).

Temporal relationships

The passage is replete with linguistic
devices used to organize events in a manner that communicates how they occurred
in relative time and location to each other.
For example, the past tense form of the
verb *had* is used twice in sentence 2, but
when embedded in the context of "all day"
versus "at night" the first occurrence of
had refers to information that is relatively
more past tense: the fun occurred before
the happy dreams. Although the sentence
taken alone can be interpreted as reference to events that happened on one
occasion, the words *every day* in the
following sentence 3 indicate that the
events took place an unspecified number
of times previous to the present. The
present, in turn, must be interpreted relative to information given in sentence 1 or a
time frame occurring "many years ago."

The verb *hop* in sentence 4 appears to
be present tense, except that in the context
of the sentence it functions as an infinitive
and part of the past tense construction
"liked to." Sentence 6 has even greater
temporal complexity: "was feeling silly"

and "hopped" are not two independent events that occurred in sequence but rather are simultaneous events, as indicated by the coordinating temporal conjunction *when*. This event itself is embedded within the temporal framework of "every day" at a time "many years ago" (Akmajian et al., 1984).

Story structure

The passage cited represents the first constituent of a complete narrative: the setting. The establishment of (1) the frog as the main character, (2) the pond as the stage, and (3) his satisfaction with his ordinary existence and his appearance as the context must be understood to recognize the significance of the second constituent (i.e., the initiating event). In this story, the initiating event occurs when a witch enters the frog's pond, casts a spell upon him, and changes him into a prince. This sets up the third constituent, or his internal response and the goal of the story: returning the character to his previously handsome state as a frog (Stein & Glenn, 1979). Each attempt (i.e., new spells) and consequence (i.e., transformations into a princess, a centaur, and a merman) represent constituents of complete episodes existing within the larger story. The constituents and hierarchical structure of stories must be understood to recognize that the many different events are in fact united in achieving the same overall goal (Applebee, 1978; Stein & Glenn, 1979).

Discourse levels

Many levels of social interaction exist within this narrative. For example, in a later sentence (i.e., "Why, oh why did you do such a thing?" the prince asked, weeping), many levels of discourse are operating. The first is reflected in the dialogue and represents the most observable social interaction, occurring between the prince and the witch. A second is reflected in the narration (i.e., the prince asked, weeping.) In conversation, this information would not be linguistic at all but visual. The listener would see the prince talking and weeping and would not be told this information. Thus the linguistic load is increased in narrative language, and the context cues that a child might ordinarily use to interpret language are now provided through the language, a discourse level existing between the narrator and the listener (Bruce, 1981). A more hidden level of discourse also is operating on an implied level. Although the prince is literally speaking the dialogue, the child must recognize the implied speaker is actually the frog.

Summary

The above analysis of a few representative sentences from the beginning of a story exemplifies many interactive levels of language structure and knowledge that are present in written text and that can be addressed in language intervention. Analyses of other forms of written language, such as expository text, will reveal similar patterns of complex syntax and morphology and different types of discourse structure. Any of these written discourse types can be used as a context for language learning. They each provide a potentially rich context for facilitating language learning in a manner that integrates meaning with function and form at levels of both sentence and discourse structure.

FACILITATING LANGUAGE LEARNING IN WRITTEN CONTEXTS

Simply reading literature, such as a story or expository text, is beneficial to language learning. Much of the vocabulary development and syntactic growth that occurs during the school years in normal development has been shown to result from reading and writing experiences (Loban, 1976; Nagy, Herman, & Anderson, 1985). Children with language and learning disorders, however, generally experience difficulty in gaining access to this source of language learning. They have difficulty reading written language, and even when they read they often fail to process and comprehend the information because of their poor mastery of semantic, syntactic, and pragmatic aspects of language. Reading, however, can be treated as an interactive and communicative exchange of information that occurs between the clinician and the child rather than a solitary experience. During the communicative exchanges that occur, the clinician can mediate language learning by assisting the child in understanding how the author of the text uses language to share meaning and accomplish goals.

Pairing oral and written language

Written language is an excellent context for this mediated language learning to occur because the print can be used to create an awareness of various elements of language without isolating the linguistic structures from a meaningful and integrated context. Furthermore, the written language paired with mediated oral interactions makes use of the advantages inherent in both the visual and the auditory modes of language. Together, written and oral language can be used to enable children to become aware of various elements of language and to learn how they function to communicate meaning.

Oral language is advantageous because it is rapid and infinitely modifiable (Sebeok, 1976). It allows for a large amount of information to be presented in a short amount of time, with revisions, elaborations, or clarifications being provided as needed. The rapid and temporary transmission of information characteristic of oral language, however, makes it difficult for children with language deficits to process the lengthy, complex, abstract, and highly transformed linguistic signals used to transmit meaning (Elliott & Hammer, 1988).

In contrast, written language presents a stable expression of language that lends itself to repeated and careful examination of its properties. Unlike spoken language, written language is a permanent record of a message. This advantage of written language allows for the same information to be repeatedly examined. Ideas or linguistic structures occurring in one context can be compared to parallel concepts in different sentences or situations. Information that is unfamiliar or that is relevant to a new context can be returned to as frequently as necessary to process the meaning, form, and function. Difficult concepts can be reviewed across time frames such as days or weeks, with each exposure being used to create greater awareness of the more abstract or complex aspects of the message as the more concrete ideas become known and easily processed (Morrow, 1985). Complex ideas can be parsed into smaller units, reorganized into topics and subtopics, and unified into superordinate relations. The written mode enables language to be examined and manipulated without the constraints of memory and changing context that are characteristic of spoken language (Sebeok, 1976).

Strategies for mediating language learning

The relative advantages of both modes of language processing can be used in language intervention. The clinician can use faciliatory strategies to mediate language learning with an individual child or a small group of children. This mediation enables the children to understand how the elements of language function to create meaning and to accomplish goals within the written language context. Bruner (1978) refers to the use of facilitatory strategies as providing a "scaffold" to the child. A scaffold can be thought of as any type of assistance that enables the child to engage successfully in language use at a level that is more complex than the child could independently comprehend and/or produce. A more elaborate scaffold is provided as the child attempts to use more unfamiliar and complex elements of language. The scaffold is reduced as the child becomes more independent in the use of the language.

The principle of scaffolding can be used to mediate language learning when written language is used as a context for intervention. A scaffold can be provided to assist a child to understand and use any element of language, including specific vocabulary words, figurative language, syntactic structures, or elements of discourse

structure. The reading is conducted as a communicative exchange between the clinician, the child, and the text and proceeds more as a conversation than oral reading. The clinician ensures that the child processes and comprehends each element of language by using the following types of assists throughout the interaction.

Preparatory sets

Children with language disorders often fail to process language because they fail to activate or retrieve the appropriate background knowledge and/or linguistic structure, even when this knowledge is possessed (Roth & Spekman, 1986, 1989). To improve processing, preparatory sets, or statements that help the child activate appropriate concepts or expectations can be provided before the child reads (Alvermann, Smith, & Readence, 1985). For example, the adult might state "Find out something about the frog" before reading sentence 1. If a child required a greater scaffold, the sentence might be parsed, and the adult might provide a series of preparatory sets, such as "This tells you what the frog looked like" (pointing to the main clause), "now find out where he lives" (pointing to the relative clause), or "how long ago was this?" (pointing to the adverbial clause). This parsing enables the

Children with language disorders often fail to process language because they fail to activate or retrieve the appropriate background knowledge and/or linguistic structure, even when this knowledge is possessed.

child to discover the component phrases or ideas within a complex sentence and to realize how they are combined to establish important facts about a topic (Nelson, 1985).

Preparatory sets also are used to link new information to previously stated ideas (Halliday & Hasan, 1985; Norris, 1989). This attention to meaning that is communicated between sentences helps the child make discoveries about how discourse structure orders events in a logical and predictable manner and how cohesive ties link different ideas to the same topic (Applebee, 1978; Halliday & Hasan, 1976). For example, the adult might say "These are some of the ways (pointing to the different ideas communicated in sentences 4 to 7) that all his days were exactly the same" (pointing to those words in sentence 3).

Preparatory sets, used by the clinician during each turn of the interaction, help the child learn to expect meaning when reading. They provide a model of how to think about the sentence and text structures as they are encountered. Their use enables the child to process the language in a manner that remains focused upon the theme or topic of the passage, that highlights elements of discourse structure, that integrates the meaning and structure of complex sentences, and that directs an abstract interpretation of language when appropriate. This type of scaffold maximizes the likelihood that the child will activate appropriate knowledge and linguistic structures that are possessed. The assistance also enables the child to process and use information and structures that may be unfamiliar.

Semantic maps

Another method that is useful in helping children retrieve and activate appropriate knowledge is the use of semantic maps (Pehrsson & Robinson, 1985). Semantic maps are used to brainstorm, or to generate possible ideas that may be related to a topic (see Figure 1). The central topic or theme is placed in a circle in the center of a piece of paper, and ideas that are associated with that concept are connected to it in general categories. For example, the word *frog* might be placed in the circle. One cluster of associated words might be generated and linked to the circle, such as "things that frogs do." Similar clusters can be formed for "things frogs eat," "what frogs look like," and "where frogs live." These ideas, generated by the children, activate needed background information that can be used to interpret the language encountered in the text (Alvermann et al., 1985).

Once created, the semantic map can be used in the process of mediated reading between the clinician and child. For example, the preparatory set "This is where (pointing to the cluster pertaining to where

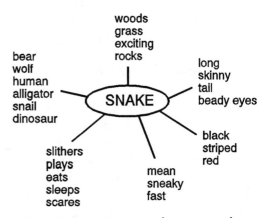

Figure 1. Semantic map used to generate ideas.

frogs live) the frog found food (pointing to the cluster relating to things frogs eat)" can be provided before sentence 7. The familiarity of the information already established by the semantic map enables the child to invest more attention to features of the language such as the complex and embedded structure of the sentence 7 used to communicate this information. Similarly, the adult can use the map to emphasize the information communicated in the text after it has been read with statements such as "That's right, *both* locations were good for finding food. Both *in the grass* and *in the pond* (pointing to the words on the map)."

In addition to assisting the child to process the language found in the text, semantic maps help accomplish other language goals. For example, the process of creating the map helps the child learn to develop a topic, form associations, categorize, compare, and make inferences (Pehrsson & Robinson, 1985).

Extensions

The mediation that the clinician provides through verbal comments can be used to elaborate upon the written language of the text. This type of scaffold is referred to as an extension (Muma, 1971). Extensions add clarification and guide more abstract interpretations. As the child reads a passage, the adult models insights or interpretations and/or invites the child to add elaborations. For example, after the reading of sentence 1 the adult might point to an accompanying picture and state "Yes, the pond looks *rather nice*. It has some rocks to sit on, a nice tree for shade, and it's not too big. What do *you* think is rather nice about the pond?"

The use of extensions is crucial to the process of facilitating the child's language learning. This type of response to the child's reading ensures that the focus is upon sharing meaning and understanding how the language communicates. Often, children with language and learning disorders do not consider reading a meaning-based act of communication but rather a process of "getting the words right" (Yaden & Templeton, 1986). If the child does not expect or comprehend meaning, then no language learning can occur from the experience of reading.

Extensions also help the child understand language by adding clarification or function to elements of syntax, morphology, or discourse structure that may not be fully understood. Many of these elements do not have meaning outside of a context of use and thus are best taught in context. For example, the adult might choose to establish in detail the temporal relationship between events to clarify how a form of the language communicates this knowledge (e.g., "He *had* dreams. He's not sleeping or dreaming now, but when he was sleeping last night he *had* dreams"). Any larger unit of meaning could similarly be focused upon and taught through extensions.

Extensions work by adding clarification or definition to an unfamiliar vocabulary word or a phrase. For example, the word *indeed* (sentence 10) is abstract and difficult to define. By pointing to the word and adding interpretations to it through statements such as "All the frogs thought so—he *really* was handsome—*of course* he was handsome," the child can begin to grasp the meaning and use of this word. A personal reaction can also be modeled, such as "Well, maybe the other frogs think he is indeed handsome, but I don't think he's very handsome. Indeed, I think he's very homely" (Rosenblatt, 1981).

Questioning

Questions are a natural part of communicating and are used to obtain information or to facilitate active problem solving. Thus the types of questions used in scaffolding are intended to extend thinking rather than to test for comprehension or factual recall (Panofsky, 1986). A recall question, such as "Who lived by the pond?" after the reading of sentence 1, diminishes communication and renders the act of reading meaningless. It is akin to an adult quizzing a child by saying "Who is visiting your house?" immediately after the child volunteered the information that Grandma was visiting to test recall.

Rather, questions such as "What is handsome about the frog?", "Why did he jump side to side only when he was feeling silly?", "What are some of the other things that the frog might eat?", "What do you think might happen to him?", "Do you think that he should have stayed there?", and other similar questions that promote prediction, role assumption, generalization, formulation of examples or exceptions, classification, justifications, solutions, and inferencing can be used to facilitate language learning (Blank et al., 1978).

Questioning also can be used in scaffolding to help the child revise misinterpretations or repair miscommunications (Goodman, 1982). For example, if the child miscued and read sentence 5 as "He hoped high and he hoped low," the adult might ask "Is that what he was doing in the grass, sitting and hoping for something to happen?" The question serves to engage the child in active problem solving, encouraging him or her to return to the text and to reexamine the language to clarify the concern and either verify or modify the initial reading (van Dijk & Kintsch, 1977). It facilitates the integration of information across sentences and helps the child consider larger units of language (Ripich & Griffith, 1988).

Old information

Many grammatical forms and structures of language refer to old or previously stated information (Halliday & Hasan, 1976, 1985). Written text enables old information to be physically located and pointed to when it is relevant to a new concept or recurs in a new context. For example, the adult can point back and forth between the pronoun *he* in sentences 2 and 4 and the word *frog* in sentence 1, stating "He, the frog, he's the one who had fun all day. He's the one who got to swim and hop" to demonstrate how this cohesive tie functions. Similarly, the relative pronoun *who* in sentence 1 can be associated with the frog ("The frog is *who* lived by the pond— the one *who* lived by the pond was the frog") to create an awareness of the grammar and how it functions to link these concepts.

Old information also can be reviewed when it is relevant to new ideas. As the physical description of the frog is encountered in sentence 8, the notion that he is considered handsome in sentence 1 can be pointed out and reread. This association is important, changing the interpretation of the new information from factual description to humor. Reference to old information can serve as a scaffold, assisting the child to associate ideas within and across sentences to interpret cohesive ties, clarify or expand upon old information, interpret new information in thematically appropriate ways, draw conclusions, or verify beliefs.

Reference to old information also can assist the child to become aware and to understand aspects of discourse structure, such as story grammar. For example, as a new episode is begun (the witch turns the character from a princess to a centaur), a previous episode can be looked at for its form. The sequence of events from the old episode (i.e., he was a prince, he asked to be changed, the witch tried a new spell, it failed, and he became a princess) can be physically pointed to in the respective written paragraphs. The child(ren) then can be asked to predict a sequence of events as the new episode is read, with assists provided when necessary, such as "Remember, he wanted to change back to a frog (returning to the page explaining that event in the previous episode). So what did he do then? What do you think he will do now?" The oral mediation, accompanied by visual reference to the written passages, can help the child process complex aspects of discourse structure.

Summarization

Summarization assists in the process of language learning by restating information, attending to the most important ideas and the relationships among them (Panofsky, 1986; van Dijk & Kintsch, 1977). Summarization can occur at any level, from the information contained within a single sentence to a synopsis of the entire

---

Summarization assists in the process of language learning by restating information, attending to the most important ideas and the relationships among them.

---

story. Sentences, phrases, or ideas in the print can be pointed to as a visual demonstration of how topically related information can be reorganized and synthesized. For example, after reading the passage above, the clinician might state "So this frog's life was pretty ordinary—he ate bugs (pointing to sentence 7), hopped in the grass (pointing to sentences 4 and 5), and swam in the pond (pointing to sentences 4 and 1)." This modeling assists the child in categorizing information and organizing events logically.

Summarization also can be used to provide the child(ren) with an opportunity to reorganize and restate information (van Dijk & Kintsch, 1977). Various prompts can be used to provide a scaffold that will maximize success. For example, the clinician can point to the relevant information in the text and assist the child to summarize important events or facts by using cloze procedures ("A frog who was very _____ lived by a _____ where he did ordinary things such as _____"), prompt additional information by using relational terms ("and then . . . ," "if . . ." or "because . . . ," "except . . ."), or prompt with questions ("What was the pond like?"; see Norris & Hoffman, 1989, for a more complete discussion of these strategies). Engaging a child in mediated summarization provides the child with the experience of talking about a topic for an extended period by using syntactically complex sentences and cohesive ties that the child may not be capable of using independently. As the child becomes more independent in the summarization process, the amount of scaffolding that the clinician uses decreases, indicating that this complex use of language is being internalized.

Flowcharts

Another method that is useful in assisting a child to organize and talk about information is the use of flowcharting (Geva, 1983). Flowcharts serve as a bridge between written language, where the organization, word choice, and syntactic structures are established by the writer, and oral language, where these linguistic choices must be independently formed by the child. Key ideas are organized hierarchically on a flowchart to conform to some goal, such as establishing the topic and supporting facts of an expository text, or the story structure of a narrative (see Figure 2).

The topic or main idea is entered in the top position of the flowchart. Constituents, supporting ideas, and important details are placed in subordinating positions, with elements that are equal in importance or structure being placed in parallel locations. When completed, the flowchart provides a visual scaffold that can be used by the child to organize language to talk about the information. The presence of key terms and the visual organization of terms on the flowchart enables the child to generate complex sentences to express these ideas.

The ideas placed on the flowchart can be used to reiterate or summarize the story as it was told by the author. The prompts described above (i.e., cloze, relational terms, or questions) can be used to scaffold the recall of the events. For example, the adult can point to a node and its constituent words while the child generates a corresponding utterance ("The frog lived

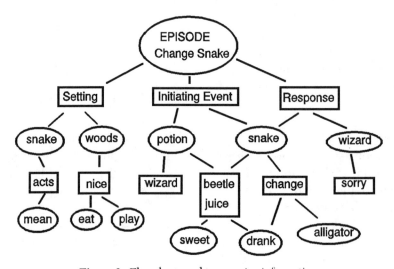

Figure 2. Flowchart used to organize information.

by a nice pond . . .") and prompt greater complexity by adding relational terms while pointing to further nodes or words (adult: "where he liked . . ." child: "to swim, hop, and eat"). A variety of different embedded and conjoined sentences can be scaffolded to help the child learn how to combine the same ideas into different relationships. Scaffolding from the flow-chart further can be used to order logically a sequence of sentences to retell the entire episode or story. Creating and then using flowcharts during the summarization process helps the child learn how to organize information, form categories, examine and use story structure, order ideas hierarchically, and generate complex sentences to express these relationships of meaning (Geva, 1983).

Metalinguistic information

Written language provides an ideal context for establishing reference to metalinguistic information (Yaden & Templeton, 1986). Patterns or regularities in the language can be explicitly referred to in context as a naturally occurring part of the interactions (Goodman, 1982). For example, the child's substitution of the word *exact* for *exactly* might indicate failure to understand the transformation of meaning that occurs as the word is changed from an adjective to an adverb. The adult can use verbal mediation to clarify this shift in meaning ("We're not talking about an *exact* day, like Tuesday. We're talking about how he lived—exactly the same, just the same every day, exactly the same"). Once the meaning has been clarified, the suffix can be explicitly pointed out with a comment such as "The *-ly* tells me that we are talking about how he did something.

Can you find or think of other words that tell *how* you do things?" Further examples can be looked for in the story or other familiar text. A notebook can be kept of these problematic linguistic forms.

Metalinguistic reference also can be used to develop concepts of wordness (Yaden & Templeton, 1986). In the natural course of discussion, the adult can point to words and refer to them metalinguistically. For example, the adult can point to the word *handsome* in sentence 1 and state "I wouldn't use an *adjective* like handsome to describe him. I might use an *adjective* like homely. What *adjective* would you use?" The naturally occurring use of these words in a context that already makes sense to the children makes these metalinguistic concepts concrete and comprehensible.

Levels of discourse also can be established by reference to cues such as punctuation. For example, the narration can be pointed to while the adult states "This tells you who is talking" followed by explicit reference to the quotation marks as the adult indicates "These quotation marks tell you that he is talking—this is exactly what he said." In addition, the dialogue offers the child opportunities to assume changing discourse roles and perspectives, varying voice and intonation to correspond to the characters and narrator (Bruce, 1981).

Theme building

The same story can be used over an extended period of time, for example as a month-long thematic unit. One constituent of the story, such as a single page or the pages related to a specific element of story structure, can be communicatively read each session. Difficult concepts presented on that page(s) can be reinforced further through collaborative activities, such as writing or drawing, or the exploration of additional resources, such as encyclopedias or nonfiction books (Harste et al., 1984).

In successive days, previously read pages can be reviewed before reading new pages. Many goals can be accomplished by reexamining old or known information. The level of the discussion regarding these pages can be increased to incorporate greater inference making and abstraction because the more factual and concrete information already is understood. Generalization of events to personal experiences or similar situations can be discussed because the significance of the event already is understood in the context of the story. The ability to organize information in large units, such as a logical story sequence, is developed as events are added gradually across sessions, each one being initially discussed as a smaller unit that becomes embedded within the larger context.

Theme building, including the use of the same story over time and the support of collaborative activities, ensures that the language encountered within the story is discussed with sufficient frequency and with enough contextual variability for generalization to occur (Gambrell, Pfeiffer, & Wilson, 1985). Theme building provides continuity of topic or theme while continuously introducing new concepts or modifying the level at which old information is presented. A variety of language behaviors are learned within the context of a dynamic activity that builds upon familiarity while maintaining interest through change and variety. This type of theme-oriented intervention is consistent with principles of whole language learning (Goodman, 1986).

• • •

Many linguistic challenges are encountered by the language- and learning-disordered child that are difficult to address through spoken language. Written language provides an alternative context for learning to recognize and use these abstract, complex, and subtle aspects of language. Meaningful contexts, such as those provided by good children's literature, are ideal for helping the child learn language in a manner that is interesting and does not artificially fragment language into subcomponents or splinter skills. Written contexts provide many naturally occurring opportunities for clinicians to assist the child in discovering how language works to share complex ideas.

The use of written language for intervention also provides a context for integrating spoken and written language. It enables the language-disordered child to acquire much of the vocabulary and the complex grammatical and discourse structures that are normally acquired through reading (Nagy et al., 1985). Thus the intervention simultaneously accomplishes multiple goals that are directly relevant to the child's school environment and provides a method for managing many of the challenges presented to the clinician by the school-age language-disordered child.

*Reprinted with permission from Horwitz, E. (1971). The Strange Story of the Frog Who Became a Prince. New York: Delacorte. © 1991 Bantam Doubleday Dell, New York, New York.

REFERENCES

Akmajian, A., Demers, R.A., & Harnish, R.M. (1984). *Linguistics: An introduction to language and communication.* Cambridge, MA: MIT Press.

Allington, R.L. (1989). Coherence or chaos? Qualitative dimensions of the literacy instruction provided to low achievement children. In A. Gartner & D. Lipsky (Eds.), *Beyond separate education* (pp. 75–99). New York: Brookes.

Alvermann, D.E., Smith, L.C., & Readence, J.E. (1985). Prior knowledge activation and the comprehension of compatible and incompatible text. *Reading Research Quarterly, 20,* 420–436.

Applebee, A.N. (1978). *The child's concept of story.* Chicago: University Park Press.

Blank, M., Rose, S.A., & Berlin, L.J. (1978). *The language of learning: The preschool years.* New York: Grune & Stratton.

Bruce, B. (1981). A social interaction model of reading. *Discourse Processes, 4,* 273–309.

Bruner, J.S. (1978). The role of dialogue in language acquisition. In A. Sinclair, R.J. Jarvella, & W.J.M. Levelt (Eds.), *The child's conception of language* (pp. 44–62). New York: Springer-Verlag.

Crais, E.R., & Chapman, R.S. (1987). Story recall and inferencing skills in language/learning-disabled and nondisabled children. *Journal of Speech and Hearing Research, 52,* 50–55.

Damico, J.S. (1989, April). *Synergy in applied linguistics: Theoretical and pedagogical implications.* Paper presented at the 18th annual University of Wisconsin–Milwaukee Linguistics Symposium, Milwaukee, WI.

Elliott, L.L., & Hammer, M.A. (1988). Longitudinal changes in auditory discrimination in normal children and children with language-learning problems. *Journal of Speech and Hearing Disorders, 4,* 467–474.

Fry, E.B. (1977). Fry's readability graph: Clarifications, validity and extension to level 17. *Journal of Reading, 21,* 242–243.

Gambrell, L.B., Pfeiffer, W.R., & Wilson, R.M. (1985). The effects of retelling upon reading comprehension and recall of text information. *Journal of Educational Research, 78,* 216–220.

Geva, E. (1983). Facilitating reading comprehension through flow charting. *Reading Research Quarterly, 28,* 384–405.

Goodman, K.S. (1982). *Language and literacy 1: Process, theory, research.* Boston: Routledge & Kegan Paul.

Goodman, K.S. (1986). *What's whole in whole language?* Portsmouth, NH: Heinemann.

Grice, H.P. (1975). Logic and conversation. In P. Cole & J. Morgan (Eds.), *Syntax and semantics 3: Speech Acts* (pp 41–58). New York: Academic Press.

Halliday, M.A.K., & Hasan, R. (1976). *Cohesion in English.* London: Longman Group.

Halliday, M.A.K., & Hasan, R. (1985). *Language, context, and text: Aspects of language in a social-semiotic perspective.* Deakin University, Victoria: Deakin University Press.

Harste, J.C., Woodward, V.A., & Burke, C.L. (1984). *Language stories and literacy lessons.* Portsmouth, NH: Heinemann.

Horwitz, E. (1971). *The strange story of the frog who became a prince.* New York: Delacorte.

Loban, W. (1976). *Language development: Kindergarten through grade twelve.* Urbana, IL: National Council of Teachers of English.

Morrow, C.M. (1985). Retelling stories: The strategy for improving children's comprehension, concept of story structure, and oral language complexity. *Elementary School Journal, 85,* 647–661.

Muma, J.R. (1971). Language intervention: Ten techniques. *Language, Speech, and Hearing Services in Schools, 2,* 7–17.

Nagy, W.E., Herman, P., & Anderson, R.C. (1985). Learning words from context. *Reading Research Quarterly, 20,* 233–253.

Nelson, K. (1985). *Making sense: The acquisition of shared meaning.* New York: Academic Press.

Norris, J.A. (1988). Using communication strategies to enhance reading acquisition. *Reading Teacher, 47,* 668–673.

Norris, J.A. (1989). Providing language remediation in the classroom: An integrated language-to-reading intervention method. *Language, Speech, and Hearing Services in Schools, 20,* 205–219.

Norris, J.A., & Hoffman, P.R. (1989). Language intervention within naturalistic environments. *Language, Speech, and Hearing Services in Schools, 21,* 72–84.

Panofsky, C. (1986, December). *The functions of language in parent-child bookreading events.* Paper presented at the National Reading Conference, Austin, TX.

Pehrsson, R.S., & Robinson, H.A. (1985). *The semantic organizer approach to writing and reading instruction.* Gaithersburg, MD: Aspen.

Ripich, D.N., & Griffith, P.L. (1988). Narrative abilities of children with learning disabilities and nondisabled children: Story structure, cohesion, and propositions. *Journal of Learning Disabilities, 21,* 165–173.

Rosenblatt, L.M. (1981). *The reader, the text, the poem: The transactional theory of the literary work.* Carbondale, IL: Southern Illinois University Press.

Roth, F.P., & Spekman, N.J. (1986). Narrative discourse: Spontaneously generated stories of learning-disabled and normally achieving students. *Journal of Speech and Hearing Disorders, 51,* 8–23.

Roth, F.P., & Spekman, N.J. (1989). The oral syntactic proficiency of learning disabled students: A spontaneous story sampling analysis. *Journal of Speech and Hearing Research, 32,* 67–77.

Sebeok, T.A. (1976). *Contributions to the doctrine of signs.* Atlantic Highlands, NJ: Humanities Press.

Stein, N., & Glenn C. (1979). An analysis of story comprehension in elementary school children. In R. Freedle (Ed.), *New directions in discourse processing.* (Vol 2, pp 53–102). Norwood, NJ: Ablex.

van Dijk, T., & Kintsch, W. (1977). Cognitive psychology and discourse: Recalling and summarizing stories. In W.U. Dressler (Ed.), *Current trends in textlinguistics.* (pp. 61–81). New York: DeGruyter.

Yaden, D.B., & Templeton, S. (1986). *Metalinguistic awareness and beginning literacy: Conceptualizing what it means to read and write.* Portsmouth, NH: Heinemann.

Semantic organizers: Implications for reading and writing

Robert S. Pehrsson, EdD
Associate Professor of Education
Director of Reading Program

Peter R. Denner, PhD
Associate Professor of Education
Department of Education
Idaho State University
Pocatello, Idaho

AMONG THE MANY and varied problems exhibited by children with language difficulties, and perhaps a basic reason for failure in reading, writing, and other academic subjects, is a lack of appropriate organizational strategies (Baker, 1982; Freston & Drew, 1974). The importance of organization as a major factor in written language is supported by a set of theories of human cognition that fall under the general rubric of schema theory (Anderson & Pearson, 1984; Mandler, 1984; Rumelhart, 1980, 1984; Rumelhart & Ortony, 1977). These theories suggest that meaning is neither realized nor expressed until some organizing structure or schema has been uncovered or imposed. Schemata are organizational constructs that enable readers and writers to integrate information about an event or topic into a referential model (Collins, Brown, & Larkin, 1980).

Basically, schemata function during reading by providing "empty slots" that

Top Lang Disord, 1988, 8(3), 24–37
© 1988 Aspen Publishers, Inc.

might be thought of as a set of expectations onto which the reader maps the segments of the text (Anderson, 1977; Anderson & Pearson, 1984). Proficient readers test their schema-based expectations by evaluating them for "goodness-of-fit" with the subsequent information (clues) supplied by the author (Rumelhart, 1984). As reading progresses, the reader's expectations are confirmed, modified, or disconfirmed as the slots become filled and the material is processed. Hence, understanding develops as the reader progressively revises an initial model of the passage until it approximates the model intended by the author of the text (Collins, Brown, & Larkin, 1980). In this way, *organization* of the clues supplied by the author via the reader's own schemata enables the proficient reader to compose a logical interpretation of the passage (Tierney & Pearson, 1983).

Schemata are essential to writing as well (Smith, 1982; Squire, 1983). Composing depends on a writer's organizational strategies (Hayes & Flower, 1983). Before writing, the author relies on prior knowledge schemata to organize what he or she will say. As writing progresses, the proficient writer develops his or her initial model of the passage, reorganizing and even creating information by filling in "slots" with particular characters, incidents, and objects. The writer's aim is to compose a written text that approximates the desired model. During the drafting and refinement stages, the proficient writer may also revise his or her initial organization. In addition, good writers take into account and are considerate of their prospective readers' organization of knowledge (background schemata).

CONSTRUCTING MEANING

Many language-disordered children demonstrate problems comprehending a story as well as producing narratives because they fail to realize the internal organization in the text (Graybeal, 1981; Hansen, 1978; Weaver & Dickenson, 1979). A rationale and some practical applications are presented here for the explicit teaching of organizational strategies to language-disordered youngsters as they learn to read and write, and for older language-disordered youngsters who are in need of remediation or advanced skills development. The method of instruction advocated here for teaching organization to all youngsters, including those with language disorders, is the *semantic organizer approach* (Pehrsson & Robinson, 1985). The approach is both preventive and remedial. It is appropriate for very young children at the readiness stage (Pehrsson & Robinson, 1985) and for older students requiring advanced skills development or remediation. In addition to facilitating reading comprehension and cohesive writing, the semantic-organizer approach improves retention and recall of information. Well-organized information that has been operated on (via organizing schemata) in a organized manner tends to be remembered well (Rumelhart & Ortony, 1977). Many language-disordered students exhibit problems remembering information they have heard or read (Wiig & Semel, 1984). Therefore, during and after reading, these youngsters should be helped to organize and reorganize the information they have understood as an aid to retention (Taylor, 1980).

Prior knowledge

A first step in the meaning-construction process of both writing and reading is activation and organization of the prior knowledge the individual brings to the activity (Squire, 1983; Tierney & Pearson, 1983). Children, however, vary greatly in how they make use of background information during reading. Some students fail to comprehend what they read because they do not develop and construct an organizational pattern of ideas similar to the one aimed at by the writer. Three styles have been identified: *fragmented, projective,* and *interactive* (Pehrsson, 1982; Pehrsson & Denner, 1985). Students who use a *fragmented* style fail to integrate new information with what they already know, and they fail to use the author's clues to develop a coherent model of the text. For example, Harry, an 11-year-old language-disordered child, was able to provide facts about a story detailing a bank robbery, but failed to integrate any of the information into a story. He recalled the story as follows: "Men got arrested. Bank robbery. Two children go home from school." Probing failed to indicate that he had organized the fragments into a coherent story. He seemed satisfied with his ability to remember fragments without organizing them in an appropriate sequence.

Other language-disordered children may be *projective* readers. They do attempt to make use of background information but draw from the wrong schemata. They appear to focus during reading on one relatively unimportant concept and build their model of the text as if the concept were the central theme. For example, Jennifer, a 9-year-old language-disordered child, read the passage about the bank robbery and retold a story about children being kidnapped. It was a good story, but not the one intended by the author.

Projective readers draw from their own experiences but fail to relate well to the organization intended by the author (Pehrsson, 1982; Pehrsson & Denner, 1985). In contrast, *interactive* readers make appropriate use of prior information. Therefore they integrate new information with old and are able to organize information effectively.

When writing, some language-disordered youngsters also have great difficulty due to poor organizational strategies (Yoshinaga-Itano & Snyder, 1985). Students who are poor writers often fail to construct an organization that follows a typical plan or is easily interpreted. Some present their ideas in a fragmented fashion. Projective writers' narratives are also difficult to interpret because they fail to take into account their intended audience's background experiences. They fail to develop pragmatic presuppositions regarding a reader's ability to organize information. In each instance, communication breaks down because of organizational differences between writer and reader.

Text structure

In addition to the organization and application of prior knowledge, successful readers and writers need to be sensitive to the ways in which texts are organized. Advances in systems for analyzing the organization or "top-level" structure of texts (Mandler & Johnson, 1977; Meyer,

1975) have contributed to increased understanding of the role text structure plays in both comprehension and composition. The "top-level" structure of a text specifies the logical organization and relations among ideas. It also identifies which ideas are more important than others. The structure can be conceived as representing the overall organizing principle or model the author uses to convey his or her message to the reader. The reader who is able to uncover the author's top-level structure can organize ideas in ways that more or less match the pattern used by the author. As a result, the reader can more readily grasp the global message the author tried to convey (Mandler & Johnson, 1977; Meyer, Brandt, & Bluth, 1980; Stein & Glenn, 1979; Taylor, 1980; Thorndyke, 1977). The writer who is capable of organizing ideas in writing so that readers will readily uncover the organizational structure will be a better communicator and, therefore, a better writer.

The reader who is able to uncover the author's top-level structure can organize ideas in ways that more or less match the pattern used by the author.

Because good readers attend to the general organization (the top-level structure) when developing their model for the text, they are good comprehenders. In contrast, poor readers, including those with language problems, are more likely to read in a fragmented fashion or to impose an organizing structure unrelated to the author's. Hence, it is important to help

these youngsters to develop strategies for organizing their schemata in relation to the top-level structures used by the author and to provide them with instructional experiences involving all types of text structures. In this way, they will be better able to comprehend and compose various forms of text organization (Squire, 1983).

Developing organizational strategies

One of the more direct ways of teaching students to be aware of their own organizational strategies for both reading and writing is through the use of *semantic organizers*, also known as semantic webs or semantic maps (Hanf, 1971; Heimlich & Pittelman, 1986; Johnson & Pearson, 1984; Pehrsson & Robinson, 1985). To construct a semantic organizer, the reader or writer must organize and sometimes reorganize ideas after either abstracting them from, or generating them for, inclusion in a prose passage, and then display them as clusters of related ideas. The major ideas are drawn in circles, rectangles, or other shapes, then lines are used to connect the ideas together in a spatial arrangement. Hence, every semantic organizer has both a verbal (semantic) component and a graphic-structure (organizer) component.

Research indicates that semantic organizers enable students to develop improved organization and recall. Several studies (Armbruster & Anderson, 1980; Dansereau, Collins, McDonald, Holley, Garland, Diekhoff, & Evans, 1977; Holly, Dansereau, McDonald, Garland, & Collins, 1979) have investigated the effects of semantic webs or maps on students' acquisition of expository text material. Other studies have examined the effects of semantic organizers on story comprehension and recall (Denner & Pehrsson, 1987; Reutzel, 1985). Results of all the studies indicate that the students who constructed maps recalled more information than students in other study conditions. Clinical practices and controlled studies (Pehrsson & Mook, 1983; Schultz, 1986) have also demonstrated that semantic organizers can improve writing when used as a prewriting strategy. As a note of caution, however, it should be pointed out that while these preliminary research findings are encouraging, many more clinical and experimental studies are needed. The possible benefits and various uses of semantic organizers are highlighted here, particularly with reference to the needs of language-disordered youngsters.

THE SEMANTIC ORGANIZER APPROACH

The use of semantic organizers as a tool for helping students display the interrelationship of ideas in both writing and reading has been explained in-depth by Pehrsson and Robinson (1985). The approach is based on the research cited earlier and extensive clinical work with students lacking appropriate organizational strategies for both writing and reading. It is a sequential approach that emphasizes prior knowlege schemas and text organization, beginning with young children, or nonreaders, and developing more complex strategies for more mature students. By using a guided-strategy approach to instruction, students are introduced to semantic organizers within the context of a metacognitive orientation (Baker & Brown, 1984; Roehler, Duffy, & Meloth, 1986).

Too frequently, students are taught skills in isolation. When students receive only skills instruction, they often fail to use the skills effectively and on their own because they are not clear about where and when to use them (Baker & Brown, 1984). As a consequence, many students fail to spontaneously transfer writing and reading skills acquired through skill instruction to real-world contexts. The guided-strategy approach (also called "metacognitive approach") attempts to help students develop generalizable strategies for learning, not isolated skills. Using this approach, students receive training in self-monitoring, or the metacognitive awareness necessary for effective use of the skills or strategies (Brown, 1982).

The major features of a successful guided-strategy approach to skill development have been delineated by Brown and her associates (Baker & Brown, 1984; Brown, 1980; Palincsar & Brown, 1987). With the semantic organizer approach to a guided-strategy lesson, the student is guided by the teacher to (a) evaluate the importance of organization to writing and reading, as well as the reasons for developing a specified type of semantic organizer; (b) observe the construction by the teacher of a particular semantic organizer; (c) participate, sometimes by finishing a partially completed organizer; and (d) gradually assume full responsibility for the development of a particular organizer. In this interactive setting, the organizing activities of the teacher are slowly adopted by the student and become internalized as a part of the student's organizational strategies. As a result, students increase their ability to construct various kinds of semantic organizers, and they develop the metacognitive awareness necessary to effectively use them during reading and writing.

ORGANIZATIONAL PATTERNS OF THE SEMANTIC ORGANIZER APPROACH

The semantic organizer approach makes use of only two basic organizational structures. Text information is graphed into either a *cluster* pattern (superordinate/subordinate), as shown in Figure 1, or an *episodic* pattern (change/sequence), as shown in Figure 2. While a variety of complex means can be used to identify different kinds of text-structure patterns (Brewer, 1980; Meyer, 1975), simplicity is a major strength of the semantic organizer approach in that any text can be reduced to two fundamental organizing principles: stasis and change. A narrative text, for example, can be thought of as a sequence (change) of causal or temporal relations across described (statis) events and states (Just & Carpenter, 1987). This simplified scheme has proved useful in clinical work with young children and with language-disordered students. Another strength of the semantic organizer approach is that it

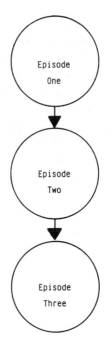

Figure 2. Episodic pattern.

can be extended to all areas of the curriculum.

Initially, students are taught to identify and use the two basic patterns of organization in their reading and writing. Later, with advancing skill, students learn to decide whether information in a text should be organized more appropriately as a cluster or as a series of episodes. For example, a unit about cities could make use of either pattern, but the purpose of the reader when interacting with the text determines the appropriateness of only one of the organizing patterns. To organize information about different areas in a city, a cluster organizer would be most appropriate. The name of the city could go in the center of the cluster, and stemming from the center the student could write the three concepts: residential, commercial, and industrial. In turn, each con-

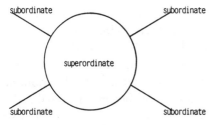

Figure 1. Cluster pattern.

cept area can serve as a center for more specific information. Figure 3 demonstrates such an organizer with pictures as graphic aids. A concept of city can also be considered episodically when growth over time rather than parts is emphasized. In this case, while each episode in turn can be treated as a cluster, the major emphasis is on the sequencing of episodes. For example, a unit about Chicago could be developed as shown in Figure 4, again with pictures to dramatize the historical changes.

A DEVELOPMENTAL SEQUENCE FOR INTRODUCING ORGANIZERS

Pehrsson and Robinson (1985) presented a developmental sequence for the introduction of cluster and episodic semantic organizers. The sequence is appropriate for all beginning readers and nonreaders, including language-disordered youngsters. With this approach, children move from realia clusters to picture clusters, verb clusters, noun clusters, concept clusters, and finally to episodic organizers of various kinds.

Realia clusters make use of real things, such as pieces of rope, pots, dishes, forks, and toy telephones, to demonstrate how things relate to a larger picture of a family eating dinner. A child places the objects around the picture and stretches the pieces of rope from the pot, dish, fork, and telephone individually to the picture. The telephone might be considered an item to be excluded from this category; therefore, another piece of rope is stretched diagonally across the first rope (this is the symbol for "not"), indicating that the telephone is not related to eating. To know what something is, it is necessary to also understand what it is not, and therefore organizers can

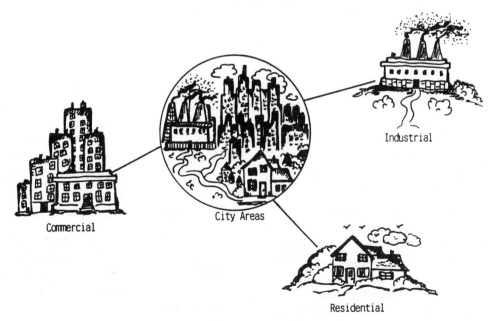

Figure 3. Cluster organizer for cities.

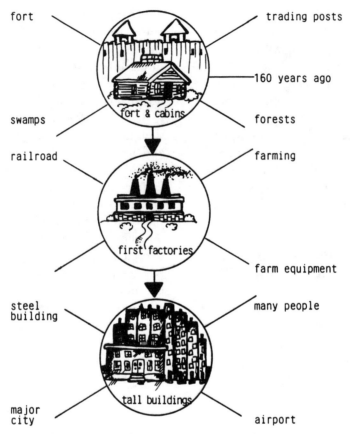

Figure 4. Episodic organizer for history of Chicago.

be developed using both inclusive and exclusive items. The telephone is an exclusive item for the dinner cluster.

Verb cluster organizers also initially make use of pictures. Pictures or stick-figure drawings represent action verbs such as walk, jump, and swim, which are labeled in the appropriate written form. Lines are drawn to connect the verbs to inclusive and exclusive agents of the specified action. With this approach, verbs rather than nouns are emphasized first (see Pehrsson & Robinson, 1985) to help students extract and express basic semantic relationships (e.g., agent–action,

agent–action–location). Hence, verb organizers depict instances and noninstances of the same basic schema. The repetition of an action schema helps to control the language of the text and provides redundancy at the semantic level, which facilitates comprehension.

The repetition of an action schema helps to control the language of the text and provides redundancy at the semantic level, which facilitates comprehension.

Verb-cluster organizers are also useful in helping to eliminate "fuzzy edges" to the application of an action schema for a language-disordered child. For example, one child stated that chairs swim because he had seen wooden chairs floating in a river. The organizer shown in Figure 5 demonstrated for him that living things swim and nonliving things float. This technique enabled him to develop the semantic features and lexical restrictions for the agents and action.

A verb-cluster organizer can be easily related to both writing and reading. A paragraph based on a verb cluster can be written by a child after modeling by the teacher or clinician, or the child might be asked to construct a verb organizer based on a paragraph that conveys the same information. As an illustration, the following paragraph could be written or read by a child based on the above verb cluster.

Fish swim. Ducks swim. Children swim. But chairs don't swim.

While verb-cluster organizers help students to construct sentences using the same basic pattern (schema) and arrange them in a simple paragraph, most paragraphs, particularly in expository passages, are better represented in the form of a *noun cluster*. In this type of cluster organizer, the noun is central and the verb phrases are subordinate (see Figure 6). The noun indicates the main topic of the paragraph. The verb phrases linked to the noun indicate events or actions that are possible for referent. In this way, students

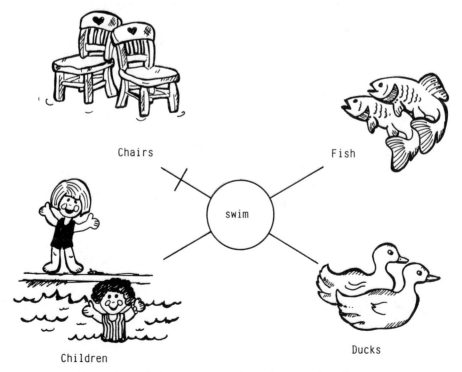

Figure 5. Verb-cluster organizer for swimming versus floating.

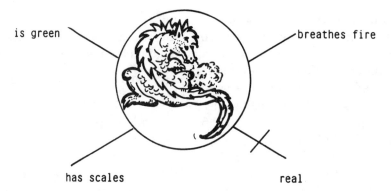

Figure 6. Noun-cluster organizer for dragon.

learn to recognize and use a common structure for the organization of a paragraph.

Noun organizers prepare children for *concept clusters*, which are similar to the more elementary noun organizers but make greater use of telegraphic language. For example, in a concept cluster the words *has* and *is* would be eliminated from the organizer about the dragon. The use of concept clusters teaches youngsters to extract meaningful information from a passage and to distinguish the less important words (e.g., function words) from the more important ones. A concept-cluster organizer, such as the one presented in Figure 7, can be particularly useful when diverse information is presented across paragraphs about a single topic, as in the following text on automobiles.

Automobiles have had some major effects on teenagers and others. Of the 110 million

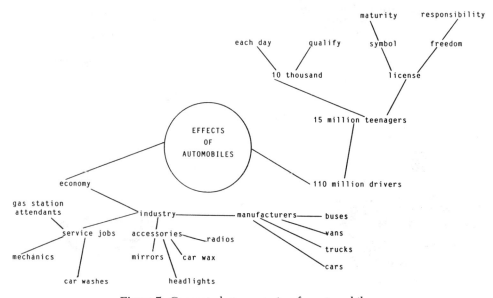

Figure 7. Concept-cluster organizer for automobiles.

drivers in this country, 15 million are teenagers, and every day 10,000 reach the qualifying age. For teenagers, a driver's license is a symbol of maturity, a modern rite of passage. A license to drive also increases freedom and the need to develop responsibility quickly.

The economy has been affected by the auto industry, which has directly and indirectly created many occupations. Auto manufacturers provide many jobs. Companies make many different kinds of cars, trucks, vans, and buses. Many people also work at making car accessories such as mirrors, headlights, radios, and car wax. The auto industry also has created service jobs, such as gas station attendants, mechanics, and car washers. Automobiles have had major effects.

Working from a concept organizer, students can be taught to write a summary of a reading passage such as this. Summarization requires both selection and elimination. Much nonessential information is eliminated during the process of developing an organizer. More important, the structure of the organizer itself can help students to decide which information is relevant. The more centrally placed within the concept organizer, the more important the information is to include as part of a written summary. In the automobile text, the specific examples given of various jobs are not as important as the job categories. Thus, after the teacher modeled the process of writing a summary using various concept clusters, Randy, a ninth-grader, independently wrote the following summary of the automobile passage using the organizer presented in Figure 7.

Automobiles effect teenagers and people. There are 110 million drivers and 15 million teenagers drivers who get freedom because

they drive. People get money from making cars and making things for cars and working on cars.

When students have acquired the basic pattern of organization involved in the clustering of ideas, they are ready to learn ways to represent change from one cluster state to the next. Causal and sequential relations connecting events or states can be represented using an *episodic organizer*. For example, Figure 8 presents an episodic organizer describing a problem and its solution. After first arranging ideas in the form of this problem–solution organizer, a language-disordered teenager wrote the following composition.

I have a problem. I have no car. I have license but I soon forget how to drive. I have friends but I don't visit because they live very far. I take subway but it takes a long time and dangerous. I shop but sometimes packages too big. My mother carry very big packages.

I have a solution. I can buy a car. I can use my license and I don't forget how to drive. I can visit friends easy and not far by car. I don't take subway. Car is fast not dangerous. I can have big packages in car an help mother carry big packages. I think it very good idea to buy a car. But I have different problem now. I have no money (Pehrsson & Robinson, 1985, pp. 124–125).

As illustrated, the episodic organizer enabled this teenager to describe an initial state of affairs—a problem—in one paragraph and to trace the changes that might transpire in a second paragraph when a new state of affairs—a solution—is achieved. Although clearly this individual's writing lags far behind the quality of writing that might be expected of his age-related peers, before his introduction

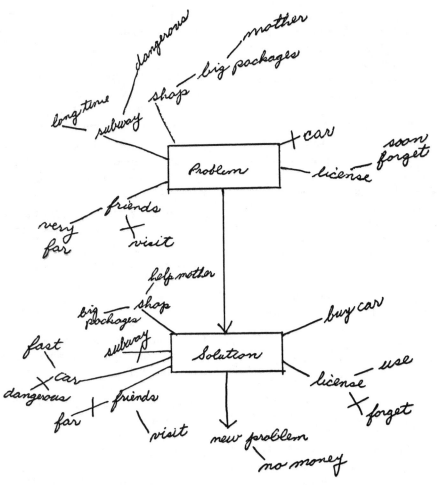

Figure 8. Problem–solution organizer. From *The Semantic Organizer Approach to Writing and Reading Instruction* (p. 125) by R.S. Pehrsson and H.A. Robinson, 1985, Rockville, MD: Aspen. Reprinted with permission of Aspen Publishers, Inc., copyright 1985.

to the use of semantic organizers, he was unable to organize, write, or even comprehend paragraphs such as these.

As the illustrations show, the semantic organizer approach supports and develops organizational strategies essential to both writing and reading. It bridges the gap between idea organization and written language structures. Young children can learn to develop organizers based on para-

graphs as a reading comprehension activity, and they can write paragraphs based on organizers. The organizer graphically displays the important relationships. With the aid of elementary structures such as verb-cluster organizers, even beginning readers and writers can learn basic organizational strategies. By developing the initial connection between writing and reading in relation to the organization of information, the semantic organizer can be a basic tool with a high degree of transfer value for language-disordered children.

• • •

A practical approach for reading and writing instruction has been presented. It is proposed that improvement in the comprehension and formulation of written language can be facilitated through the use of semantic organizers. The approach can be viewed as both preventive and remedial. Clinical experience with language-disordered students suggests that the semantic-organizer approach has considerable merit. Semantic organizers, used as graphic tools and taught within a guided-strategy (metacognitive) approach to instruction, can help students not only improve organizational skills, but also instill the awareness (metacognition) necessary to transfer these skills to new contexts, thereby enhancing students' reading and writing competence.

REFERENCES

Anderson, R.C. (1977). The notion of schemata and the educational enterprise: General discussions of the conference. In R.C. Anderson, R.J. Spiro, & W.E. Montague (Eds.), *Schooling and the acquisition of knowledge*. Hillsdale, NJ: Erlbaum.

Anderson, R.C., & Pearson, P.D. (1984). A schema-theoretic view of basic processes in reading. In P.D. Pearson (Ed.), *Handbook of reading research*. New York: Longman.

Armbruster, B., & Anderson, T. (1980). *The effect of mapping on the free recall of expository text* (Technical Report No. 160). Urbana, IL: Center for the Study of Reading, University of Illinois.

Baker, L. (1982). An evaluation of the role of metacognitive deficits in learning disabilities. *Topics in Learning and Learning Disabilities, 2(1)*, 27–35.

Baker, L., & Brown, A.L. (1984). Cognitive monitoring in reading. In J. Flood (Ed.), *Understanding reading comprehension*. Newark, DE: International Reading Association.

Brewer, W.F. (1980). Literary theory, rhetoric, and stylistics: Implications for psychology. In R.J. Spiro, B.C. Bruce, & W.F. Brewer (Eds.), *Theoretical issues in reading comprehension*. Hillsdale, NJ: Erlbaum.

Brown, A.L. (1980). Metacognitive development and reading. In R.J. Spiro, B.C. Bruce, & W.F. Brewer (Eds.), *Theoretical issues in reading comprehension*. Hillsdale, NJ: Erlbaum.

Brown, A.L. (1982). Learning to learn how to read. In J. Langer & T. Smith-Burke (Eds.), *Reader meets author, bridging the gap: A psycholinguistic and social linguistic perspective*. Newark, DE: International Reading Association.

Collins, A., Brown, J.S., & Larkin, K.M. (1980). Inference in text understanding. In R.J. Spiro, B.C. Bruce, & W.F. Brewer (Eds.), *Theoretical issues in reading comprehension*. Hillsdale, NJ: Erlbaum.

Dansereau, D., Collins, K., McDonald, B., Holley, C., Garland, U., Diekhoff, G., & Evans, S. (1979). Development and evaluation of a learning strategy training program. *Journal of Educational Psychology, 71*, 64–73.

Denner, P.R., & Pehrsson, R.S. (1987, April). *A comparison of the effects of episodic organizers and traditional notetaking on story recall*. Paper presented at the annual meeting of the American Educational Research Association, Washington, DC.

Freston, C.W., & Drew, C.J. (1974). Verbal performance of learning disabled children as a function of input organization. *Journal of Learning Disabilities, 7*, 424–428.

Graybeal, C.M. (1981). Memory for stories in language-impaired children. *Applied Psycholinguistics, 2*, 269–283.

Hanf, M.B. (1971). Mapping: A technique for translating reading into thinking. *Journal of Reading, 14*, 225–230, 270.

Hansen C. (1978). Story retelling used with average and learning disabled readers as measure of reading comprehension. *Learning Disabilities Quarterly, 1*, 62–69.

Hayes, J.R., & Flower, L.S. (1983). Uncovering cognitive processes in writing: An introduction to protocol analysis. In P. Mosenthal, L. Tamor, & S.A. Walmsley (Eds.), *Research on writing: Principles and methods* (pp. 207–220). New York: Longman.

Heimlich, J.E., & Pittelman, S.D. (1986). *Semantic mapping: Classroom applications*. Newark, DE: International Reading Association.

Holley, C.D., Dansereau, D.F., McDonald, B.A., Garland, J.C., & Collins, K.W. (1979). Evaluation of a hierarchical mapping technique as an aid to prose processing. *Contemporary Educational Psychology, 4,* 227–237.

Johnson, D.D., & Pearson, P.D. (1984). *Teaching reading vocabulary* (2nd ed.). New York: Holt, Rinehart & Winston.

Just, M.A., & Carpenter, P.A. (1987). *The psychology of reading and language comprehension.* Boston: Allyn & Bacon.

Mandler, J.M. (1984). *Stories, scripts, and scenes: Aspects of schema theory.* Hillsdale, NJ: Erlbaum.

Mandler, J.M., & Johnson, N.S. (1977). Remembrance of things parsed: Story structure and recall. *Cognitive Psychology, 9,* 111–151.

Meyer, B.J.F. (1975). *The organization of prose and its effects on memory.* Amsterdam: North-Holland.

Meyer, B.J.F., Brandt, D.M., & Bluth, G.J. (1980). Use of the top-level structure in text: Key for reading comprehension of ninth-grade students. *Reading Research Quarterly, 16,* 72–103.

Palincsar, A.S., & Brown, D. (1987). Enhancing instructional time through attention to metacognition. *Journal of Learning Disabilities, 20,* 66–75.

Pehrsson, R.S. (1982). *An investigation of comprehending during the process of silent reading: The op-in procedure* (Final Report, Grant No. 486). Pocatello, ID: Idaho State University. (ERIC Document Reproduction Service No. ED 236 573)

Pehrsson, R.S., & Denner, P.R. (1985). *Assessing silent reading during the process: An investigation of the op-in procedure.* Paper presented at the annual meeting of the Northern Rocky Mountain Educational Research Association, Jackson, WY. (ERIC Document Reproduction Service No. ED 265 529)

Pehrsson, R.S., & Mook, J.E. (1983). *A model of curriculum development in rural schools.* (ERIC Document Reproduction Service No. ED 230 361)

Pehrsson, R.S., & Robinson, H.A. (1985). *The semantic organizer approach to writing and reading instruction.* Rockville, MD: Aspen Systems Corp.

Reutzel, D.R. (1985). Story maps improve comprehension. *The Reading Teacher, 38,* 400–404.

Roehler, L.R., Duffy, G.G., & Meloth, M.S. (1986). What to be direct about in direct instruction in reading: Content-only versus process-into-content. In T.E. Raphael (Ed.), The contexts of school-based literacy. New York: Random House.

Rumelhart, D.E. (1980). Schemata: The building blocks of cognition. In R.J. Spiro, B.C. Bruce, & W.F. Brewer (Eds.), *Theoretical issues in reading comprehension.* Hillsdale, NJ: Erlbaum.

Rumelhart, D.E. (1984). Understanding understanding. In J. Flood (Ed.), *Understanding reading comprehension: Cognition, language and the structure of prose.* Newark, DE: International Reading Association.

Rumelhart, D.E. & Ortony, A. (1977). The representation of knowledge in memory. In R.C. Anderson, R.J. Spiro, & W.E. Montague (Eds.), *Schooling and the acquisition of knowledge.* Hillsdale, NJ: Erlbaum.

Schultz, M.M. (1986). *The semantic organizer: A prewriting strategy for first grade students.* Unpublished doctoral dissertation, University of Connecticut, Storrs, CT.

Smith, F. (1982). *Writing and the writer.* New York: Holt, Rinehart, & Winston.

Squire, J.R. (1983). Composing and comprehending: Two sides of the same basic process. *Language Arts, 60,* 581–589.

Stein, N.L., & Glenn, C.G. (1979). Analysis of story comprehension in elementary school children. In R. Freedle (Ed.), *New directions in discourse processing* (Vol. 2). Norwood, NJ: Ablex.

Taylor, B. (1980). Children's memory for expository text after reading. *Reading Research Quarterly, 15,* 399–411.

Thorndyke, P.W. (1977). Cognitive structures in comprehension and memory of narrative discourse. *Cognitive Psychology, 9,* 77–110.

Tierney, R.S., & Pearson, P.D. (1983). Toward a composing model of reading. *Language Arts, 60,* 568–580.

Weaver, R., & Dickenson, D. (1979). Story comprehension and recall in dyslexic students. *Bulletin of the Orton Society, 29,* 157–171.

Wiig, E., & Semel, E. (1984). *Language assessment and intervention for the learning disabled.* Columbus, OH: Merrill.

Yoshinaga-Itano, C., & Snyder, L. (1985). Form and meaning in the written language of hearing impaired children. *Volta Review, 87*(5), 75–90.

Part II
From Clinic to Classroom: Intervention Scenarios Among and Between

Early intervention for children's reading problems: Clinical applications of the research in phonological awareness

Benita A. Blachman, PhD
Associate Professor
Division of Special Education and
*   Rehabilitation*
Syracuse University
Syracuse, New York

PERHAPS NO OTHER educational debate is as politically charged as the controversy that surrounds the teaching of beginning reading (Adams, 1990). Some would like us to believe that learning to read is as natural as learning to speak (Goodman, 1986; Goodman & Goodman, 1979). As we consider this premise, however, we must also consider the following facts about language (Liberman & Liberman, 1990):

1. All communities of humans have a fully developed spoken language, but only a minority of these exists in a written form. Where there is a written form, many competent speakers do not, and indeed, cannot use it effectively, no matter how strong the pressure to do so.
2. In the history of the race, as in the development of the child, speech comes first, reading second. Apparently, speech is as old as the human species, having evolved with it as perhaps the most important of its species-typical characteristics; alphabets, on the other hand, are developments of the last three or four thousand years, and they are

Top Lang Disord, 1991,12(1),51–65
© 1991 Aspen Publishers, Inc.

cultural achievements, not the primary products of biological evolution. . . .

4. In order to develop speech, the normal child need only be in an environment where language is spoken; reading, on the other hand, almost always requires explicit tuition.[(p.55)]

Given these facts and the estimated 35 million American adults (20% of the adult population) who continue to have severe problems with even the most common reading activities (Stedman & Kaestle, 1987), it seems reasonable to conclude that, although reading is clearly a language-based activity, reading and speech are not "equivalent forms of development" and that all children do not learn both "in the same natural, unconscious way" (Liberman & Liberman, 1990, p. 56). Consequently, it is imperative that we continue to explore exactly what it is that children must understand about the connections between print and speech to become literate.

Despite the sometimes acrimonious debate regarding the best way to teach beginning reading, we have actually learned a great deal in the last two decades about the language factors important in early reading acquisition (Kamhi & Catts, 1989; Liberman, 1971, 1983; Perfetti, 1985; Shankweiler & Liberman, 1989; Vellutino, 1979, 1987). As research evidence converges from a variety of disciplines, a consensus is beginning to emerge about some of the basic precursors of literacy development (Adams, 1990; Stanovich, 1987). Perhaps the most successful area of inquiry has been research in phonological awareness (Stanovich, 1987). We now know that an awareness of the phonological segments in words and the ability to manipu-

late these segments are of crucial importance in reading acquisition. As Williams (1987) points out, one of the most important insights in beginning reading has been the realization that "sometimes children have trouble learning to decode because they are completely unaware of the fact that spoken language is segmented . . ." (pp. 25–26). It is these phonemic segments, after all, that are more or less represented by the letters in an alphabetic writing system. As we know, however, it is the complex relationship among the phonemes in the speech stream that makes it difficult for the young child to gain access to these phonemic segments. Research in speech perception has shown that the phonemes are coarticulated or merged during speech production (the consonants are folded into the vowels; Liberman, Cooper, Shankweiler, & Studdert-Kennedy, 1967; Liberman, 1971). Thus speech, unlike writing, "does not consist of separate phonemes" produced one after the other "in a row over time" (Gleitman & Rozin, 1973, p. 460). Consequently, an awareness of the phonological segments in words, and of the relationship of these segments to print, cannot be taken for granted in the preliterate child. Neither can we assume that the older disabled reader has achieved this awareness. Although exposure to print may trigger phonological awareness for some children, even before formal reading instruction begins, we also know that other children who have had formal instruction in reading fail to develop even the most rudimentary connections between print and speech (Rozin, Bressman, & Taft, 1974).

Children have been asked to demonstrate their phonological awareness, for example, by counting the sounds in words, deleting sounds (e.g., say *sun* without the /s/), manipulating sounds (e.g., reversing phonemes), and categorizing sounds (categorizing words by the beginning, middle, or ending sounds). Regardless of how phonological awareness has been measured, the research indicates that phonological awareness is related to success in learning to read (for reviews see Blachman, 1984a, 1989; Wagner & Torgesen, 1987; Williams, 1986). Not only has phonological awareness been determined to be a powerful predictor of reading ability (Blachman, 1984b; Blachman & James, 1986; Bradley & Bryant, 1983; Juel, 1988; Juel, Griffith, & Gough, 1986: Lundberg, Olofsson, & Wall, 1980; Mann, 1984; Mann & Liberman, 1984; Share, Jorm, Maclean, & Matthews, 1984; Stanovich, Cunningham, & Cramer, 1984; Torneus, 1984; Vellutino & Scanlon, 1987), but we now have results from training studies conducted here and abroad that indicate that phonological awareness can be trained and that such training makes a difference in beginning reading and spelling achievement (see, for example, Ball & Blachman, 1988, 1991; Bradley & Bryant, 1983; Cunningham, 1990; Fox & Routh, 1984; Lundberg, Frost, & Peterson, 1988; Treiman & Baron, 1983; Williams, 1980). Indeed, after a thorough review of the research in beginning reading, Adams (1990) concludes that "The evidence is compelling: Toward the goal of efficient and effective reading instruction, explicit training of phonemic awareness is invaluable" (p. 331).

Unfortunately, despite the evidence, activities to build phonological awareness have not routinely been integrated into

> *Despite the evidence, activities to build phonological awareness have not routinely been integrated into our kindergarten and first grade classrooms.*

our kindergarten and first grade classrooms. What, exactly, should the classroom teacher or the language or learning specialist do to heighten phonological awareness? This article attempts to answer this question by reviewing the results of selected training studies and describing research-based intervention and assessment activities that are applicable to the classroom and other clinical settings.

INTERVENTION APPLICATIONS

Among the many researchers who have investigated the effectiveness of explicitly training phoneme awareness (see Blachman, 1989, for a review), several investigators have developed experimental programs that can be adapted for use in the classroom with kindergarten and low-readiness first grade children (Ball & Blachman, 1988, 1991; Blachman, Ball, Black, & Tangel, 1991; Bradley & Bryant, 1983, 1985; Cunningham, 1990; Lundberg et al., 1988; Olofsson & Lundberg, 1983, 1985). Others have focused their phoneme awareness intervention efforts on older learning-disabled students (Williams, 1979, 1980). Researchers have explored a variety of intervention models (i.e., whole class, small group, or one-to-one instruction), varying the duration of the intervention and the choice of activities. The activities described in the following studies can be used and/or modified by classroom teachers and language, reading, and learning specialists.

An intervention built around sound categorization activities

Bradley and Bryant (1983, 1985) conducted one of the first large-scale training studies and demonstrated a causal relationship between phoneme awareness and reading and spelling acquisition. Their study, conducted in England, utilized a simple, but elegant, sound categorization task as the primary phoneme awareness training activity. In this activity, children were taught to categorize or group pictures together on the basis of shared sounds. For example, *hen* could be grouped with *men* and *pen* because they rhymed. In addition, the children were taught that *hen* could be grouped with *hat* and *hill* because they shared the initial sound; that *hen* could be grouped with *pin* and *sun* because they shared the end sound; and finally that *hen* could be grouped with *leg* and *net* because the middle sound was shared. Eventually, the children learned to play a game called "the odd one out." Several picture cards that rhymed or that shared a sound in the initial, middle, or final position would be placed on the table along with one picture that did not share this sound. The child was asked to identify the "odd one out" and to explain his or her choice.

After 65 kindergarten and first-grade children who had low scores on a sound categorization pretest were selected, the children were divided into four groups matched on IQ, age, sex, and sound categorization ability. The children in the first

group learned to categorize words on the basis of common sounds. In the second group, children also learned to categorize words on the basis of common sounds but, in addition, were taught to represent the common sounds with plastic letters. They were able to see, for example, that when *hen* was changed to *pen* only one letter needed to be changed. The plastic letters that represented the shared sounds stayed in place on the table, while the child changed the *h* to a *p*. The children in a third group were taught to categorize the identical pictures on the basis of semantic categories (e.g., *hen* and *dog* were grouped together because both are animals). The children in the first two treatment groups and the semantic categorization control group each participated in 40 individual lessons over a 2-year period. A fourth group received no intervention.

After the intervention, the children who were trained in sound categorization consistently outperformed the untrained children in reading and spelling. The results indicated, however, that the children who were the most successful on measures of reading and spelling were the children who learned both to categorize words by their common sounds and to represent the sounds with plastic letters. Four years after the original study ended, a follow-up study found that the children who learned to make the connections between letters and sounds as part of their training in sound categorization were still the most successful in reading and spelling (Bradley, 1988).

The study by Bradley and Bryant (1983, 1985) provides support for a causal relationship between phonological awareness and reading and spelling and has clear practical, as well as theoretical, significance. Of particular importance was the demonstration that the benefits of training in phonological awareness can be increased when the connections between the phonological segments and letters are made quite explicit in the training. One question that could not be answered by their study, however, was whether training in the letter sound connections, without training in phonological awareness, also would have resulted in superior reading and spelling performance. Another unanswered question was whether children would benefit as much from small group instruction in phoneme awareness as they had benefitted from the one-to-one instruction provided by Bradley and Bryant. To answer these questions, Ball and Blachman (1988, 1991) recently conducted a study to evaluate the effects of providing training in phonological awareness to groups of kindergarten children.

An intervention built around instruction in phoneme segmentation

In the study by Ball and Blachman (1988, 1991), 90 kindergarten children were randomly assigned to either a treatment group or one of two control groups. Children in the treatment group learned to segment one-, two-, and three-phoneme items and also learned letter sound associations. Children in the first control group engaged in a variety of language activities (e.g., listening to stories and general vocabulary development) and also learned letter sound associations by using the same letter sound stimuli as the phoneme awareness treatment group. The children in the phoneme awareness treatment group and the language activities control group met in groups of four or five, outside the regular classroom with specially trained teachers, for 15 to 20 minutes a day, 4 days a week, for 7 weeks. The children in the third group received no intervention.

Before the treatment, the children in these groups did not differ in age, sex, race, socioeconomic status (SES) levels, Peabody Picture Vocabulary Test scores, phoneme segmentation ability, letter name and letter sound knowledge, and reading as measured by the Word Identification Subtest of the Woodcock Reading Mastery Tests. After the intervention, the treatment children significantly outperformed the children in both control groups in phoneme segmentation, reading, and spelling.

It is also important to note that after the intervention the treatment group and the language activities control group had equivalent letter sound knowledge (just as we hoped they would) because both groups were exposed to the same letter sound stimuli for the same period of time. As might have been expected, both these groups significantly outperformed the no intervention control group on letter sound knowledge. Despite the equivalent letter sound knowledge of the treatment group and the language activities group after the intervention, however, the treatment group significantly outperformed the language activities control group in phoneme awareness and reading and spelling. Thus from the results of this study, it appears that increasing letter sound knowledge, in and of itself, does not improve initial reading and spelling. On the other hand, phoneme awareness training, coupled with instruction in letter sounds, does have a positive effect on beginning reading and spelling.

The study by Ball and Blachman (1988, 1991) also provided evidence that training in phonological awareness can be effective when provided to groups of kindergarten children, an intervention model that may have more practical utility than one-to-one instruction. It should be remembered, however, that the group instruction was provided to the children outside the regular classroom by specially trained teachers. The next logical question was whether phoneme awareness activities were as effective when provided to groups of children in the regular classroom by their kindergarten teachers. If educators are going to heed the advice of numerous researchers (see, for example, Adams, 1990; Blachman, 1989; Juel, 1988) to provide instruction in phoneme awareness in regular classrooms before children have experienced failure, we need more direct evidence that this model of instruction is effective.

To evaluate this model, we (Blachman et al., 1991) trained teachers and teaching assistants in urban schools to provide instruction in phoneme awareness and sound-symbol associations to small groups of children in their kindergarten classrooms. The 84 treatment children met in groups of 4 or 5, 4 days a week, 15 to 20 minutes a day, for 11 weeks, completing a total of 41 lessons (adapted from Ball & Blachman, 1988). The 75 control children received no special intervention, although they continued to participate in kindergarten classrooms where the teaching of letter names and letter sounds was a standard part of the curriculum.

Before the intervention, the children in the treatment and the control groups did not differ in age, sex, race, SES levels, Peabody Picture Vocabulary Test scores, phoneme segmentation ability, letter name knowledge, letter sound knowledge, or reading. After the intervention, the treatment children significantly outperformed the control children on measures of phoneme segmentation, letter sound knowledge, reading phonetically regular real words, reading phonetically regular nonsense words, and invented spelling. Thus it was clear from the results of this study that kindergarten teachers and their teaching assistants could effectively incorporate activities to enhance phonological awareness into regular classroom instruction. In addition, these language awareness activities improved the beginning reading and spelling ability of the children who participated in them.

The intervention model evaluated in these two studies (Ball & Blachman, 1991; Blachman et al., 1991) utilized a simple, three-step lesson plan. At the beginning of each lesson there was a phoneme segmentation activity called say-it-and-move-it (adapted from Elkonin, 1963, 1973). This was followed by one of several activities that reinforced phoneme awareness; we referred to these as segmentation-related activities. Finally, one of several games was selected to teach letter names and sounds.

During say-it-and-move-it, children were taught to represent the sounds in one-, two-, and three-phoneme words by using manipulatives, such as disks, tiles, buttons, or blocks. In this activity, each child and the teacher had a laminated 8½ × 11-inch sheet of paper with a clown, boat, square, circle, triangle, or rectangle in the top half. A thick black line separated the top half of the sheet from the bottom

---

During say-it-and-move-it, children were taught to represent the sounds in one-, two-, and three-phoneme words by using manipulatives, such as disks, tiles, buttons, or blocks.

---

half; a 4-inch arrow pointing from left to right was depicted on the bottom half of the sheet. Several disks (or other manipulatives) were placed in the picture in the top half of the paper. (This picture was used simply as a place to store the disks when they were not actually being used to segment an item. Because kindergarten children like to play with the disks, the pictures or geometric shapes were added to the sheets to make it easier for teachers to indicate where the disks were to be "stored" between items. For example, a teacher might say "All aboard" to let the children know it was time to put the disks on the boat and get ready for the next word to be segmented.)

The order of presentation of items to be segmented followed a relatively fixed sequence. First, after modeling by the teacher, the teacher said to the children "Show me /a/." The children were taught to represent one sound (e.g., /a/ or /s/) with one disk. One finger was used to move one disk from the top half of the sheet to the left hand part of the arrow at the bottom, and the children were taught to say the sound as the disk was moved. Next, the teacher repeated a single sound twice (e.g., /i/ /i/), and the children learned to move one disk to represent each sound. When children demonstrated success with single sounds repeated twice,

two-phoneme real words were introduced, such as *up*, *it*, and *am*. Children were taught to say the word slowly and to move one disk to represent each sound. Eventually, three-phoneme items were introduced, such as *sun*, *fat*, *zip*, and *leg*. Initially, words were carefully selected so that only those beginning with continuous sound letters—letters that can be held with a minimum of distortion—were used, as in the examples above. The words were pronounced slowly, as in *sssuuunnn*, and children moved one disk per sound. Eventually children also learned to segment words that begin with stop consonants (e.g., *bat* and *cup*).

After completing the say-it-and-move-it activity, one segmentation-related activity was selected for the second step in the lesson. These included, for example, teaching children to categorize words on the basis of their common sounds, specifically rhyme and alliteration (modified from Bradley & Bryant, 1983, 1985, described previously). In another lesson, children practiced segmentation by using materials modeled after the sound analysis activities developed by the Soviet psychologist Elkonin (1963, 1973). In this activity, a picture of the word to be segmented (e.g., *sun* or *fan*) was illustrated at the top of an 8½ × 11-inch sheet. Beneath the picture were a series of connected boxes representing the number of phonemes in the word to be segmented. (Again, it should be noted that at first only pictures of objects that begin with a continuous sound letter were used.) As in the say-it-and-move-it activity, children practicing with the Elkonin cards were taught to say the word slowly as they moved a disk into a corresponding square to represent each sound in the word.

Other activities used during the segmentation-related portion of the intervention included having children practice saying words slowly while, at the same time, holding up one finger to represent each sound in the word. Still another activity emphasized sound blending. A puppet with a moveable mouth was used to tell the children a story. At several points in the story the puppet would mispronounce a word by segmenting it into its constituent phonemes. The bashful puppet would turn away from the group of children until the children fixed the mispronounced word by pronouncing or "blending" it correctly.

The third part of each lesson focused on teaching letter names and letter sounds. Children learned keywords and phrases to help them remember the sound of each letter. The letters of the alphabet, as well as illustrations of these keywords and phrases, were depicted on 8½ × 11-inch cards. For example, the *t* card had a picture of *two teenagers talking* on a *telephone*, and the *f* card was illustrated with *five funny faces*. To reinforce letter name and letter sound knowledge, children engaged in one letter name and letter sound activity during each phoneme awareness lesson. For example, one day the children played "Post Office," selecting a picture, identifying the letter that represented its first sound, and "mailing" the picture card in the appropriate letter pouch. On another day, a Bingo game might be selected, with cards being used that illustrated a subset of letter names and pictures representing those sounds (e.g., one set of cards reinforced the letters *a, m, b,* and *t*).

After children have mastered several letter names and their corresponding sounds, these letters can be put on the manipulatives (e.g., disks, buttons, tiles, or blocks) and used in the say-it-and-move-it activity. At first, only one letter tile should be provided, and the remainder should be blank tiles. For example, the child might have an *a* tile and three blank tiles, and the teacher would ask the children to segment *man,* then *fat,* and then *am*. After the child has successfully segmented with one letter tile, other letter tiles can be added as new letter sounds are mastered. Some children in the group may continue to use only blank tiles, and this should be encouraged for those children who are not ready to use letters.

Although the teachers in our studies used scripted lessons and played a particular game on a particular day, it is not always necessary to follow a scripted lesson plan format. The basic idea behind these lessons is that children should receive direct instruction in segmenting one-, two-, and three-phoneme items (using concrete manipulatives to represent successive sounds) and that they should be given structured opportunities to learn sound-symbol associations.

The activities described were developed to be used with heterogeneous groups of children. Although children need to understand the concept of one-to-one correspondence to represent one sound with one disk, children in the group may vary greatly in their knowledge of letter names and sounds and in their awareness of the phonological segments in words. Within the structure of the group, it is possible to give some children a two-phoneme word to segment with blank tiles, whereas others are comfortable segmenting three-phoneme items with letter tiles. We found that the kindergarten children who were not ready to use letter tiles in kindergarten quickly attained this level of mastery when these activities were continued in first grade. Blank tiles and later Scrabble tiles with letters can also be used quite successfully with older remedial students.

An intervention built around metalinguistic games

The studies reviewed so far have demonstrated that teaching phoneme awareness, and making the connections between letters and the sound segments in the words, have a positive influence on reading and spelling acquisition. It should be noted that other successful training studies have reported a positive effect on reading (Cunningham, 1990; Lundberg et al., 1988) by providing training in phonological awareness that did not include explicit instruction in sound-symbol associations.

Lundberg and colleagues (1988), for example, provided 8 months of such metalinguistic instruction to nonreading kindergarten children in Denmark. Although these children were a year older than their counterparts in the United States, according to custom "preschool children are seldom subjected to informal literacy socialization by parents or older peers" (p. 266). Consequently, by providing a program in metalinguistic awareness that did not include making connections between the sound segments in words and letters, Lundberg and associates were able to investigate whether phonemic awareness could be developed outside the context of literacy instruction. They were also able to "challenge the notion that metalinguistic skills are only a consequence of reading instruction" (p. 267).

A wide variety of games, starting with rhyming activities followed by the segmentation of sentences into word units and the segmentation of multisyllabic words into syllables, were conducted for the first 2 months of training. Phonemes were introduced during the third month of training by helping children identify the initial phonemes in words, starting with words that begin with continuous sound letters. Two months later, activities progressed to two-phoneme items and then to more complex words. Whole groups of children (15 to 20) participated in these activities, and the program proceeded at a slow pace to make sure that all the children experienced some level of success.

The results indicated that children who participated in this program had significantly greater metaphonological awareness than the control children, although there were no differences between the two groups on post-tests of prereading skills. By the end of first grade, however, the treatment children outperformed the control children in spelling, and by the end of second grade the treatment children outperformed the control children in reading and spelling. Thus Lundberg and colleagues (1988) were able to increase phonological awareness outside the context of formal literacy instruction by using group games and whole-class instruction provided by regular classroom teachers. Once formal reading instruction began, it appears that this heightened awareness of the phonological structure of language gave children an edge that was evident in their superior scores in reading and spelling at the end of grade 2.

Given the results of these studies as well as others not reviewed here (see

Blachman, 1989, for a review of this literature), it seems reasonable to conclude that training in phonological awareness that does not emphasize the connections between sound segments and letters can make a difference in reading and spelling. As illustrated so compellingly in the study by Bradley and Bryant (1983), however, the value of instruction in phoneme awareness is enhanced when the connections between the sound segments in words and the printed alphabet symbols are made explicit during training. Thus in planning a program for young children, whether in a classroom or some other clinical setting, it makes sense to start with language games that do not involve written symbols. Nevertheless, the instructional sequence should progress to the point where connections are made between the sound segments in one-, two-, and three-phoneme items and the written symbols that represent those sound segments. Ideally, these activities should be available in the classrooms of all our prereading children (Adams, 1990; Blachman, 1989; Juel, 1988) as part of creating the kind of rich oral language and print-rich environment that fosters literacy acquisition (Anderson, Hiebert, Scott, & Wilkinson, 1985).

ASSESSMENT APPLICATIONS

As indicated earlier, researchers have used a variety of tasks to measure phonological awareness, including, for example, categorizing or matching words on the basis of common sounds, counting phonemes, segmenting words into phonemes, deleting phonemes, and manipulating phonemes. The literature is remarkably consistent in demonstrating that, almost regardless of how phoneme awareness has been measured, it is related to reading achievement. In two studies of task comparability (Stanovich et al., 1984; Yopp, 1988), a variety of phoneme awareness tasks were administered to kindergarten children. Both studies found that, despite the variety in task demands, the phonological awareness tasks shared a large amount of variance, thus supporting the construct validity of the concept of phonological awareness (see also Vellutino & Scanlon, 1987). Stanovich et al. (1984) found, for example, that of the 10 tasks they administered the 7 nonrhyming phoneme awareness tasks all loaded heavily on one factor, and all were significant predictors of first grade reading ability. The tasks used by Yopp (1988) sampled an even broader range of behaviors thought to measure the child's phonological awareness, including, for example, rhyme, phoneme counting and segmenting, and phoneme deletion. Yopp found two highly related factors, simple phonemic awareness and compound phoneme awareness. Tasks in the first category required only one step: blending, isolating, or segmenting sounds. Tasks in the second category required more than one step, such as deleting a sound, holding the remaining sounds in memory, and blending the remaining sounds to form a word. A hierarchy of task difficulty was also confirmed in these two studies, indicating that rhyming tasks were the easiest for the end of kindergarten child and phoneme deletion the most difficult. In the study by Yopp (1988), phoneme segmentation and phoneme counting (tasks not used in the study by Stanovich et al., 1989) ranked between rhyming and deletion in the hierarchy of task difficulty.

Rhyme detection and production are among the easiest phoneme awareness tasks for kindergarten children.

Although researchers have begun to explore how the varying cognitive demands of the different tasks influence performance, there are, as yet, no definitive answers for the clinician who wants to know which phoneme awareness tasks to administer to which child. Rhyme detection and production are among the easiest phoneme awareness tasks for kindergarten children. Because of their relative ease, performance on tasks that assess rhyming at the end of kindergarten have not been found to be as closely associated with reading achievement as other measures of phonological awareness (Blachman, 1984b; Stanovich et al., 1984; Yopp, 1988). Nevertheless, there are data (Bryant, Bradley, Maclean, & Crossland, 1989; Maclean, Bryant, & Bradley, 1987) to indicate that knowledge of nursery rhymes at age 3 is related to the ability to detect rhyme 1 year later and that performance on rhyme detection tasks among these 3 and 4 year olds is related to beginning word reading. Thus rhyming may have a particularly valuable place as an early indicator of phonological awareness and, as such, needs to be evaluated more thoroughly as an assessment tool with preschool children. Kindergarten children who are unable to identify words that rhyme or who cannot produce rhyme should be given more explicit instruction in this and other phonological awareness tasks.

What do we know about kindergarten

performance on the more conceptually complex measures of phoneme awareness, such as phoneme segmentation? The findings from one of the earliest developmental studies (Liberman, Shankweiler, Fischer, & Carter, 1974) indicated that only 17% of a group of kindergarten children were successful when asked to tap out the individual phonemes in words, whereas by the end of first grade 70% of the children were successful on this task. Thus it is to be expected that the majority of kindergarteners will not be able to demonstrate awareness of the phonological structure of words, on a segmentation task, for example, despite their ability to rhyme and gain access to the more readily identifiable syllabic unit (Blachman, 1984b; Liberman et al., 1974; Stanovich et al., 1984; Yopp, 1988).

Unfortunately, kindergarten performance on measures of phonological awareness is being used to make unwarranted decisions about instruction. For example, in some cases "failure" on a test of phoneme segmentation in kindergarten is used to indicate that a whole word approach to reading might be more appropriate than an approach that emphasizes the alphabetic code. Nothing could be further from the truth; there is simply no research evidence to support this premise. Not only can children who have not yet learned to read be taught to segment words into phonemes (see, for example, Olofsson & Lundberg, 1983), but studies have also shown that this instruction in kindergarten and first grade may, in fact, have the greatest benefit for those with low phoneme awareness pretest scores (Bradley & Bryant, 1983, 1985; Stanovich, 1986; Torneus, 1984). The benefits of instruction in phonological awareness have been demonstrated not only in terms of improved performance on measures of phonological awareness but also on measures of subsequent reading and spelling performance. Thus to eliminate a child from activities that could increase his or her phonological awareness, because the child has "failed" a phonological awareness test in kindergarten or first grade, not only is not warranted but is likely to be detrimental to the child's reading development.

When phoneme segmentation tests have been administered in kindergarten in intervention research, it is important to remember that these tests have not been used for the purpose of deciding who should and who should not have instruction in phonological awareness. Rather, they have been used to measure preintervention performance in phonological awareness. This is a more appropriate use for these measures in kindergarten (see, for example, the phoneme segmentation used by Ball & Blachman, 1988). Such measures can, of course, indicate which children already have a high degree of phonological awareness and therefore do not need explicit instruction.

What do we do about assessment of phonological awareness with the older remedial student? Given the hierarchy of task difficulty and developmental data on end of first grade children, it appears appropriate to expect most end of first grade children who have had a year of formal reading instruction to be able to count phonemes, segment phonemes, or delete initial phonemes in one-, two-, and three-phoneme items. Thus these might be appropriate assessment tasks to use to identify those who need explicit instruc-

tion in phoneme awareness. With older children (e.g., end of third grade), it might be more useful diagnostically to assess phonological awareness with a more complex task, such as phoneme deletion and/or phoneme manipulation (see, for example, Pratt & Brady, 1988, for data on tasks used with third-grade children). These broad guidelines for assessment await further research regarding their clinical utility.

WHERE DO WE GO FROM HERE?

The research in phonological awareness has been described as a "scientific success story" (Stanovich, 1987). Not only has a predictive relationship between phonological awareness and reading success been demonstrated, but a causal relationship has been demonstrated as well. Training studies here and abroad have shown that providing systematic instruction in phonological awareness to kindergarten and first-grade children can have a positive impact on beginning reading and spelling acquisition, especially when the instruction includes helping children make the connections between the sound segments of the word and the letters representing those segments.

For those of us interested in improving early reading instruction and reducing reading failure, however, the real challenge is to ensure that this "scientific success story" becomes a reality for the many children who could benefit from its findings. Teachers and clinicians need to be supported in their efforts to incorporate these activities into kindergarten and first-grade classrooms and into the instruction provided to older remedial students. Unfortunately, there are some educators who argue against the inclusion in the curriculum of direct instruction in phoneme awareness. Goodman and Goodman (1979), for example, who are proponents of whole language instruction, argue that the use of written language does not require a "high level of conscious awareness of the units ..." (p. 139). More recently, Goodman (1986) has suggested that "breaking whole (natural) language into bite-size, abstract little pieces ... words, syllables, and isolated sounds" (p. 7), makes learning to read more difficult. It is important to recognize that, despite a lack of research to support their premise, some of the most vocal proponents of whole language are telling teachers to avoid doing exactly that which research has shown promotes literacy acquisition.

It is also important to remember that in the majority of phonological awareness training studies the instructional activities required only 15- to 20-minute lessons. Thus, although these activities appear to be a crucial ingredient in the instructional

environment created to foster literacy acquisition, no one has suggested that these activities provide a complete diet or encompass the child's entire day. Ideally, one would want phonological awareness activities to be incorporated into a classroom where storybook reading was commonplace, oral language experiences were valued, basic concepts about print (e.g., how to hold a book) and the functions of reading and writing were developed, and children had opportunities both to talk and to write about their experiences (for a more detailed discussion of these ideas, see Anderson et al., 1985). Fortunately, many of these more general ideas to foster literacy are gaining popularity and are now shared by whole language proponents and those with a more traditional orientation to beginning reading. We now need to make a more concerted effort to work together to integrate phonological awareness activities into the rich, oral language environments we are creating for our children.

REFERENCES

Adams, M.J. (1990). *Beginning to read: Thinking and learning about print.* Cambridge, MA: MIT Press.

Anderson, R., Hiebert, E., Scott, J., & Wilkinson, I. (Eds.). (1985). *Becoming a nation of readers: The report of the Commission on Reading.* Washington, DC: National Institute of Education.

Ball, E.W., & Blachman, B.A. (1988). Phoneme segmentation training: Effect on reading readiness. *Annals of Dyslexia, 38,* 208–225.

Ball, E.W., & Blachman, B.A. (1991). Does phoneme awareness training in kindergarten make a difference in early word recognition and developmental spelling? *Reading Research Quarterly, 26,* 49–66.

Blachman, B. (1984a). Language analysis skills and early reading acquisition. In G. Wallach & K. Butler (Eds.), *Language learning disabilities in school-age children* (pp. 271–287). Baltimore: Williams & Wilkins.

Blachman, B. (1984b). Relationship of rapid naming ability

and language analysis skill to kindergarten and first-grade reading achievement. *Journal of Educational Psychology, 76,* 610–622.

Blachman, B. (1989). Phonological awareness and word recognition: Assessment and intervention. In A.G. Kamhi & H.W. Catts (Eds.), *Reading disabilities: A developmental language perspective* (pp. 133–158). Boston: College-Hill.

Blachman, B., Ball, E., Black, S., & Tangel, D. (1991). *Promising practices for improving beginning reading instruction: Teaching phoneme awareness in the kindergarten classroom.* Manuscript submitted for publication.

Blachman, B., & James, S. (1986, October). *A longitudinal study of metalinguistic abilities and reading achievement in primary grade children.* Paper presented at the meeting of the International Academy for Research in Learning Disabilities, Northwestern University, Evanston, IL.

Bradley, L. (1988). Making connections in learning to read and spell. *Applied Cognitive Psychology, 2,* 3–18.

Bradley, L., & Bryant, P. (1983). Categorizing sounds and learning to read: A causal connection. *Nature, 30,* 419–421.

Bradley, L., & Bryant, P. (1985). *Rhyme and reason in reading and spelling.* Ann Arbor: University of Michigan Press.

Bryant, P.E., Bradley, L., Maclean, M., & Crossland, J. (1989). Nursery rhymes, phonological skills, and reading. *Journal of Child Language, 16,* 407–428.

Cunningham, A.E. (1990). Explicit v. implicit instruction in phonemic awareness. *Journal of Experimental Child Psychology, 50,* 429–444.

Elkonin, D.B. (1963). The psychology of mastering the elements of reading. In B. Simon & J. Simon (Eds.), *Educational psychology in the USSR* (pp. 165–179). London, England: Rutledge & Kegan Paul.

Elkonin, D.B. (1973). USSR. In J. Downing (Ed.), *Comparative reading* (pp. 551–580). New York: Macmillan.

Fox, B., & Routh, D.K. (1984). Phonemic analysis and synthesis as word attack skills: Revisited. *Journal of Educational Psychology, 76,* 1059–1061.

Gleitman, L.R., & Rozin, P. (1973). Teaching reading by use of a syllabary. *Reading Research Quarterly, 8,* 447–483.

Goodman, K.S. (1986). *What's whole in whole language: A parent-teacher guide.* Portsmouth, NH: Heinemann.

Goodman, K.S., & Goodman, Y.M. (1979). Learning to read is natural. In L.B. Resnick & P.A. Weaver (Eds.), *Theory and practice of early reading* (Vol. 1, pp. 137–154). Hillsdale, NJ: Lawrence Erlbaum.

Juel, C. (1988). Learning to read and write: A longitudinal study of 54 children from first through fourth grades. *Journal of Educational Psychology, 80,* 437–447.

Juel, C., Griffith, P., & Gough, P. (1986). Acquisition of literacy: A longitudinal study of children in first and second grade. *Journal of Educational Psychology, 78,* 243–255.

Kamhi, A.G., & Catts, H.W. (Eds.). (1989). *Reading disabilities: A developmental language perspective.* Boston: College-Hill.

Liberman, A.M., Cooper, F.S., Shankweiler, D., & Studdert-Kennedy, M. (1967). Perception of the speech code. *Psychological Review, 74,* 731–761.

Liberman, I.Y. (1971). Basic research in speech and lateralization of language: Some implications for reading disability. *Bulletin of the Orton Society, 21,* 72–87.

Liberman, I.Y. (1983). A language-oriented view of reading and its disabilities. In H. Myklebust (Ed.), *Progress in learning disabilities* (Vol. 5, pp. 81–101). New York: Grune & Stratton.

Liberman, I.Y., & Liberman, A.M. (1990). Whole language vs. code emphasis: Underlying assumptions and their implications for reading instruction. *Annals of Dyslexia, 40,* 51–76.

Liberman, I.Y., Shankweiler, D., Fischer, F.W., & Carter, B. (1974). Explicit syllable and phoneme segmentation in the young child. *Journal of Experimental Child Psychology, 18,* 201–212.

Lundberg, I., Frost, J., & Peterson, O. (1988). Effects of an extensive program for stimulating phonological awareness in preschool children. *Reading Research Quarterly, 23,* 263–284.

Lundberg, I., Olofsson, A., & Wall, S. (1980). Reading and spelling skill in the first school years predicted from phonemic awareness skills in kindergarten. *Scandinavian Journal of Psychology, 21,* 159–173.

Maclean, M., Bryant, P., & Bradley, L. (1987). Rhymes, nursery rhymes, and reading in early childhood. *Merrill-Palmer Quarterly, 33,* 255–281.

Mann, V. (1984). Longitudinal prediction and prevention of early reading difficulty. *Annals of Dyslexia, 34,* 117–136.

Mann, V.A., & Liberman, I.Y. (1984). Phonological awareness and verbal short-term memory: Can they presage early reading problems? *Journal of Learning Disabilities, 17,* 592–599.

Olofsson, A., & Lundberg, I. (1983). Can phonemic awareness be trained in kindergarten? *Scandinavian Journal of Psychology, 24,* 35–44.

Olofsson, A., & Lundberg, I. (1985). Evaluation of long term effects of phonemic awareness training in kindergarten: Illustrations of some methodological problems in evaluation research. *Scandinavian Journal of Psychology, 26,* 21–34.

Perfetti, C. (1985). *Reading ability.* New York: Oxford University Press.

Pratt, A.C., & Brady, S. (1988). Relation of phonological awareness to reading disability in children and adults. *Journal of Educational Psychology, 80,* 319–323.

Rozin, P., Bressman, B., & Taft, M. (1974). Do children understand the basic relationship between speech and writing? The mow-motorcycle test. *Journal of Reading Behavior, 6,* 327–334.

Shankweiler, D., & Liberman, I.Y. (1989). *Phonology and reading disability: Solving the reading puzzle.* Ann Arbor: University of Michigan Press.

Share, D.J., Jorm, A.F., Maclean, R., & Matthews, R. (1984). Sources of individual differences in reading achievement. *Journal of Educational Psychology, 76,* 466–477.

Stanovich, K.E. (1986). Matthew effects in reading: Some consequences of individual differences in the acquisition of literacy. *Reading Research Quarterly, 21,* 360–407.

Stanovich, K.E. (Ed.). (1987). Introduction [Special issue]. *Merrill-Palmer Quarterly, 33.*

Stanovich, K.E., Cunningham, A.E., & Cramer, B.B. (1984). Assessing phonological awareness in kindergarten children: Issues of task comparability. *Journal of Experimental Child Psychology, 38,* 175–190.

Stedman, L.C., & Kaestle, C.E. (1987). Literacy and reading performance in the United States from 1880 to the present. *Reading Research Quarterly, 22,* 8–46.

Torneus, M. (1984). Phonological awareness and reading: A chicken and egg problem? *Journal of Educational Psychology, 76,* 1346–1358.

Treiman, R., & Baron, J. (1983). Phonemic-analysis training helps children benefit from spelling-sound rules. *Memory & Cognition, 11,* 382–389.

Vellutino, F.R. (1979). *Dyslexia: Theory and research.* Cambridge, MA: MIT Press.

Vellutino, F.R. (1987). Dyslexia. *Scientific American, 256,* 34–41.

Vellutino, F.R., & Scanlon, D.M. (1987). Phonological coding, phonological awareness, and reading ability: Evidence from a longitudinal and experimental study. *Merrill-Palmer Quarterly, 33,* 321–363.

Wagner, R., & Torgesen, J. (1987). The nature of phonological processing and its causal role in the acquisition of reading skills. *Psychological Bulletin, 101,* 192–212.

Williams, J. (1979). The ABD's of reading: A program for the learning disabled. In L.B. Resnick & P.A. Weaver (Eds.), *Theory and practice of early reading* (Vol. 3, pp. 179–195). Hillsdale, NJ: Lawrence Erlbaum.

Williams, J. (1980). Teaching decoding with an emphasis on phoneme analysis and phoneme blending. *Journal of Educational Psychology, 72,* 1–15.

Williams, J. (1986). The role of phonemic analysis in reading. In J. Torgesen and B. Wong (Eds.), *Psychological and educational perspectives on learning disabilities* (pp. 399–416). Orlando, FL: Academic Press.

Williams, J. (1987). Educational treatments for dyslexia at the elementary and secondary levels. In R. Bowler (Ed.), *Intimacy with language: A forgotten basic in teacher education.* Baltimore: Orton Dyslexia Society.

Yopp, H.K. (1988). The validity and reliability of phonemic awareness tests. *Reading Research Quarterly, 23,* 159–177.

Integrating microcomputers into language intervention with children

Sylvia Steiner, PhD
Professor
Department of Communication Disorders
University of Wisconsin–Eau Claire

Vicki Lord Larson, PhD
Professor
Department of Communication Disorders
Associate Dean
School of Graduate Studies and University
  Research
University of Wisconsin–Eau Claire
Eau Claire, Wisconsin

COMPUTER applications for language intervention with children require minimal technical expertise. According to Cochran (1987),

However, all successful applications require *clinical* expertise on the part of clinicians. . . . Such clinical expertise is just as important for the successful use of computers in therapy as it is for the success of any other approach to intervention. (p. 2)

As microcomputers infiltrate the profession, new technology must be integrated optimally with established procedures. The microcomputer can change clinical speech-language pathology positively or negatively, depending on decisions made by clinicians.

This article describes guidelines for the integration of microcomputers into language intervention with children, employing case examples to illustrate vital principles. Specialized applications, such as word processing and augmentative systems, are reviewed elsewhere in this issue (Bull & Cochran) or in other publications (Black-

Top Lang Disord, 1991,11(2),18–30
© 1991 Aspen Publishers, Inc.

stone & Cassatt-James, 1988; Silverman, 1989).

GUIDELINES FOR INTEGRATION

The seven guidelines discussed in this article are of particular importance for integrating computer technology into language intervention with children. Additional guidelines for microcomputer applications in this profession are discussed elsewhere by Larson and Steiner (1985, 1988).

Focus of intervention

The focus of effective intervention is the client. The current model of teaching and learning is marked by technology that is "ubiquitous, yet invisible, and computers become one of many powerful tools to enhance learning." (November, 1989, p. 8) When clinicians begin to use computers clinically, one tendency is for the computers to become a focal point for intervention (Schwartz, Brown, DelCalzo, & Kunicki, 1989). The computer itself becomes a topic of discussion, which may detract from intervention effectiveness. Software and hardware employed should be transparent during intervention, allowing clients to focus on the program's content rather than on the computer (Schwartz et al., 1989). Only when intervention for a client would be enhanced by using a computer should it be integrated into the client's program.

Embedding computerized activities in the total language program

This article emphasizes integrating the computer with other intervention practices into cohesive, effective total language programs. Several models have been employed for children to incorporate computers clinically in this profession:

- an additive model, in which computerized activities are merely appended to procedures a clinician has been using;
- a replacement model, in which clinicians replace more traditional methodology with computerized activities; and
- an integrative model, in which computerized activities are blended with other activities.

The integrative model supplies a philosophical foundation for this article, which advocates embedding computerized activities in the context of a client's total language program.

After clinical goals are delineated for a child, intervention plans should be developed, because it is not appropriate to identify goals to fit the tools available. Although this is an era of professional exploration with the computer, clinicians should not seek for occasions to use computer technology, but better ways to accomplish goals. They should evaluate computers as one alternative available. The power, flexibility, and adaptability of computers provide innovative ways to address clinical goals. Increasing variety of intervention activities to enhance the motivational or attentional level of a client provides sufficient reason to integrate computers into intervention.

During the past decade, speech-language pathologists started to flirt with the computer as a potential clinical tool, and the computer has been highlighted in information disseminated to practitioners (Larson & Steiner, 1985). Early publications about computer technology discussed *microcomputer-based intervention,* acknowledging that optimal clinical practice would involve combinations of computer-based activities with other activities (Larson & Steiner, 1988). The computer is just another tool for intervention; therefore, it is no more sensible to talk about microcomputer-based intervention than about *crayon-based* or *workbook-based* intervention.

Theoretical considerations

Theoretical principles guiding intervention do not change when the microcomputer is employed as a clinical tool. Clinicians are unlikely to violate sound theoretical principles if they first ask what is good language intervention for a child and then ask if a computer might enhance intervention plans.

During an era when clinicians are experimenting with the computer to discover its possible contributions, clinicians need to reaffirm their theoretical principles and ensure that planned computer applications are consistent with those principles. For example, drill and practice work inherent in software should not be accepted as appropriate for a child if drill and practice employing other materials would be unacceptable. Because software frequently presents drill and practice work, this violation of principles is common. Although articulating that the ultimate goal of language intervention is enhancing functional communication behavior, clinicians lose sight of that when making choices about integrating computers into language intervention. While advocating that vocabulary development should concentrate on words important in a child's daily environment, clinicians may employ software characterized by a fixed vocabulary, nonadaptable for individual students. Sound principles should not be discarded when the computer is employed clinically. The computer should be approached as a clinical tool with open-mindedness, curiosity, and optimism, tempered by scientific skepticism.

Stimuli, responses, and reinforcements

Computers often are suggested for facilitating learning to control stimulus delivery and reinforcements, to ensure consistency of required responses. However, the computer must be evaluated not only regarding consistency and control, but also regarding appropriateness of stimuli, responses, and reinforcements for each client.

Computer-delivered stimuli can generate excitement from children through use of colorful and animated graphics, simulations of real-world and imaginative events, and combinations of auditory with visual stimuli. However, a program may be rejected because graphic items cannot be identified by a child or because nonoptional sounds or fast-moving graphics coexisting with on-screen stimuli distract another child.

Software should be evaluated to determine whether responses required by the program are reasonable. One aspect of computer technology is that its use may permit a child to demonstrate appropriate language knowledge by activating a speech synthesizer to produce speech signals before the child can do so. A clinician may be able to modify response requirements to fit the situation (e.g., a clinician might operate the keyboard, based on oral comments from the child, to give a response required by the program).

Part of the reinforcement available through computer usage is clients' realization of the ability to control events, the magical and motivating experience of commanding the machine. However, consequent events supplied by software often have limited value as reinforcers (e.g., the software may lack power or variety, may be too time-consuming, may always employ a 100% reinforcement schedule, or may be distracting to students).

Some clinicians employ computer activities as reinforcement, promising that a client may perform some enjoyable activity on the computer as a reward for hard work during an intervention session. If this is the only way a computer is employed, the power of this clinical tool is wasted, because the computer really is not being integrated into language intervention.

Roles of client, aide, and clinician

Computers may be integrated into both individual and group language intervention activities. Whether the activity is group or individual, a clinical decision must be made regarding who should be present during each computer application and what type of participation should occur. That decision depends on the goal to be addressed, the nature of the activity, and the child's language/computer capabilities.

It is the experiential position of many clinicians, and it is a philosophical premise of the authors, that functional communication behavior is enhanced best when both clinician and child are active participants. However, few data are available to support

or refute this position as it applies to computer usage during language intervention (Hoover & Thompson, 1990). Some clinicians using computers in language intervention believe in employing the computer as a surrogate clinician while the clinician works with other children. Wilson and Fox (1989) state they select computer usage ". . . over live tutoring whenever appropriate software is available" (p. 38) to foster student self-esteem. These software developers believe that clinician-child interaction ". . . should be reserved for extending and expanding knowledge gained through using the computer" (p. 39). Goals may be achieved through a client's independent endeavors, mainly when software is tutorial or drill-and-practice. Other applications, such as a student's independent construction of documents with a word processor, might be useful to supplement intervention involving direct interaction between clinician and student. However, the most effective integration of computer technology generally occurs when the clinician is present, engages actively in the session, comments on the content of software, and assists the child to extract maximum value from the program. Human/human interaction is needed to build functional interpersonal communication behavior. However, intrapersonal communication skills might be enhanced by human/machine interaction.

When computers are employed in language intervention, the child's role should not always include providing input directly to the computer. Although children enjoy controlling computers, sometimes it is most productive if child and clinician interact while the clinician controls the computer, the primary activity being a dialogue between them. Children less than 2 years old can operate a computer (Meyers, 1987), but optimal learning often will not place the child at the keyboard.

Reaching decisions about paraprofessional involvement in intervention should be based on the same guidelines (Helmick et al., 1981) whether a computer is employed or not. Because computer programs automate activities, aides need to make fewer clinical judgments; thus involving aides in computer activities is tempting. Careful planning can yield effective aide participation, but their roles must be designed equally carefully when computers and other tools are selected.

Few data are available to indicate how effective it may be to supplement face-to-face intervention with computer applications, or to document the impact of involving an aide rather than a clinician in intervention (Schetz, 1989). The question-comment-question (QCQ) approach (A.H. Schwartz, personal communication, November 13, 1989) employs clinician-client interaction during computer applications. To extract maximum power from a computer during intervention, a clinician's presence is needed so observations of the moment can serve as foundation for continual, appropriate readjustment of events. Rapid, intelligent decision making by a clinician permits maintenance of an appropriate context for interpersonal dialogue. Information exchanges with computers may be interactive, but they are not interpersonal.

Individualization

Although clinicians realize the need to individualize intervention, computer hardware and software frequently are not individualized appropriately. When planning purchases of hardware for use with children, a color monitor, a printer to generate output, and a single-switch input device or joystick should be considered essential. Dual disk drives may be important for certain intended applications. The value of adding other features to increase adaptability of the system depends on the caseload and the frequency with which those features are needed to provide appropriate services, as well as on the software selected.

Software often is flexible, serving multiple purposes with a number of clients, even when it cannot be individualized. Flexibility is shown when a single program is applicable for multiple goals and when a single goal may be addressed with multiple programs. Most software can be employed for various clinical goals, regardless of the software authors' intentions. For example, developers of software such as *The Stickybear ABC* (Hefter, Worthington, Worthington, & Howe, 1982) may suggest specific goals for that program (e.g., teaching children to recognize letters of the alphabet), whereas clinicians might employ the program to meet other goals such as:

- production of appropriate answers to Wh-questions;
- generation of subject-verb utterances; and
- production of discourse to tell a story about events displayed.

Individualization and variety can be enhanced clinically by using software, blended with other activities, to address a clinical goal. All of the programs listed below and others could address a goal involving discourse generation: *Where in the World is Carmen Sandiego?* (Bigham, Portwood, & Elliott, 1986); *Mystery at Pinecrest Manor* (Klug, 1983); *Walt Disney Comic Strip Maker* (The Walt Disney Company, 1983); and *Tiger's Tales* (Hermann, 1986). Language intervention goals may be addressed with many activities, some involving the computer.

Clinicians who use computers for delivery of services usually employ commercially available software. Although clinicians rarely develop their own computer programs, some speech-language pathologists have developed and distributed designer software for language intervention. While it is not reasonable to expect most clinicians to become sophisticated software developers who market programs, it is possible for many clinicians to develop software on a limited scale. Authoring programs such as *SuperPILOT* (Apple Computers, Inc., 1982) and *Create Your Own Lessons* (Hartley Courseware, 1983) are simple to learn to use, require little knowledge of computer programming, permit software construction to be individualized, and are comparatively inexpensive (Venkatagiri, 1987). In this issue, Clymer describes uses of hypermedia that clinicians could employ to develop software for clients. Even clinicians who do not develop software for the commercial market and do not use authoring programs may individualize computer programs by inserting stimuli for clients. Word lists may be inserted in programs such as *Wizard of Words* (Neely & Aaronson, 1983); questions and answers may be inserted into programs such as *The Game Show* (Zawolkow, Rowe, & Perry, 1982).

Generic and designer software

Designer software, developed for use with individuals with communication problems, is relatively sparse. Less than 300 of more than 5,000 educational programs available commercially are designed for persons with communication problems. However, some programs have been created for children who display language disorders, including software such as *Representational Play* (Meyers & Fogel, 1985a), *Micro-LADS* (Wilson & Fox, 1983a), *Speak Up* (Wilson & Fox, 1983b), and *Language Carnival* (Ertmer, 1986). Often, documentation for designer software is more thorough regarding a program's theoretical rationale, procedures to be employed during program usage, data recording and analysis, and results of field testing. Language content usually is planned carefully for designer software. It is laudable that some clinicians have developed high-quality software for language intervention. However, designer software often is expensive, having a limited market and a limited variety of individuals with whom it is useful.

A generic program, developed for a mass market, is usually less expensive. Generic programs such as *The Stickybear ABC* (Hefter, Worthington, Worthington, & Howe, 1982) and *The Factory* (Kosel & Fish, 1984) also possess other advantages for clinicians, such as (a) often they can be used with larger numbers of children, (b) they may be bought with funds external to a clinician's budget for use with students not receiving special services, and (c) they are more adaptable to meet individual needs. Color graphics and animation are more often present and polished in generic programs than in designer software.

Regardless of the software developer's description of the intended use and user, a clinician must consider whether to employ that program with a child and how to employ it. Clinicians find designer and generic software yield appropriate applications with children displaying language disorders. As Schwartz (1989) commented, "Generic software programs do not, nor should they, replace software designed for speech, language, and hearing." (p. 47)

CASE EXAMPLES

In early educational applications of computers, it was suggested that the best way to evaluate computer-based activities involves examining "instructional scenarios in which the computer is embedded in a skill- or knowledge-learning sequence" (Budoff, Thormann, & Gras, 1984, p. 100). The following case examples are instructional scenarios about children with language disorders, supplying a context within which the computer is embedded as a tool for accomplishing clinical goals and illustrating the integration guidelines described previously. For each example, language intervention goals are identified, and activities that could assist in reaching goals are presented. On-the-computer and off-the-computer activities are described to illustrate how computer technology can be integrated into language intervention. Each example is an amalgamation of many clients. No example represents a single real client. Case examples evolved from numerous conversations with practitioners over the years and from personal experience with real children.

Case example 1: Mark

Mark is 3 years old and attends a preschool program, receiving individual intervention for 30 minutes daily. He is impulsive and displays difficulty following simple directions, but understands basic functional words and short sentences. After formal and informal assessment, goals were generated to:

- increase Mark's following of simple directives;
- increase his use of functional short utterances in play and real situations; and
- decrease incidence of impulsive behaviors.

To increase Mark's ability to follow simple directions, intervention began with Mark matching real objects to photographs and then pointing to objects upon command. He experimented with cause and effect actions such as blowing bubbles. Using computer software entitled *Exploratory Play* (Meyers & Fogel, 1985b), Mark learned new vocabulary for labeling objects while involved both in computer-related and other activities. *Exploratory Play,* which encourages the child to use language to talk about selected play routines, is accompanied by related toys to be used in activities not involving the computer. Mark learned quickly to produce computer pictures of the toys. With a single keystroke, a color graphic of the object appeared and the speech synthesizer said the object's name, acting as Mark's voice until he learned to produce the words. Used in this manner, the computer functions as a language scaffold, ". . . supporting children's use of language to communicate meaning while they are developing the language skills needed to communicate on their own." (Meyers, 1987, p. 1)

Software, *First Words* (Wilson & Fox, 1982), was used to increase comprehension of 50 early-developing nouns. Although initially the program was used to increase Mark's word comprehension, it was even more helpful in decreasing Mark's impulsive behavior. Several pictures were presented, then the speech synthesizer said the word for a pictured noun. Because Mark wanted to show he knew the right answer, he had to wait patiently for the program to present the correct choice and then respond. Using *First Words* (Wilson & Fox, 1982), it became clear that a program could be used to work on several goals simultaneously and that it could be used in a meaningful way unintended by its authors.

Case example 2: Mary

Mary, a 6-year-old in first grade, has difficulty following simple directions, and in understanding basic concepts needed for academic tasks. She uses short sentences and questions that are often ungrammatical. She is passive and demonstrates learned helplessness. After testing and observing her performance in the classroom and at home, language intervention goals were selected to:

- increase ability to follow directions,
- increase use and variety of grammatically correct utterances,
- increase understanding of basic concepts needed for academic success, and
- decrease the incidence of learned helplessness behaviors.

To increase Mary's understanding of concepts for following directions, an early procedure was for her to manipulate her body in space in relationship to objects. Later, she manipulated real objects in relationship to each other. As progress occurred, worksheets from the Boehm Concept Kit (Boehm, 1976) were used to reinforce and elaborate on concepts. Simultaneously, she was introduced to software such as the *Concept Understanding Program* (Blum, Kavaloski, Irwin, Olsen, & Schippits, 1983), *Juggles' Rainbow* (Piestrup, 1982) Speech-Language Activities Booklet (Bramschreiber & Wiegert, 1984), and *Stickybear Opposites* (Hefter, Worthington, & Worthington, 1983) to provide variety and to improve her interest in applying the concepts. The software was particularly helpful because Mary's parents had a home computer, so she could take the program home to show her parents the new concepts. Since Mary started using the computer and realized that she could control the machine, she demonstrated less tendency to engage in learned helplessness.

During intervention addressing concept development, Mary was also learning to follow more complex directions through use of Simon Says activities, barrier games, and meal-planning activities. When it was learned that Mary liked to help with meal preparation at home, generic software entitled *Bake & Taste* (Mindplay, 1986) was introduced. This program used colorful animated graphics to guide Mary in planning, organizing, reading for detail, and following directions. Recipes on the disk can be printed, so Mary could take them home and use them with her mother in the kitchen. Her mother first observed Mary using this program during intervention sessions, then had Mary perform similarly in the real kitchen.

Case example 3: Juan

Juan, an 11-year-old, is in an open-concept middle-school classroom. He displayed more interest in learning during cooperative learning situations. He has difficulty producing and understanding multiple-meaning words, prefixes, and suffixes. Frequently, he does not understand humor in a situation, and has poor social communication skills. He is a poor problem solver and cannot follow teachers' directives readily. Juan is in a small language intervention class meeting for 3 hour-long sessions a week. The following goals were established:

- increase understanding of multiple-meaning words, prefixes, suffixes, and humor;
- improve problem-solving skills;
- increase understanding of classroom directives; and
- increase social communication skills in conversations.

Software was selected to provide a context for

Juan to be a more successful problem solver and to improve his conversational skills. The software required group members to engage in decision making, to take turns, and to maintain conversations to solve a problem. Using simulation software, *The Whitewater Canoe Race* (Decision Development Corporation, 1985a), group members cooperatively made decisions. While making decisions, students had to abide by rules of good conversation, under the clinician's guidance. Using a simple adventure game, *Mystery at Pinecrest Manor* (Klug, 1983), students worked cooperatively and communicatively to make decisions, including strategies for recording data provided by the program. Other software, such as *Gnee and Not Gnee* (Stanger, 1986) and *The Factory* (Kosel & Fish, 1984), was employed in problem-solving activities to engage Juan and others in effective use of conversational rules. *Gnee and Not Gnee* involves geometric classification. In *The Factory* students created a machine assembly line to generate products.

In addition to performing software-based activities, the students discussed and practiced rules of a good conversation. They learned how to identify a problem, generate alternative solutions, select the best solution, implement it, and evaluate its effectiveness. Combining traditional intervention procedures with selected software, Juan progressed as a conversationalist and problem-solver while participating as a cooperative member of a small group.

Case example 4: Susan

Susan is in 10th grade and attends regular senior high courses, working with the English teacher and a consulting speech-language pathologist to modify language problems. The clinician drew upon concepts and software described in *Communication Assessment and Intervention Strategies for Adolescents* (Larson & McKinley, 1987). Susan has minor word retrieval problems, uses many low information words, and has difficulty solving problems and organizing activities. Goals addressed daily in Susan's English classroom included activities designed:
- to decrease word retrieval problems,
- to increase use of specific words,
- to improve problem-solving behavior in daily life, and
- to increase use of organizational skills in planning daily activities.

To increase Susan's ability to organize daily living situations, she was given everyday events to plan. She decided what to do in each situation and indicated the best order for accomplishing tasks. After a series of scenarios of this type, Susan was introduced to a software/videotape package, *Plan Ahead* (Decision Development Corporation, 1985b), which teaches students to manage time during a school week. The program was first introduced to Susan's entire English class, because all students could benefit from its principles. Then selected class members, including Susan, were encouraged to use the program independently. With the clinician's assistance, Susan planned 1-week personal schedules and reviewed them. Susan's class investigated other time management software. Students discussed books about time management and visited office supply stores to examine planning devices that might help in organizing daily activities. Using a wide array of materials, Susan became a better time manager in daily functional living situations.

CURRENT STATUS

It is reasonable to characterize current computer usage in the profession as sporadic and computer technology as underutilized (Olson, 1989; Shewan, 1989). As computer technology is integrated appropriately for delivery of speech-language services, computers will be used daily and perhaps hourly by clinicians.

Shriberg, Kwiatkowski, and Snyder

(1989) mention that "Few controlled data are available on the efficacy of microcomputers for speech management with children." (p. 233) That comment applies equally to language intervention. Meyers (1987) published descriptive information about the success of computer applications in language intervention with very young children. She demonstrated how the computer can be incorporated into language activities so that toddlers can immediately be successful communicators. Meyers affirms that it is not always necessary for a clinician to guide the child through sequential learning of prerequisite skills that might characterize more traditional language therapy without the computer. Traditional approaches might attempt to teach cause/effect notions, picture recognition, and understanding of word meaning before having the child produce meaningful utterances. Meyers (1987) reports that if the child can touch a keyboard, producing an intended picture on the monitor and activating a speech synthesizer that expresses ideas the child wants to communicate, then all the important prerequisite skills can be learned simultaneously through the child's natural language-learning medium (i.e., play).

Schetz (1989) described a study conducted in a public school setting where aides employed software to enhance conceptual/linguistic skills of children not on the speech-language pathologist's caseload. O'Connor and Schery (1986) examined semantic and social growth of severely handicapped children in infant intervention programs, reporting significant progress with both traditional and computer-aided approaches. More recently, O'Connor and Schery (1989) completed a grant project about the effects of computer technology on communication development, reporting that "Data analyses showed discernible effect of the additional computer training when compared to regular classroom communication training alone." (p. 1)

Harn (1986) compared the relative effects of teaching children between the ages of 24 and 41 months to produce subject-verb utterances with three different types of stimuli (i.e., ongoing live action, computer animation, and pictures). He reported that children in the computer-animation condition and children in the live-action condition learned at similar rates, whereas those in the picture condition progressed less rapidly.

Schetz and Sheese (1989) reviewed "software that works in school settings" (p. 65), considering program applicability within four service delivery models, but presented no data about the efficacy of employing the reviewed programs as suggested. However, it is reassuring that a number of publications presenting data about efficacy of computer technology for language intervention have appeared recently.

As clinicians explore applications of computer technology to language intervention, valuable data and insights about relative efficacy of computer applications will be gathered. Sharing of these insights and data through professional dissemination would compound their value. There is a demonstrated need to learn specifics about when, with whom, how long, and in what ways it is beneficial to use computer applications. It is equally important to learn the limitations of computer utilization and the disadvantages of specific applications. It is crucial that professionals share information about both successful and unsuccessful attempts to integrate the computer into language intervention.

• • •

As access to hardware and software improves, and as clinicians integrate computer applications with other intervention activities, it will become difficult for clinicians to imagine functioning without the computer as a clinical tool. Eventually, clinicians may find it hard to estimate how many hours per week they are using the computer, just as it would be difficult now to estimate how many hours per week one employs a ballpoint pen as a tool. The November 1989 issue of the *Journal for Computer Users in Speech and Hearing* (Seaton, 1989) presents a fascinating and provocative view of microcomputer applications in communication disorders during the 1990s.

Access to hardware and software is only part of the answer to the question of how computers can be integrated into the clinical domain. The remaining necessary aspect of the solution is the design of the intervention environment by a clinician to permit appropriate integration of the computer into language protocols for individual children. Decisions about integration

of computer technology must be made by clinicians who are proficient with hardware, knowledgeable about software, and capable of making the technology transparent in the context of language intervention.

As the case examples in this article illustrate, the computer is a valuable clinical tool, but should not become the focus of intervention. Computer technology can contribute effectively to group and individual language intervention in working toward goals established for children from the early preschool age range through adolescence. Each clinician has a responsibility to assist the profession toward an increasingly technological future. As Cochran (1989) states,

The time is past for tip-toeing around computer technology and assuming it . . . is available only to a chosen few. If the clinicians of the 1990s expect computer access and request it without apology, employers will also begin to think of computers . . . as standard equipment for professionals in communication disorders. (p. 113)

Optimal integration of computer technology into language intervention will occur only when the most sophisticated tool, the clinician's expertise, activates the electronic tools of today and tomorrow.

REFERENCES

Apple Computers, Inc. (1982). *SuperPILOT* [Computer program]. Cupertino, CA: Author.

Bigham, D., Portwood, G., & Elliott, L. (1986). *Where in the world is Carmen Sandiego?* [Computer program]. San Rafael, CA: Broderbund Software.

Blackstone, S.W., & Cassatt-James, E.L. (1988). Augmentative communication. In N.J. Lass, L.V. McReynolds, J.L. Northern, & D.E. Yoder, (Eds.), *Handbook of*

speech-language pathology and audiology. Toronto, Ontario: B.C. Decker.

Blum, P., Kavaloski, R., Irwin, S., Olsen, J.S., & Schippits, S. (1983). *Concept understanding program* [Computer program]. St. Paul, MN: Amidon Publications.

Boehm, A. (1976). *Boehm resource guide for basic concept teaching.* New York, NY: The Psychological Corporation.

Bramschreiber, J., & Wiegert, J. (1984). *Juggles' rainbow:*

Speech-language activity booklet. Tucson, AZ: Communication Skill Builders.

Budoff, M., Thormann, J., & Gras, A. (1984). *Microcomputers in special education.* Cambridge, MA: Brookline Books.

Cochran, P.S. (1987). How to use a computer in therapy: For a clinician, by a clinician. *Synergy '87: Proceedings of the ASHF Computer Conference.* Houston, TX: American Speech-Language-Hearing Foundation.

Cochran, P.S. (1989). Clinical computing in the 1990s: There's more to it than which key to press. *Journal for Computer Users in Speech and Hearing, 5*(2), 110–113.

Decision Development Corporation. (1985b). *Plan ahead* [Computer program]. Bloomington, IN: Agency for Instructional Television.

Decision Development Corporation (1985a). *The whitewater canoe race* [Computer program]. Bloomington, IN: Agency for Instructional Television.

Ertmer, D.J. (1986). *Language carnival* [Computer program]. Moline, IL: Linguisystems.

Harn, W.E. (1986). Facilitating acquisition of subject-verb utterances in children: Actions, animation, and pictures. *Journal for Computer Users in Speech and Hearing, 2*(2), 95–101.

Hartley Courseware. (1983). *Create your own lessons* [Computer program]. Dimondale, MI: Author.

Hefter, R., Worthington, J., & Worthington, S. (1983). *Stickybear opposites* [Computer program]. Middletown, CT: Xerox Education Publications.

Hefter, R., Worthington, J., Worthington, S., & Howe, S. (1982). *The stickybear ABC* [Computer program]. Middletown, CT: Xerox Education Publications.

Helmick, J.W., Alpiner, J.G., Bender, D.R., Montague, J.C., Rosenberg, J.S., Snyder, J.M., Talbot, C.A., & Maisel, C.G. (1981). Guidelines for the employment and utilization of supportive personnel. *ASHA, 23*(3), 165–169.

Hermann, M.A. (1986). *Tiger's tales* [Computer program]. Pleasantville, NY: Sunburst Communications.

Hoover, J.H., & Thompson, R.H. (1990). Teaching skills via CAI: Does generalization occur in real world settings? *Closing the Gap, 9*(2), 8–9.

Klug, R. (1983). *Mystery at Pinecrest Manor—microzine #3* [Computer program]. New York, NY: Scholastic.

Kosel, M., & Fish, M. (1984). *The factory* [Computer program]. Pleasantville, NY: Sunburst Communications.

Larson, V.L., & McKinley, N. (1987). *Communication assessment and intervention strategies for adolescents.* Eau Claire, WI: Thinking Publications.

Larson, V.L., & Steiner, S. (1985). Language intervention using microcomputers. *Topics in Language Disorders, 6*(1), 41–55.

Larson, V.L., & Steiner, S. (1988). Microcomputer use in assessment and intervention with speech and language

disorders. In N.J. Lass, L.V. McReynolds, J.L. Northern, & D.E. Yoder (Eds.), *Handbook of speech-language pathology and audiology.* Toronto, Ontario: B.C. Decker.

Meyers, L.F. (1987). Bypassing the prerequisites: The computer as a language scaffold. *Closing the Gap, 5*(6), 1, 20.

Meyers, L.F., & Fogel, P. (1985a). *Representational play* [Computer program]. Santa Monica, CA: Peal Software.

Meyers, L.F., & Fogel, P. (1985b). *Exploratory play* [Computer program]. Santa Monica, CA: Peal Software.

Mindplay. (1986). *Bake & taste* [Computer program]. Stoneham, MA: Author.

Neely, A., & Aaronson, T. (1983). *Wizard of words* [Computer program]. Berkeley, CA: Advanced Ideas.

November, A. (1989). What kind of learning environment do students need? *Sunburst Solutions: News for Computer Educators, 4*(1), 8.

O'Connor, L., & Schery, T.K. (1986). A comparison of microcomputer-assisted and traditional language therapy for developing communications skills in nonoral toddlers. *Journal of Speech and Hearing Disorders, 51*(4), 356–361.

O'Connor, L., & Schery, T.K. (1989). *Using microprocessors to develop communication skills in young severely handicapped children* (Unpublished Final Project Report, Grant No. G008730283). Washington, DC: U.S. Department of Education.

Olson, C.G. (1989). Microcomputer applications in the Wisconsin public schools by speech-language clinicians, psychologists, and teachers of the learning disabled. Unpublished master's thesis, University of Wisconsin-Eau Claire, Eau Claire, WI.

Piestrup, A. (1982). *Juggles' rainbow* [Computer program]. Menlo Park, CA: The Learning Company.

Schetz, K.F. (1989). Computer-aided language/concept enrichment in kindergarten: Consultation program model. *Language, Speech, and Hearing Services in the Schools, 20,* 2–10.

Schetz, K.F., & Sheese, R.J. (1989). Software that works in school settings. *ASHA, 31*(1), 65–68.

Schwartz, A.H. (1989, Spring). Generic software: Increasing your options for integrating microcomputers into clinical practice. *HEARSAY,* pp. 46–47.

Schwartz, A.H., Brown, V., DelCalzo, P., & Kunicki, E. (1989). *Integrating microcomputers into clinical practice* [Videotape]. Cleveland, OH: Cleveland State University.

Seaton, W.H. (1989). *Journal for Computer Users in Speech and Hearing, 3*(2).

Shewan, C.M. (1989). Quality is not a four letter word. *ASHA, 31*(8), 51–55.

Shriberg, L.D., Kwiatkowski, J., & Snyder, T. (1989). Tabletop versus microcomputer-assisted speech management: Stabilization phase. *Journal of Speech and Hearing Disorders, 54*(2), 233–248.

Silverman, F.H. (1989). *Communication for the speechless.* Englewood Cliffs, NJ: Prentice-Hall.

Stanger, D. (1986). *Gnee or not gnee* [Computer program]. Pleasantville, NY: Sunburst Communications.

The Walt Disney Company. (1983). *Walt Disney comic strip maker* [Computer program]. New York, NY: Bantam Software.

Venkatagiri, H.S. (1987). Writing your own software: What are the options? *ASHA, 29*(6), 27–29.

Wilson, M., & Fox, B. (1982). *First words* [Computer program]. Burlington, VT: Laureate Learning Systems.

Wilson, M., & Fox, B. (1983a). *Microcomputer language assessment and development systems (Micro-LADS)* [Computer program]. Burlington, VT: Laureate Learning Systems.

Wilson, M., & Fox, B. (1983b). *Speak up* [Computer program]. Burlington, VT: Laureate Learning Systems.

Wilson, M., & Fox, B. (1989). Developer's response to a review by Vicki L. Brown of *Twenty Categories. Journal for Computer Users in Speech and Hearing, 5,* 38–39.

Zawolkow, G., Rowe, P., & Perry, T. (1982). *The game show* [Computer program]. Berkeley, CA: Advanced Ideas.

Emerging literacy and children with severe speech and physical impairments (SSPI): Issues and possible intervention strategies

Patsy L. Pierce, PhD
Research Assistant Professor

P. J. McWilliam, PhD
Research Associate
The Carolina Literacy Center
Department of Medical Allied Health
  Professions
The University of North Carolina at
  Chapel Hill
Chapel Hill, North Carolina

THE EFFECTS OF early experiences related to literacy development have been a particular focus of research and practice in regular and special education over the past decade. Parents, practitioners, researchers, and politicians across our nation have become increasingly aware of the important contributions of children's experiences in the first five years of life to their later achievement in school and adult life. While much remains to be learned, there is now sufficient evidence (Sulzby & Teale, 1991) to conclude that the accumulated experiences of children during the preschool years have a significant impact on their ability to learn to read and write upon entering school and on school achievement in general. Such findings have been cause for the emergence of a number of programs aimed specifically at enhancing the literacy-related experiences of children who might otherwise not have such opportunities during their preschool years (e.g., *Reach Out and Read: A*

Top Lang Disord, 1993,13(2),47–57
© 1993 Aspen Publishers, Inc.

Pediatric Program to Support Emergent Literacy, Fitzgerald & Needlman, 1991).

The recent focus on literacy and early life experiences is further reflected in two of the six national goals established by America 2000, former President George Bush's 1990 blueprint for educational reform. According to one goal, all children in America will start school ready to learn, and another advocates that every adult American will be literate (U.S. Department of Education, 1991). It is hoped that this federal sanctioning of early intervention efforts related to literacy development will serve to support and enhance programs designed to facilitate the development of emergent literacy skills for children from disadvantaged environments and those who are otherwise at risk for school achievement.

What implications does our growing knowledge about emergent literacy have for children who have severe speech and physical impairments (SSPI)? Are these children to be included in the President's America 2000 plan? And, if they are, how should early intervention be provided for these children to ensure that they start school ready to learn and become literate adults? These are the questions that are addressed in the pages that follow. First, an overview of the factors that have been shown to have the greatest influence in the development of emerging literacy skills from research with typically developing preschoolers is provided. At the same time, we will explore how the experiences of preschoolers with SSPI may differ from other children's experiences. Second, suggestions are offered for facilitating the development of emergent literacy skills

with this population of children based on our own research and clinical experiences.

EARLY LITERACY INTERACTIONS AND POTENTIAL DIFFERENCES

All pathways of language development from birth occur in environments where language is used for functional purposes. Children must be exposed to and use language for different reasons to make it their own. Written language, like spoken language, develops when it is used to accomplish tasks and through exposure to its varied purposes. Children learn about written language in the same way they learn to communicate through speech, gestures, and other means. In other words, "*all* processes of communication are influenced by immersion in stimulating and meaningful environments" (Katims, in press, p. 4). Specifically, children's early literate understandings and behaviors emerge in environments offering exposure to and direct experience with activities that include

- using reading and writing artifacts (e.g., books, paper, pencils; Smith, 1983),
- observing and interacting with literate models who use print for functional purposes (Baghban, 1984; Greany, 1986; Strickland & Taylor, 1989), and
- being involved in storybook reading (Durkin, 1975; Hall, 1987; Sulzby & Teale, 1991).

Using literacy artifacts

Children who are consistently and regularly engaged in literacy-rich environments learn about written language through handling books, drawing pictures, and scribbling down their ideas (Katims, in press). Playing with reading and writing artifacts is one way in which they learn about written language and its use (McLane & McNamee, 1991). Several recent research efforts have investigated the effects of incorporating literacy-related events and materials into children's play areas (Christie & Enz, 1991; Hall, May, Moores, Shearer, & Williams, 1987; Morrow & Rand, 1991; Neuman & Roskos, 1991; Vukelich, 1991). These studies indicate increases in children's literacy-related play and early literacy skills, especially when adult models are involved in the play.

Play is the "work" of children and is an opportunity for them to incorporate culturally valued activities, such as reading and writing, into their own experience. When children play with literacy artifacts, they develop a sense of the purpose and usefulness of such materials. Through play, children can acquire a wide range of concepts about print and skills related to reading and writing by becoming familiar with the tools of literacy and how to use and control them (McLane & McNamee, 1991).

In addition to acquiring knowledge and skills related to literacy, children may also begin to consider themselves "readers" and "writers" by playing with the artifacts of our literate society (i.e., they can develop feelings and expectations for themselves as potential readers and writers). Through pretend play, children can create a sense of ownership for the roles of people who use reading and writing for functional purposes, for example, mommy using a recipe, a policeman writing a ticket, a reporter writing and reading the news (McLane & McNamee, 1991).

Also through play, children begin to develop a sense of story construction. By pretending, children often develop characters and act out the beginning, middle, and endings of stories in their play. Children's play often incorporates aspects of actual stories that have been read to them (Edmiaston, 1989). This pretend-story-making is essential to the development of understanding the metastructures children will encounter throughout literature as literacy learning develops (McLane & McNamee, 1991).

For children with SSPI, play is often difficult as well as different because of their fine and gross motor impairments. They may have difficulty playing with literacy artifacts because of their special motor needs. Children with SSPI may be unable to grasp a crayon or piece of chalk so that they can begin to develop scribbling and drawing. They may also be unable to ask for books, hold them, or even turn a page. These seemingly simple behaviors are necessary to develop the independent book interactions that support the emergence of concepts about print.

In addition to motor and access differences, another potential difference between children with SSPI and nondisabled children is their level of language development. Because language and play are linked, children with difficulties expressing themselves may have underdeveloped pretend play skills. The underlying language and cognitive factors associated with "acting out" stories or pretending to read and write may develop later or differently in children who do not have easy or ready access to the motor or speech abilities necessary to carry out these activities.

With their potential motor, access, and language differences, children with SSPI may have fewer opportunities to engage in play with books, typewriters, and other literacy-related items. It is often difficult to adapt these types of items for children with SSPI to use during play. They may require additional interactions with nondisabled adults or peers in order to interact with any reading or writing toy. Because of this difficulty, opportunities for literacy-related play may not be as frequent or as interactive as the opportunities afforded children who are nondisabled.

Participating with literate models

Children learn about reading and writing long before formal schooling by "participating with adults in holistic, meaningful literacy activities, and ultimately by independently practicing what they have learned" through play and other interactions (Katims, in press, p. 4). Family members and other caregivers play critical roles in early literacy development by serving as models using reading and writing (e.g., looking up a program in a television guide or writing a thank-you note), providing printed materials, offering support in using these materials, and communicating values and expectations about the use of literacy and the child's potential development into a reader and a writer (Gundlach, McLane, Stott, & McNamee, 1985; McLane & McNamee, 1991).

Children with SSPI may not have the incidental opportunities to take advantage

of literate models in their environments. In our clinical experience, the physical mobility and positioning needs of some children with SSPI often make it necessary to be more purposeful or at least more conscious in setting up modeling opportunities. Parents of children with SSPI who indicated that they did expect their children to become literate to some degree made purposeful efforts to include their children in their own uses of print (e.g., reading magazines and newspapers, reading directions on a microwave oven) and pointed out print in the environment (labels on food containers, notes on the refrigerator). Many other incidental opportunities for modeling the use of print were missed, however, because the child was often in another room in his prone stander or another piece of adaptive equipment (Coleman, 1991).

Reading storybooks

One of the most extensively studied aspects of emergent literacy over the past decade has been storybook reading. This research has provided compelling evidence indicating that parents' reading of storybooks to their children during the preschool years enriches language development (Heath, 1982; Whitehurst et al., 1988) and is significantly associated with reading comprehension in the early school years (Wells, 1985). Still other evidence has suggested that it is not the reading of storybooks alone that produces positive outcomes related to language and literacy development. The impact of storybook reading is also dependent on the nature and quality of conversational interactions between parent and child that occur during reading episodes. The extent to which parents adapt storybook text and dialogue to the child's level of understanding, encourage the child's active participation in the reading process (e.g., asking questions), reinforce the child's attempts to participate, and relate the text to the child's personal experiences (Altwerger, Diehl-Faxon, & Dockstader-Anderson, 1985; DeLoache, 1984; Flood, 1977; Ninio, 1980; Phillips & McNaughton, 1990) affects what the child gains from the experience. The child's behavior also contributes to the outcome of storybook reading (Flood, 1977; Yaden, Smolkin, & Conlon, 1989). For example, Flood (1977) found that the following child behaviors, exhibited during storybook reading episodes with three- and four-year-olds, were most highly correlated with developing reading skills: total number of words spoken by the child, the number of parent questions answered by the child, and the number of questions asked by the child.

Perhaps the most obvious difference in storybook reading experiences for children with SSPI is the relative lack of control they have in parent–child interactions compared with their typically developing peers. For many, asking questions or making comments about the illustrations, text, or the relationship between the story and their own experiences is impossible. For others, it is difficult or limited at best. Similarly, responding to parents' questions is severely restricted. In addition to the barriers imposed by severe speech impairments, these children often have little to no control over the selection of the book, the turning of pages, the pace

at which the text is read to them, the position of the book for their viewing, or the length of the reading session. We have further noted, from our own experiences with children with SSPI, that many have an accompanying visual impairment. The combination of positioning difficulties attributable to the motor and visual impairments makes it next to impossible for some children to even see the illustrations in the book as it is read.

The children's lack of control over the reading experience has its effect on the parents. First, parents become the dominant partner as most of the dialogue is left to them. Even if the parent asks questions or otherwise encourages the child's participation, the limited physical and vocal–verbal abilities of the child to respond result in the quick return of turn-taking responsibility to the parent. Second, it can be extremely difficult for the parent to "read" the child. The lack of verbal responsiveness on the part of the child and the lack of clarity of nonverbal cues as a function of motor involvement make it extremely difficult for parents to know what the child understands, his or her preferences, or even if the child is interested in the book being read to him or her. Consequently, parents may not be able to make adaptations in the text or elaborate on the story to support the child's understanding of vocabulary, concepts, or storyline. Third, holding the child can be very cumbersome and tiring when the child is severely physically disabled. In our own observations of parent–child dyads, repositioning occurred frequently to ensure that the child could see the book, to allow for the turning of pages and to see the text, and to improve the comfort of both parent and child (McWilliam, Coleman, Koppenhaver, & Yoder, 1992).

POSSIBLE INTERVENTION STRATEGIES

We are just beginning to address the issues of literacy surrounding individuals with SSPI and, therefore, have little data on which to base recommendations for alleviating or preventing the problems encountered. We do know, however, that a large percentage of persons with SSPI have significant reading and writing difficulties (Berninger & Gans, 1986a, 1986b; Kelford Smith, Thurston, Light, Parnes, & O'Keefe, 1989). Further evidence (Koppenhaver, Evans, & Yoder, 1991) suggests that the early home literacy experiences of individuals with SSPI may significantly influence later reading and writing skills. Koppenhaver and colleagues (1991b) surveyed 22 adults with SSPI and found that these individuals grew up in "homes where literacy materials and literate models were abundantly available ... were immersed in environments of varied reading materials, [and] surrounded by a variety of readers who were eager to share their expertise" (p. 28). These findings, combined with our growing knowledge of emergent literacy skill development in typically developing children, suggest that we should not ignore the development of emergent literacy skills in our interventions with very young children with SSPI. Even so, enthusiasm should perhaps be tempered with caution in light of our limited knowledge in this area. We offer

the following suggestions and discussion with this caveat.

An emphasis on literacy

The experiences of children with SSPI during infancy and their preschool years are qualitatively different from those of typically developing children, as are the experiences of their parents. Multiple appointments with doctors and clinicians as well as daily regimes of therapies are not uncommon for these families. Consequently, activities such as storybook reading, that might otherwise be engaged in by these families, may easily fall by the wayside. They may not be seen as priorities by the family in light of the child's other needs, or parents may not have the time or energy to devote to them in the course of the family's hectic schedule. Clinicians working with these children and families may also lose sight of the importance of early literacy experiences as they help to establish priorities for intervention.

The extreme difficulty of predicting the developmental potential of infants and preschoolers with SSPI may also contribute to the limited provision of early literacy experiences to these children. All too often, these children appear far more cognitively disabled in their early years than may actually be the case, and, at present, we are at a loss for accurate methods of assessment and prediction with this young population. A lack of responsiveness or unclear communication signals on the part of the children may be cause for parents and professionals alike to misinterpret the children's interest in or understanding of the kinds of reading and writing activities that typically developing children relish.

Perhaps we should heed the advice of others (Butler, 1979; Katims, 1991; Koppenhaver, Coleman, Kalman, & Yoder, 1991; van Kleeck, 1990) who propose that no child is too cognitively, physically, or communicatively disabled to benefit from experiences with written language. We can remind both ourselves and the families we serve of the importance of early experiences with written language that are a part of the everyday lives of so many young children. Furthermore, when reading and writing activities are a high priority for a family, we should support them in their efforts and may even need to reduce the intensity of other therapeutic interventions to allow families to act on this priority.

Access and opportunity

There are many light-tech and high-tech ways to adapt books so that children with SSPI may access and independently interact with them. Books can be entered onto disks, slides, videos, and tapes or placed in page turners. Each of these adaptations can, in turn, be accessed through single-switch input. Writing and drawing can be accessed through a variety of light-tech holders and surfaces or through any number of computer software and hardware options.

Improving access to play involving literacy artifacts may be a matter of increasing opportunities and providing the environmental support to help children with SSPI to become engaged in pretend play and to use books, papers, and pens for their literate purposes. Entire thematic play areas surrounding literacy and stories have been developed for both nondisabled children (Christie & Enz, 1991) and for children with SSPI (Coleman, Steelman, Koppenhaver, & Yoder, 1991). For nonspeaking children, communication boards have been developed for children to act out stories and to pretend to read and write for functional purposes (e.g., to order from a menu, to write a prescription, or to dictate a letter). In both of these studies, the children showed increases in their understandings of the early concepts about print.

Interactive storybook readings

To assist children with SSPI in becoming more active participants during storybook reading, caregivers may want to use some light-tech applications, such as providing a few communication symbols for their children to ask them to read, to turn the page, to act out, and to repeat parts of stories. To support their language development, symbols could also be added that would allow children to make simple comments about pictures, to ask simple "what's that?" questions, and to begin to retell aspects of stories as they reach four to five years of age. In addition to providing communication symbols, readers should consider the following suggestions for making story reading as interactive as possible for children. These approaches and materials have been found to have significant effects on the interactive nature of children's responsiveness during story reading (Katims, in press).

Multiple readings

Multiple readings of favorite books encourage varied exploration and independent reenactments of the stories (Hoskisson, 1979; Sulzby & Teale, 1991). Multiple readings provide ample opportunities for children to assimilate and accommodate the language and event of the story into their own experience. Familiarity with the story helps to build a child's confidence and, thus, encourages independent interactions with the book (Katims, in press).

Type of book

Children with special needs have also been found to interact with greater frequency and in more sophisticated ways with predictable books (Katims, in press). Predictable stories, those containing "rhythmical, repetitive patterns, and/or natural sounding dependable story structure and plots" (Katims, in press, p. 10), may afford children a special kind of access because their features facilitate independent reenactments (Teale & Martinez, 1988). Predictable, repetitive stories offer the regularity needed by children who have learning disabilities (McClure, 1985).

Large, clear illustrations and large print may also help to facilitate engaging the child with SSPI since many of these children often have visual impairments. Books that are conducive to gestures and sound effects also seem to provide support for interactive communication (McWilliam et al., 1992).

Dyadic readings

Katims (in press) found significant differences in the independent reenactments of stories by children with cognitive disabilities when caregivers used a dyadic process of reading with the children. In this process, stories were read repeatedly until the children became familiar with the text. A cloze procedure was then used wherein simple nouns, verbs, and eventually phrases were filled in by the children. This same technique could easily be adapted for use in reading to children with SSPI by placing symbols with words and short phrases on an augmentative communication device or a simple loop tape system.

Other language characteristics of the reader that have been found to facilitate engagement and interaction during storybook reading among nondisabled children include

- using developmentally appropriate language,
- relating story events to the child's real-life experiences,
- encouraging the child to be an active participant,
- structuring linguistic/nonlinguistic language to meet the child's developmental needs, and
- using predictable and repetitive language (Snow, 1983).

• • •

There is ever-increasing evidence indicating that a child's home experiences during the first five years of life have a significant effect on the development of literacy skills in later life. Access to literacy artifacts in the presence of literate adults who value and support the development of reading and writing skills provide preschoolers with a foundation for success in school. We can only assume that children with SSPI can benefit from similar experiences, and retrospective reports of literate adults with SSPI give credence to this assumption (Koppenhaver et al., 1991b).

The authors propose that more attention be given to the literacy experiences of preschoolers with SSPI and that efforts be made to support interested families in providing their children with these experiences. Although the methods by which this may be accomplished are not yet clear, our knowledge of emergent literacy development with typically developing children and the availability of new technology for individuals with SSPI provide us with a number of options for getting started. Ensuring that preschool-aged children with SSPI have experiences with written language may be at least one method by which we can support the America 2000 goals for all children to start school ready to learn and for all American adults to be literate.

As mentioned earlier, enthusiasm toward achieving these tasks should be tempered with caution. Perhaps the most important thing to keep in mind is that literacy learning is a complex sociocultural process (Bloome & Green, 1984; Teale & Sulzby, 1986). The values placed on reading and writing, as well as the methods by which concepts about written communication are introduced to children, vary considerably from culture to culture and from one family to the next within a culture. To be truly supportive of families, we should find out which skills and activities are important to them and provide appropriate assistance to meet the families' goals rather than our own.

In closing, we offer one final caution based on our direct observation of young children with SSPI and their parents during storybook reading (McWilliam et al., 1992). We have been awestruck by the ability of the parents we observed to adapt storybook reading to their children's physical disabilities, sensory impairments, and level of cognitive functioning. Even more impressive is the obvious enjoyment of the reading activity by parents and children alike. It is an intimate activity filled with laughter, conversation, and physical affection. Although many of the children observed have adaptive seating equipment, and some have augmentative communication devices, these are seldom used during storybook reading. The parents prefer the more traditional mode of reading stories to their children—on their lap or snuggled beside them on the sofa. We have come to realize that more is gained from storybook reading than emergent literacy skills. Even though we may be tempted to add communication systems into the storyreading process to make it more interactive, introducing too much technology and "teaching" into this family activity may, in some cases, cause more loss than gain. Once again, family values should dictate the nature of our interventions.

REFERENCES

Altwerger, B., Diehl-Faxon, J., & Dockstader-Anderson, K. (1985). Read-aloud events as meaning construction. *Language Arts, 62,* 476–484.

Baghban, M. (1984). *Our daughter learns to read and write: A case study from birth to three.* Newark, DE: International Reading Association.

Berninger, V., & Gans, B. (1986a). Assessing word processing capability of the nonvocal, nonwriting. *Augmentative and Alternative Communication, 2,* 56–63.

Berninger, V., & Gans, B. (1986b). Language profiles in nonspeaking individuals of normal intelligence with severe cerebral palsy. *Augmentative and Alternative Communication, 2,* 45–50.

Bloome, D., & Green, J. (1984). Directions in the sociolinguistic study of reading. In P.D. Pearson (Ed.), *Handbook of reading research.* New York, NY: Longman.

Butler, D. (1979). *Cushla and her books.* Boston, MA: Horn Books.

Christie, J., & Enz, B. (1991, December). *Literacy play interventions: A follow-up study.* Paper presented at the meeting of the National Reading Conference, Palm Springs, CA.

Coleman, P. (1991). *Literacy lost: A qualitative analysis of the early literacy experiences of preschool children with severe speech and physical impairments.* Unpublished doctoral dissertation, University of North Carolina at Chapel Hill.

Coleman, P., Steelman, J., Koppenhaver, D., & Yoder, D. (1991). *Augmented O.W.L.: An oral and written language preschool curriculum.* Unpublished manuscript, Carolina Literacy Center, University of North Carolina at Chapel Hill.

DeLoache, J.S. (1984). What's this? Maternal questions in joint picture book reading with toddlers. *The Quarterly Newsletter of The Laboratory of Comparative Human Cognition, 6,* 87–95.

Durkin, D. (1975). A six year study of children who learned to read in school at the age of four. *Reading Research Quarterly, 10,* 9–61.

Edmiaston, R. (1989). Preschool literacy assessment. *Seminars in Speech and Language, 9*(1), 27–37.

Fitzgerald, K., & Needlman, R. (1991). Reach out and read: A pediatric program to support emergent literacy. *Zero to Three, XII*(1), 17–20.

Flood, J.E. (1977). Parental styles in reading episodes with young children. *The Reading Teacher, 30,* 846–867.

Greany, V. (1986). Parental influences on reading. *The Reading Teacher, 39,* 813–818.

Gundlach, R., McLane, J., Stott, F., & McNamee, G. (Eds.) (1985). The social foundation of children's early writing development. In *Advances in Writing, 1.* Norwood, NJ: Ablex.

Hall, N. (1987). *The emergence of literacy.* Portsmouth, NH: Heinemann.

Hall, N., May, E., Moores, J., Shearer, J., & Williams, S. (1987). The literate home corner. In P. Smith (Ed.), *Parents and teachers together.* London, England: MacMillan.

Heath, S. (1982). What no bedtime story means. *Language and Society, 2,* 49–76.

Hoskisson, K. (1979). Learning to read naturally. *Language Arts 56*(5), 489–496.

Katims, D. (1991). Emergent literacy in early childhood special education: Curriculum and instruction. *Topics in Early Childhood Special Education, 11*(1), 69–84.

Katims, D. (in press). How preschool children with handicaps become literate. *Learning Disabilities Quarterly.*

Kelford Smith, A., Thurston, S., Light, J., Parnes, P., & O'Keefe, B. (1989). The form and use of written communication produced by physically disabled individuals using microcomputers. *Augmentative and Alternative Communication, 5,* 115–124.

Koppenhaver, D., Coleman, P., Kalman, S., & Yoder, D. (1991a). The implications of emergent literacy research for children with developmental disabilities. *American Journal of Speech-Language Pathology, 1*(1), 38–44.

Koppenhaver, D., Evans, D., & Yoder, D. (1991b). Childhood reading and writing experiences of literate adults with severe speech and motor impairments. *Augmentative and Alternative Communication, 7,* 20–33.

McClure, A. (1985). Predictable books. *Teaching Exceptional Children, 17,* 267–273.

McLane, J., & McNamee, G. (1991). The beginnings of literacy. *Zero to Three, XII*(1), 1–8.

McWilliam, P., Coleman, P., Koppenhaver, D., & Yoder, D. (1992). *Interactions between parents and young, nonspeaking children with physical impairments during storybook reading.* Unpublished raw data.

Morrow, L., & Rand, M. (1991). Preparing the classroom environment to promote literacy during play. In J.F. Christie (Ed.), *Play and early literacy development.* Albany, NY: State University of New York Press.

Neuman, S., & Roskos, K. (1991). The influence of literacy-enriched play centers on preschoolers' conceptions of the functions of print. In J.F. Christie (Ed.), *Play and early literacy development.* Albany, NY: State University of New York Press.

Ninio, A. (1980). Picture-book reading in mother-infant dyads belonging to two subgroups in Israel. *Child Development, 51,* 587–590.

Phillips, G., & McNaughton, S. (1990). The practice of storybook reading to preschool children in mainstream New Zealand families. *Reading Research Quarterly, 25,* 196–212.

Smith, F. (1983). *Essays into literacy.* Portsmouth, NH: Heinemann.

Snow, C. (1983). Literacy and language: Relationships during the preschool years. *Harvard Educational Review, 53*(2), 165–189.

Strickland, D., & Taylor, D. (1989). Family storybook reading: Implications for children, families, and curriculum. In D. Strickland & L. Morrow (Eds.), *Emerging literacy: Young children learn to read and write.* Newark, DE: International Reading Association.

Sulzby, E., & Teale, W. (1991). Emergent literacy. In R. Barr, M. Kammil, P. Mosenthal, & D. Pearson (Eds.), *Handbook of reading research (Vol II)*. White Plains, NY: Longman.

Teale, W., & Martinez, M. (1988). Getting on the right road to reading: Bringing books and young children together in the classroom. *Young Children, 44*(1), 10–15.

Teale, W., & Sulzby, E. (Eds.). (1986). *Emergent literacy: Writing and reading*. Norwood, NJ: Ablex.

U.S. Department of Education. (1991). *America 2000: An education strategy sourcebook*. Washington, DC: Department of Education.

van Kleeck, A. (1990). Emergent literacy: Learning about print before learning to read. *Topics in Language Disorders, 10*(2), 25–45.

Vukelich, C. (1991). Materials and modeling: Promoting literacy during play. In J.F. Christie (Ed.), *Play and early literacy development*. Albany, NY: State University of New York Press.

Wells, G. (1985). Preschool literacy-related activities and success in school. In D.R. Olson, N. Torrance, & A. Hildyard (Eds.), *Literacy, language, and learning: The nature and consequences of reading and writing*. New York, NY: Cambridge University Press.

Whitehurst, G.J., Falco, F.L., Lonigan, C.J., Fischel, J.E., DeBaryshe, B.D., Valdez-Menchaca, M.C., & Caulfield, M. (1988). Accelerating language development through picture book reading. *Developmental Psychology, 24*(4), 552–559.

Yaden, D.B., Smolkin, L.B., & Conlon, A. (1989). Preschoolers' questions about pictures, print conventions, and story text during reading aloud at home. *Reading Research Quarterly, 24*, 189–213.

Ethnography and the clinical setting: Communicative expectancies in clinical discourse

Dana Kovarsky, PhD
Assistant Professor
Department of Language, Reading, and
*   Exceptionalities*
Appalachian State University
Boone, North Carolina

Madeline M. Maxwell, PhD
Associate Professor
Department of Speech Communication
The University of Texas at Austin
Austin, Texas

ETHNOGRAPHIES of communication reveal that communities develop their own communicative norms and expectancies for how to participate in various events and activities (Crago, 1988; Heath, 1983; Philips, 1983; Schieffelin, 1990). Our concern in this article is with the different expectancies and assumptions associated with clinical discourse. We begin by describing some of the communicative norms for participation associated with two clinical discourse styles—adult centered and child centered. Next, the ethnographic concept of thick description and the procedure of indefinite triangulation to explore how such communicative expectancies impact on utterance interpretations are discussed. Finally, it is suggested that intervention may be enriched when clinicians seek to apprehend client utterances from multiple communicative perspectives.

COMMUNICATIVE EXPECTANCIES IN THERAPY DISCOURSE

Although there are hybrids that combine aspects of both adult-centered and

Top Lang Disord, 1992,12(3),76–84
© 1992 Aspen Publishers, Inc.

child-centered intervention (Fey, 1986), each approach is discussed in its most distinctive form, focusing on their respective ways of interpreting children's communications.

Adult-centered clinical discourse

The handful of studies reported in the literature paint a consistent picture of adult-centered therapy discourse. Prutting, Bagshaw, Goldstein, Juskowitz, and Umen (1978) audiotaped eight clinician–child dyads during therapy and found that the clinicians made many requests for known information, evaded children's efforts to initiate conversations, and were in charge of introducing new topics into the lessons. Bobkoff and Panagos (1986) reported that nonverbal behaviors, such as leaning, touching, and pointing, are used by clinicians to allocate speaker turns, highlight specific linguistic forms, and capture the child's attention. Analyzing the conversations of six therapists conducting articulation or language lessons with second-grade children, Ripich, Hambrecht, Panagos, and Prelock (1984) discovered, similar to Prutting et al. (1978), that clinicians made many requests for known information, provided evaluative feedback of children's performances, and controlled the topics of conversation.

Ripich and Panagos (1985) videorecorded eight dyads of phonologically impaired children, ranging from six to nine years of age, after asking them to role play a therapy lesson. One child took the part of the clinician while the other played the child. The researchers discovered that child clinicians "explained instructional tasks, selected materials, pointed at pic-

tures, gave directions, requested responses, and commented on errors" (p. 338). On the other hand, child clients tended to acquiesce to the child clinicians' demands.

In general, interactional asymmetries exist in the communicative roles assumed by participants in adult-centered therapy. Clinicians regulate the distribution and evaluation of information, control conclusions drawn from lesson discourse, and direct activity transitions during therapy (Kovarsky, 1990). In contrast, children tend to assume a relatively passive role, willing participants in clinicians' efforts to regulate therapy discourse at a variety of levels.

Another aspect of this therapy register, closely related to the manner in which information is evaluated by the clinician, is the child's role as error maker. Because clients are typically enrolled in speech-language therapy because of perceived problems or weaknesses, *both* intervention participants expect to focus on the child's communicative mistakes. Consider the following interview with a child therapy participant (Ripich & Panagos, 1985):

Ripich: What do you usually do in therapy?
Child: Well, I'm supposed to make the bad *r* sounds, and Mrs. Smith is supposed to make the good *r* sounds.
Ripich: Don't you ever make good *r* sounds?
Child: No! I'm supposed to make the bad *rs*. (p. 343)

Although the child's statement does not necessarily mean that only incorrect sounds are produced during therapy, it does suggest that she views her mistakes as an expected aspect of therapy activity.

Clinicians also place a great deal of emphasis on the remediation of child errors in therapy. As van Kleeck and Richardson (1986) state:

We will change anything and everything in an effort to get that ultimate plum of teaching—the correct response.

We believe that the clinician who consciously thinks about errors—what causes them and how to respond to them—will be a much more effective language facilitator.... It is time to add to our lesson plans—along with our goals, activities, methods for measuring progress, and plans for generalization—a serious consideration of how we plan to deal with child errors. (p. 25)

Under certain circumstances, this type of adult-controlled intervention, in which child mistakes are remediated in terms of the clinician's conception of what constitutes correct responses, may be perfectly appropriate. There are times, for example, when one of the objectives of therapy is to provide a child with opportunities to practice a new articulatory behavior. In contrast, in a child-centered framework, the clinician focuses on following the client's communicative lead, and thus the evaluative stance of an adult-centered framework may require modification.

Child-centered clinical discourse

Motivated to a large extent by the pragmatics movement within speech-language pathology in the 1980s, concerns have surfaced regarding the appropriateness of adult-centered therapy. It has been suggested, for example, that traditional adult-centered patterns of language use common to the therapy room may be far enough removed from how communication develops and proceeds in other contexts as to have a negative impact on generalization (Muma, 1978; Ripich & Panagos, 1985).

As one alternative to traditional trainer-oriented practices, child-centered models have emerged in which the clinician's role is to follow and regard positively the child's communicative lead (Hubbell, 1981). Similar to certain aspects of Western style "motherese" (Ochs & Schieffelen, 1984), emphasis is placed on an adult who accommodates to the child's communicative intentions (Norris & Hoffman, 1990). Instead of "the traditional focus on right answers that are defined beforehand by the language clinician ... the approach require[s] that the clinician fine tune to what the child is saying and doing" (Duchan, 1986, p. 194).

The focus on understanding communicative acts from the child's frame of reference requires clinicians to reinterpret what sorts of behaviors constitute errors during therapy:

A child who calls stacking rings "bagels" in response to the question "What are these?" is wrong from the adult frame of reference. They are not bagels, they are rings. But the rings, in fact, do look like bagels, and the child's sense of the event is appropriate in that he understands that he is being asked to label the object and that he even offered a sensible label, when seen from his point of view. (Duchan, 1986, p. 197)

When responses like "bagels" are counted as errors, therapy may become a guessing game in which answers considered appropriate by the adult, but not necessarily sensible to the child, become the goal of the lesson. On the other hand, in a child-centered approach the clinician's role is to negotiate meaning from the child's point of view, no longer defining mistakes from the perspective of what constitutes correct responses to adult requests for known information.

Within a child-centered intervention

framework, the clinician would treat "bagels" as an act of communicative competence rather than as a mistake to be evaluated negatively. In this particular case, the clinician could rely on her own understanding of the perceptual similarity between "rings" and "bagels" and then construct a reply that is plausible from the child's point of view. Sometimes, however, interpreting utterances from an alternative frame of reference is far more difficult. The clinical discourse data presented next are considered with an eye toward those instances in which child-centered interpretation is problematic.

PARTICIPANT INTERPRETATIONS OF CLINICAL DISCOURSE

The clinical discourse data to be discussed come from child language therapy lessons, as well as intervention and assessment situations involving deaf children. Vignettes from these contexts for analysis are in accordance with the ethnographer's concept of *thick description.* Ethnographers construct thick, layered descriptions that reflect not only behavior but also its possible interpretations by community members. Geertz (1973), borrowing from philosopher Gilbert Ryle, explains thick description through an example involving eye twitches and winks. From a behavioral point of view, twitches and winks are both eye blinks that involve the same rapid contraction of the eyelids. Within the flow of social discourse, however, an eye blink becomes layered with potential meanings. It may be a simple response to a gust of wind (a twitch), or an act of conspiracy (a wink), or even a mock act of conspiracy (a mock wink). Winks that mock conspiratorial winks may also be produced. A thick

description is one that would interpret all layers of meaning.

To construct valid thick interpretations, ethnographers seek to triangulate (compare and contrast) information from a variety of data sources (Fielding & Fielding, 1986; Hammersley & Atkinson, 1983). Techniques used for triangulation include interviews, participant observation, and written documents (Briggs, 1986; Spradley, 1979, 1980). As part of the data collection process, social events may be preserved on audiotape or videotape, allowing them to be studied at length and shown to different audiences. In other words, the recorded data can be *indefinitely triangulated* by replaying it to any number of audiences (Circourel, 1974).

Participant interpretations of intervention discourse

Presenting recorded events to different audiences demonstrates how participant expectancies for communicative interaction influence the manner in which utterances are interpreted in child language intervention and assessment contexts. The two illustrations that follow are from a therapy session involving a nine-year-old boy and a speech-language clinician. They are presented to illustrate how ethnographic understanding emerges from the process of indefinite triangulation.

The lesson revolves around a crystal garden, which is constructed by mixing a series of chemicals into a liquid solution (Kovarsky, 1989). As shown below, the therapist (T) asks the child (C) to define the word *solution:*

1. T: What is a solution (T crinkling nose)
2. C: Um an idea
3. T: Oh (T raising eyebrows, nodding head

up and down) a solution to a problem would be an idea you come up with
4. C: An idea
5. T: Okay (T raising index finger) that's good thinking
6. T: When you talk about adding vinegar to the salt solution what did you just do
7. C: Put salt in the water
8. T: Okay you brought (T interlacing her fingers) those two together and you (T looking at C)
9. C: Slowly I stirred 'em
10. T: Um hm and when you did (T interlacing fingers) that you made a solution
11. C: Solution
12. T: Okay let me put that word over here (T writing on separate sheet of paper)

The child's definition of a solution as "an idea" receives a positive evaluation (utterance #5). As the teacher and clinician independently viewed this segment, they indicated that the child's definition was consistent with how the term was used during classroom activities. The therapist added, however, that she was seeking an alternative meaning of this homonym, in which *solution* refers to the combining of elements to form a liquid mixture, as evidenced by her repair initiation (utterance #6).

In other words, the clinician's prior awareness of how this term was used in the classroom, along with her knowledge that "solution" has an alternative meaning, resulted in a positive evaluation of the child's response (utterance #5), even though this was not the definition being sought. The clinician's awareness of the appropriateness of the child's alternative interpretation is then turned into a learning opportunity in which the different meanings of solution are discussed (utterances #6 to #12).

In the next example, however, the clinician could not rely on prior linguistic knowledge of a term or information about other contexts of language use when interpreting the child's response. In this case, the prior information needed to interpret utterances thickly was lacking and may have resulted in a negative evaluation and a lost learning opportunity. Here, the child prepares to write his story about building the crystal garden. Before responding in the example presented below, he had expressed uncertainty about how to begin his composition. The therapist had replied by asking, "What did you do first?" In response, the child stated that he "made a crystal garden" (utterance #3):

1. C: First we XX
2. T: (T looks at C's paper) Did what?
3. C: Um made a crystal garden
4. T: First we did that?
5. T: What did we do when we STARTED the crystal garden
6. C: Um
7. C: We got the ingredients (C looks at T)
8. T: GOOD (T nodding her head up and down)

The initiation of repair work (utterance #5) coupled with the subsequent approval (utterance #8) indicate that the child's initial response (utterance #3) was evaluated negatively by the clinician. She reported, during our review of the videotape, that the child was to begin his story by listing the first step taken in constructing the crystal garden.

On the other hand, the mother's reaction when viewing the tape was different. She mentioned that her husband had received college training in journalism and that their son engaged in writing activities at home. On these occasions, her son was encouraged to begin his stories with a main idea summarizing the topic for the entire composition. From the mother's point of view, the child's initial response (utterance #3) was acceptable because he was writing down what he was supposed to do "first," and that was to begin his story with a general topic statement about making the crystal garden.

The mother's perspective on structured writing activities in the home was shared with the clinician. On reflection, the clinician indicated she would have responded more positively to the child's initial efforts to begin his story. Unlike the first example, in which this therapist had enough background information to evaluate the child's definition of "solution" positively, here the therapist was unaware of how writing was being taught at home. Not only was the plausibility of the child's initial response discarded, a learning opportunity focusing on different ways of writing was lost. Unfortunately, no skilled clinician is capable of triangulating enough background information to interpret thickly all a child's utterances during therapy.

It would be a mistake, however, to conclude that a lack of background information fully accounts for the therapist's negative evaluation during the writing exercise. After viewing the videotape, the therapist was asked to imagine that instead of having a communicatively impaired youngster saying he "made a crystal garden," it was someone with expertise in writing, such as a famous novelist. The therapist replied that she probably would have accepted the response as appropriate and requested further explanation.

In other words, the clinician's reinterpretation of the child's response as more appropriate was based on expectancies associated with a communicatively competent writing expert. The children in this investigation, however, were enrolled in therapy because of academic language

difficulties. It was *expected* that they would make errors. Unlike the famous novelist, when the child's response differed from the therapist's perspective on what constituted an appropriate reply, the onus for the misunderstanding was placed on the "communicatively incompetent" child.

At this point, one could ask why the child does not take steps to correct the misunderstanding and explain how writing activities are conducted at home. On the basis of results from a larger investigation (Kovarsky, 1989), the child clearly possesses the communicative abilities to express this alternative point of view. To answer this question it is necessary to consider the children's general audience reactions while viewing the videotapes. For the most part, the children were silent viewers. When they did comment, it was common for them to note places in which they "messed up," saying things like "I'm not understanding." These self-evaluations always occurred at the same time the therapist was negatively judging their performances on the videotapes. In other words, the children's comments mirrored the evaluative stance taken by the clinician on the videotape. They added that the clinician's role was "to help [them] correct [their] mistakes."

The children's comments revealed that they conceived of themselves as error makers, similar to the child interviewed by Ripich and Panagos (1985) who stated that her responsibility was "to make the bad *r* sounds" (p. 343) during therapy. Given the error maker expectancy held by both lesson participants in this investigation, it is reasonable for the child, who believes himself to be at fault in the therapy context, to accept the clinician's view as to what constitutes an appropriate way to begin his story without any disagreement. That is, because he assumes responsibility for mistakes and accepts the clinician's authority in deciding when responses are correct, it makes little sense to justify explicitly an alternative interpretation. Unfortunately, this type of "collusion" (Dore & McDermott, 1982) on the part of both lesson participants is particularly problematic when operating within a child-centered intervention framework in which an attempt is made to follow and regard positively the client's communicative lead.

In general, assuming a critical stance that views the child as an error maker appears to involve, at least, two expectancies: (1) the child is incompetent and (2) the adult is to interpret behavior as evidence of that incompetence. The following examples present even more striking contrasts that emerge when such adult-centered discourse practices are operating.

Participant interpretations of sign language

The two conversational excerpts described below involve deaf children who are signing with hearing clinicians. In both instances, the hearing clinicians interpret signs as secondary representations of English words, whereas the children view them as direct conduits of meaning (Maxwell, 1990). The children attend schools in which the policy is to use signs to represent English words and morphemes. The clinicians are skilled in this mode of communication. In the first example, a clinician working on "social skills" asks a deaf boy how he handles himself when "unsure" of what to do. She signs and writes the word "unsure" and, when the boy expresses confusion, she signs "NOT SURE."

He looks puzzled and then signs, "OH LIE." She shakes her head and signs, "NO, NOT LIE, NOT SURE." She then proceeds to give examples of social uncertainty while he continues to talk about lying.

What happened in this situation is that the sign NOT SURE can also be taken to mean "not true." The sign the clinician used as SURE means "true," "really," or "sure" in the sense of "surely true" or "oh, sure" but not in the sense of "confident." To the clinician, the signs are for English words that have meaning. In contrast, for the deaf boy, the signs are what have meaning and the English words may stand for them. The boy saw NOT TRUE and plausibly thought about lying. The clinician, focusing on signs as representations of English words, did not see the connection between lying and insecurity and ended up abandoning the discussion of social uncertainty.

The same communicative expectancy contrasts about signs as direct conveyors of meaning versus signs as standing for English led to a disastrous informal language assessment. A signing child starts the interaction in competent ASL (American Sign Language), talking about the movie *Star Wars*. Two clinician-evaluators voice the English words for the signs he is using when they can identify them.

To them, a great deal of the time he appears to be signing "a bunch of structureless words." As he signs, the clinicians, who are hearing, try to assign the child's talk sequences a label, as if he were trying to describe things because he does not know the English referents and they need to supply them, instead of looking for the sequence of images in forms and movements. (Maxwell, 1990, p. 218)

That is, their primary activity is to attach English word labels to signs. They assume the child is communicatively incompetent. On the other hand, when the child is not understood, he repeats himself through pantomime, gradually abandoning language altogether and communicating nonverbally through gesture. Apparently, the clinicians have located the communicative breakdown in the child instead of in the linguistic mode of representation.

This language assessment session was videorecorded and shown informally to ASL signers. They viewed this interaction as lack of communicative competence on the part of the evaluators, not the child. Unfortunately, the completed evaluation report indicated that the child was linguistically immature because he used little language and communicated primarily by nonverbal means during the evaluation.

• • •

Although the child-as-error-maker expectancy is compatible with adult-centered clinical models in which the therapist's authority and own frame of reference determines the appropriateness of the interactants' communications, it is inconsistent with child-centered discourse practices. Furthermore, it may lead the adult to see errors that are not there and to underestimate children's abilities. In a child-centered approach, children's utterances are not selected out for scrutiny as right or wrong from the adult's evaluative point of view. Instead, communicative appropriateness is established by the ability of participants to engage in and sustain a mutually intelligible conversation from the child's frame of reference.

In a child-centered approach, every effort is made to treat children's comments as appropriate even when, on the surface,

they may appear inappropriate. This becomes difficult without sufficient background information to access the potential interpretations of a particular utterance. As in some of the preceding illustrations, there is not always enough information to suggest how a child's comment can be most appropriately construed. Although the recovery of thick descriptions during a lesson may not always be possible (nor even desirable), a step toward this end is to change one's expectancies regarding the child's communicative role during therapy.

Similar to the therapist who was asked to imagine that the child in therapy was a famous novelist, *treating* children as competent communicators can counteract the adult-centered tendency to assign them culpability for misunderstandings that occur during clinical interactions. Shifting the responsibility for potential misunderstandings to the professional increases the capacity to reinterpret utterances from the child's perspective. In a similar vein, Malinowski discusses how outside audiences reading ethnographic texts can be helped to view culture from the native point of view (cited in Thornton, 1985). Building on the work of scientist Ernst Mach, Malinowski proposes that the imagination must be stimulated, allowing others to apprehend different cultural perspectives:

The ethnographer must undertake the work of convincing readers by managing their imaginations in a way that would allow them to conceptualize in images what the text could not present in full. (Thornton, 1985, p. 8)

Although speech-language pathologists may never be able to triangulate enough information to create thick descriptions of all utterances, the imagination could help clinicians to interpret child communications in their best possible light and capitalize on learning opportunities. Furthermore, this should caution them against many obvious negative interpretations. Constructing an image of the child as a competent (rather than incompetent) communicator minimizes the client-as-error-maker expectancy, which, in turn, helps

the therapist accommodate to the child's point of view. Such a strategy enables the clinician to follow and regard positively the child's communicative intentions. Adapting the ethnographic notions of thick description, triangulation, and Malinowski's "imagination" to the clinical process will enhance the therapist's ability to interact with children.

REFERENCES

Bobkoff, K., & Panagos, J.M. (1986). The "point" of language intervention lessons. *Child Language Teaching and Therapy, 2,* 50–62.

Briggs, C.L. (1986). Learning how to ask. New York: Cambridge University Press.

Circourel, A. (1974). *Sociology: Language and meaning in social interaction.* New York: Free Press.

Crago, M.B. (1988). *Cultural context in communicative interaction of young Inuit children.* Unpublished doctoral dissertation, McGill University, Montreal.

Dore, J., & McDermott, R. (1982). Linguistic determinancy and social context in utterance interpretation. *Language, 58,* 376–398.

Duchan, J.F. (1986). Language intervention through sense-making and fine tuning. In R.L. Schiefelbusch (Ed.), *Language competence: Assessment and intervention* (pp. 187–212). San Diego: College-Hill Press.

Fey, M.E. (1986). *Language intervention with young children.* San Diego: College-Hill Press.

Fielding, N.G., & Fielding, J.L. (1986). Linking data. Qualitative research methods series (Vol. 4). Newbury Park, CA: Sage.

Geertz, C. (1973). *The interpretation of cultures.* New York: Basic Books.

Hammersley, M., & Atkinson, P. (1983). *Ethnography principles and practise.* London: Tavistock.

Heath, S.B. (1983). *Ways with words.* New York: Cambridge University Press.

Hubbell, R. (1981). *Children's language disorders.* Englewood Cliffs, NJ: Prentice-Hall.

Kovarsky, D. (1989). *An ethnography of communication in child language therapy.* Unpublished doctoral dissertation, The University of Texas at Austin.

Kovarsky, D. (1990). Discourse markers in adult-controlled therapy: Implications for child-centered intervention. *Journal of Childhood Communication Disorders, 13,* 29–41.

Maxwell, M. (1990). Visual-centered narratives of the deaf. *Linguistics and Education, 2,* 213–229.

Mehan, H. (1979). *Learning lessons.* Cambridge: Harvard University Press.

Muma, J. (1978). *Language handbook: Concepts, assessment, intervention.* Englewood Cliffs, NJ: Prentice-Hall.

Norris, J.A., & Hoffman, P.R. (1990). Language intervention within naturalistic environments. *Language, Speech, and Hearing Services in Schools, 21,* 72–84.

Ochs, E., & Schieffelin, B.B. (1984). Language acquisition and socialization: Three developmental stories and their implications. In R. Shweder & R. LeVine (Eds.), *Culture theory: Essays on mind, self, and emotion.* New York: Cambridge University Press.

Philips, S.U. (1983). *The invisible culture.* White Plains, NY: Longman.

Prutting, C.A., Bagshaw, N., Goldstein, H., Juskowitz, S., & Umen, I. (1978). Clinician-child discourse: Some preliminary questions. *Journal of Speech and Hearing Disorders, 43,* 123–139.

Ripich, D.N., Hambrecht, G., Panagos, J.M., & Prelock, P. (1984). An analysis of articulation and language remediation discourse patterns. *Journal of Childhood Communication Disorders, 7,* 17–26.

Ripich, D.N., & Panagos, J.M. (1985). Accessing children's knowledge of sociolinguistic rules for speech therapy lessons. *Journal of Speech and Hearing Disorders, 50,* 335–346.

Schieffelen, B.B. (1990). *The give and take of everyday life.* New York: Cambridge University Press.

Spradley, J.P. (1979). *The ethnographic interview.* Orlando, FL: Holt, Rinehart & Winston.

Spradley, J.P. (1980). *Participant observation.* Orlando, FL: Holt, Rinehart & Winston.

Thornton, R.J. (1985). Imagine yourself set down. *Anthropology Today, 1,* 7–14.

van Kleeck, A., & Richardson, A. (1986). What's in an error? Using children's wrong responses as teaching opportunities. *NSSLHA Journal, 14,* 25–50.

Part III
Older Children: Changing Needs

Magic buries Celtics: Looking for broader interpretations of language learning and literacy

Geraldine Wallach, PhD
Director, Los Angeles Center
Professor of Communication Disorders
Emerson College—Los Angeles
Los Angeles, California

DURING a language acquisition class, Anthony Bashir fielded questions from graduate students about word finding and retrieval problems, two classic symptoms associated with language-learning disabilities (German, 1987; Kail & Leonard, 1986). After listening to a number of proposals about the appropriateness of various assessment and intervention methods, he said reflectively: "It is not only a matter of asking what a word means, it's a matter of asking *what else* could it mean?" (Wallach & Miller, 1988, p. 181). Bashir's words, although focused on a specific topic, characterized the notion of flexibility in learning—flexibility that enables individuals to go beyond one-sided interpretations and consider the different dimensions of something or someone.

Bashir's remarks also bring to mind the double-edged mandate facing professionals working with children and adolescents with language-learning disabilities. One part of the mandate relates to the students

Top Lang Disord, 1990,10(2),63–80
© 1990 Aspen Publishers, Inc.

these professionals serve; the other part relates to the professionals' specializations. As the profession moves away from 1960s, categorizations of children as having auditory or visual strengths and weaknesses, language specialists move toward an understanding of the importance of each individual's experience as a learner and as a language user. As the profession grows away from rigid interpretations about what disciplines do or do not represent, language specialists come closer to building meaningful intervention programs. Indeed, one-dimensional interpretations of children and the professionals who serve them are now avoided.

More sophisticated interpretations of some of the connections among language proficiency, literacy, and academic success have been developed (Kamhi & Catts, 1989; Wallach & Miller, 1988). The new body of research provides a broad base from which integrated language and literacy programs may evolve. One consummate language intervention or reading program may never be identified as the best, but language specialists have started to exploit and apply to practice some of the excellent research currently available.

Teaching children and adolescents with language-learning disabilities is a complex business that requires constant reevaluation of interpretations about what it means to be literate and what it takes to help children acquire literacy. As concerned professionals examine their own interpretations of learning and literacy and propose various strategies that might help children learn to read, they must keep in mind that even proficient and highly skilled readers may be wondering: "What *does* 'Magic buries Celtics' really mean?"

The first professional responsibility is to remain open and flexible in one's own thinking. The second responsibility is to recognize that answers to questions like, "What can I do to help children learn to read?" will never be simple.

The value of theory-driven intervention will be emphasized throughout this article (Wallach, 1989). However, practitioners are reminded to evaluate carefully intervention suggestions gleaned from this and other research. Professionals who take an either/or approach to reading, espousing either whole language or phonics approaches, ignore the reality that what they do with children has more to do with what the children are ready for rather than what a language or reading program promises.

A number of topics are covered in this article that bear on attempts to look at language learning and literacy within a broad framework. The differences that exist between oral and written communication are explored in the first section. Some of the content and form requirements of written language are discussed in the sections that follow. The article will show how the processing, form, and content requirements of written language pose challenges to professionals trying to design and implement educational programs, regular or remedial.

DIFFERENCES BETWEEN ORAL AND WRITTEN LANGUAGE

Learning to read is not the same thing as learning to speak. Whereas language specialists tended to focus on the similarities between spoken and written language in the past, they now recognize that spoken and written communication are somewhat different. For example, some degree of explicit language knowledge, or metalinguistic awareness, is recognized as necessary to become a reader and writer of one's language. The style of language changes when one moves from oral to written text. As with many aspects of language study, attempts to oversimplify relations among systems, although well meaning, have created problems. Liberman, Shankweiler, Camp, Blachman, and Werfelman (1980) have been reminding us for a long time that reading is not just speech written down. Gee's (1988) and Westby's (1984, 1985) work have taken Liberman et al.'s notion even further by delineating some of the differences between oral and print-oriented cultures.

Two examples of the difference between spoken and written language illustrate why making the transition to literacy is difficult for some children. The first example involves consideration of the processing requirements of written language (e.g., written language is explicit and metalinguistic); the second example involves consideration of the style and form requirements of written language (e.g., written language is literate in form).

Process differences

To state the complex in simple terms, "the speech signal is more or less continuous, whereas letters are presented individually on the page" (Stark & Wallach, 1982, p. 9; also, see Liberman et al., 1980). This difference between speech (continuous) and print (segmented) presents the beginning reader with an immediate dilemma.

The words and sounds of oral language are spoken, more or less, in connected chunks. For example, when the word *bat* is spoken, initial and final consonants blend with the medial vowel so that even though the word *bat* has three phonemes, it represents only *one* acoustic segment (Liberman, 1973; Rubin, 1986; Stark & Wallach, 1982). People speak (and process) individual phonemes simultaneously. During the normal flow of conversation, one rarely focuses on the individual units of a message, unless there is a communication breakdown, the speaker has an accent, or there is a particular purpose for stopping on a word or sound. Requests like: "Was that precede or proceed?" and "Did you say her name was Gerry or Terry?" reflect reasons for shifting the focus of a conversation to a smaller linguistic unit, the phoneme.

By contrast, the printed word is segmented, that is, represented by discrete letter units. Unlike oral words, printed word boundaries are marked explicitly by spaces on the page. Young children have to come to terms with speech versus print discrepancies. They must figure out how individual letters on a page represent the continuous sound that has been coming out of their mouths. Unlike spontaneous conversations, which occur in contexts and which tap into implicit language knowledge, reading and writing are decontextualized, and they tap into metalinguistic knowledge. Young readers must become linguists. They must bring their spoken language knowledge to the surface and develop a more analytical sense about language and its parts. Beginning reading is the time when the implicit becomes explicit and the linguistic becomes metalinguistic.

Experiences with second-language learning may help illustrate the young child's speech versus print confusion. Processing breakdowns occur when one listens to a foreign language that is newly learned or unfamiliar. The auditory stream that goes by sounds like an unending and unsegmented garble of information. Naive listeners are usually unable to discern where one word ends and another begins. The French novice might be surprised to learn that *il y a* (there is) is represented by three separate characters in print, rather than something like *illya* (one character).

Younger English-speaking children make similar errors when they indicate that "thehouse" is one word (van Kleeck & Schuele, 1987). Van Kleeck and Schuele point out that preschoolers begin their experimentation with words and sounds before learning to read. They say that "language curiosity," reflected in word and sound games with oral language, may be an aspect of preliteracy practice. Van Kleeck and Schuele provide many examples, one of which comes from a 3-year-old girl who made her confusion with word boundaries quite explicit by asking, "Mommy, is it an *A-dult* or a *NUH-dult?*"

The writing errors of children also show literal-like translations from the auditory, as reflected in the written "stoppid" for *stop it*. Indeed, many examples in the literature demonstrate young children's appropriate auditory confusions and mirror mistakes that adults might make about phrase, word, or sound boundaries in foreign languages. These mistakes are evidence of the continuous and unsegmented nature of oral language. They also indicate

Many examples in the literature demonstrate young children's appropriate auditory confusions and mirror mistakes that adults might make about phrase, word, or sound boundaries in foreign languages.

that oral language is somewhat different from written language and bring to mind the linguistic sensitivity needed to make oral-to-written or speech-to-print translations.

Two points should be underlined from the previous discussion of speech and print differences. First, awareness of phrase, word, syllable, and sound boundaries is part of explicit language knowledge, or metalinguistic awareness, which develops over time and, in some cases, improves after exposure to reading (Allan, 1982; Backman, 1983; Wallach & Miller, 1988). Children do not automatically come to the task of reading with an understanding of word, syllable, and sound boundaries. Second, spoken English is represented on the printed page by a series of letter segments, better known as the alphabet (Rubin, 1986). Alphabetic systems like English present young children with a particular challenge because individual letters are indirectly connected to meaningful speech by virtue of their connection to individual phonemes—the most abstract piece of language structure. In the word *bat*, for example, three written symbols represent one word. Some writing systems, such as Japanese kanji, connect to spoken language in different ways. In kanji, one written symbol represents a complete word. Similarly, in the Japanese kana (a syllabary system), one symbol represents a syllable. Both kanji and kana writing symbols represent bigger pieces of speech than the English alphabet, making them, in one sense, more direct representations of spoken language (Liberman et al., 1980; Rubin, 1986; Wallach & Miller, 1988). As might be implied from the previous statements, the English writing system presents young readers of English with quite an analytical challenge.

Young children are generally nonanalytical (Tunmer, Herman, & Nesdale, 1988). Novice Japanese, French, and Spanish speakers might have the same nonanalytical sense about a new language that young children have about their first language. Research suggests that one gets better at figuring out Japanese, French, and Spanish syllabic and phonemic boundaries after some experience as a speaker and listener of those languages (Blachman, 1984; Rubin, 1986).

Children develop a more conscious awareness of some of the structural boundaries of their language at about 5 or 6 years of age. It is suggested that children who enter school already having a metalinguistic sensitivity about words and sounds make smoother transitions to reading and writing. While researchers disagree about the role of reading in facilitating structural awareness, most recognize the importance of at least some degree of word and sound awareness for reading and writing proficiency. Warren-Leubecker (1987) found that 5- and 6-year-olds who understood word order in sentences, as demonstrated by role playing activities with puppets who spoke "good sentences" and "mixed up sentences," were more advanced in reading, vocabulary, and reading readiness than children who had difficulty making judgments about word order (Wallach & Miller, 1988). Blachman (1984), Bradley and Bryant (1983), and Liberman et al. (1980), among others, report that children who are sensitive to word, syllable, and sound boundaries tend to be the better readers in their groups by the end of grade 2. Tunmer, Herman, and Nesdale (1988) say that children who have a sense of syntactic and sound segments of language recognize that print reflects certain structural features of spoken language earlier than children who do not. They go on to say that phonological and structural awareness may play a more important role in beginning reading than pragmatic awareness. Although the ultimate goal is to enable students to handle text-level and discourse-level processes in reading, children need to have some strategies for engaging with print before they can shift to inferring about text, figuring out the intent of the author, and so forth (Bashir, 1988; Chall, 1983). In one sense, children may need to do the opposite of what they do in spoken language acquisition at the beginning stages of reading. That is, they may need to come to terms with the smaller elements initially, gaining some degree of automaticity with words and sounds, so that they are free to focus on the larger units of text 2 or 3 years later.

What can professionals do? They can question their assumptions about what children bring with them to the task of reading. They can also question their assumptions about reading programs. More careful tailoring of analytic tasks to the abilities and developmental levels of children is needed. Phonics may be a bad idea if recommended without any consideration of children's communicative and metalinguistic abilities. Starting with print activities may be inappropriate for children without a sense of what reading means, what words are, or what events are being discussed in print (Miller, 1988). Van Kleeck and Schuele (1987) provide numerous examples of preschoolers' early metalinguistic behaviors in three areas: word consciousness, word segments, and phonological awareness. They indicate that verbal play in these areas, which occurs spontaneously in young, normal language users, may be useful to include in the language activities in preschool and early school language programs.

Van Kleeck (1984a, 1984b) encourages professionals to assess reading (and language) programs from a developmental perspective. She says that early reading programs that focus on word and structural analysis may be appropriate if children are ready to make structural judgments about language. Liberman and colleagues (1980), Blachman (1984, 1989), and Catts (1989) provide suggestions for metalinguistic development in the speech segmentation area. They include phrase, word, syllable, and sound awareness activities in their sequences and use developmental information as a guide. For example, Liberman et al. point out that whole word approaches to reading, sometimes characterized as *sight* approaches, are misnamed. They say that regardless of the unit of language being analyzed, readers have to access verbal information from print. Reading words, as well as naming words, requires coming up with their phonological representations. Thus, it is illogical to say that word recognition is *sight* and phonics is *sound*. Liberman

(personal communication, 1986) says that word recognition activities, such as naming words printed on flash cards, are not more visual than phonics activities. Rather, whole-word approaches represent an earlier stage of structural awareness. Words can generally be segmented from the speech stream earlier than syllables, and syllables can generally be segmented before phonemes. Four-year-olds are more likely to think that "ahouse" is one word than 6-year-olds (van Kleeck, 1984b). Five- and 6-year-olds improve dramatically in their ability to segment words into syllables and sounds, but even some 7- and 8-year-olds have difficulty with phonemic segmentation (Fox & Routh, 1975).

A wide range of activities, including sound blending, phoneme deletion, and rhyming, fall under the general heading of *speech segmentation activities*. Auditory discrimination, auditory blending, auditory analysis, and auditory closure tasks, among others in the auditory perceptual area, may actually be speech segmentation activities. The segmentation activities span the continuum from easy to very difficult. It is important for practitioners working with language-impaired and non–language-impaired students to recognize and understand the developmental, cognitive, and metalinguistic demands involved in such tasks (Catts, 1989; Hallie, 1988; van Kleeck & Schuele, 1987).

Form and style differences

Consider the following examples:
1. and then this guy here comes along from behind the building and he scares the kids ...
    and then the good guys come along and save the kids

2. The man [who came from behind the building] scared the children . . .
   However, the police came along and saved them . . .

In the broadest sense, the two samples impart the same message in different styles. The first example represents what Westby (1984) calls an oral style of communication, whereas the second sample represents a literate style. Gee (1988) uses the terms *pragmatic mode* and *syntactic mode* to discuss oral and literate style variations. Pragmatic modes, reflected in oral cultures, have strong ties to face-to-face interactions. Westby (1984, 1988) says the same thing when she points out that oral styles of communication tend to be participant and situation oriented. Gee (1988) adds that pragmatic modes of communication force the listener to figure out what goes together (as can be seen in Example 1). However, prosody, gesture, and facial cues usually help listeners comprehend messages. Syntactic modes, on the other hand, are less personal than pragmatic modes. Syntactic modes are the communications that go on in the public sphere. The connection between sentences and thoughts is made more explicit in syntactic modes (as evidenced in Example 2). Literate styles of communication, such as this article, are syntactically heavy. Embedded clauses, transitional phrases, active and passive sentence changes, and conditional and causal conjunctions, among other structural devices, make meanings explicit in print. By contrast, "although speakers can choose any number of conjunctions, *and* or *and then*, accompanied by gesture and situation, usually work well to join thoughts and describe event sequences in oral exchanges" (Wallach & Miller, 1988, p. 7).

The implications from the research in oral versus literate communication (pragmatic and syntactic modes respectively) are tremendous. For one thing, syntactic or literate styles of communication are the ones rewarded in school. Children who come to school from high-print homes (see Miller article in this issue) generally have an easier time making the transition to literacy, in part because they talk like books; that is, they use syntactic modes of communicating in oral language. Moreover, they learn which styles of language are appropriate for which situations. As implied in the previous statements, literate styles of communication can be spoken. Formal lectures, meetings, and classroom instructional language, although oral, are characteristic of literate or syntactic modes. We can talk like books when the situation demands it. Similarly, we can write conversations. Casual notes to best friends and letters to close family members, although written, tend to be closer to the style one might use in face-to-face encounters. Children whose styles of communication are primarily oral or pragmatic and whose cultures reflect "strong historical ties to rich oral cultures" may be at a disadvantage when they come to school, because schools and texts present themselves almost exclusively in literate or syntactic modes (Gee, 1988, p. 9).

The implications from the research in oral versus literate communication are tremendous. For one thing, syntactic or literate styles of communication are the ones rewarded in school.

Gee (1988) provides some stunning examples of children's stories that illustrate the organization of their spoken language and the mismatches that can occur among child, teacher, and textbook. The following example is part of a spoken story from a 7-year-old African American girl:

Today
it's Friday the thirteen
an' it's bad luck day
an' my grandmother's birthday is on bad luck
    day

an' my mother's a bakin' a cake
an' I went up my grandmother's house while
    my mother's bakin' a cake
an' my mother was bakin' a cheese cake
an' my grandmother was bakin' a whipped
    cream cup cakes

Gee (1988) notes the rhythmic style reflective in the child's speech, which loses its musical quality when presented in written form. He states that her language demonstrates a number of things. It is completely organized into thought units that are like poetry stanzas. Each stanza has one perspective, and the stanzas are set apart by being focused on a main idea. The repetitive use of "an" creates a pattern, and the phrase "a whipped cream cup cakes," which might be awkward out of context, fits nicely into the pattern being developed. The story goes on for 12 stanzas and reflects an elaborate discussion of the various events surrounding the cakes for grandmother's birthday. Gee (1988) points out that different stanzas in the story could be misinterpreted as "rambling" or "disorganized" when, in fact, the stanzas are part of a sophisticated and rule-governed narrative. This example, while at variance with some story grammar formulas (e.g., Stein & Glenn's,

1979), is highly systematic and representative of a culture with a rich oral tradition (Gee, 1988).

What can professionals do? They might think about ways to structure language assessment and intervention programs for students in light of the information discussed in the previous section. Evaluation of children and their textbooks from oral or pragmatic and literate or syntactic points of view requires greater integration of services across disciplines. The mandate that disciplines work together (a case that could be made throughout this article) is strengthened by the need to focus on side-by-side analyses of oral and literate communication. The examples from Gee (1988) and Westby (1988) demonstrate that speech–language pathologists must do more than assess pragmatics and syntax as separate categories. Pragmatic and syntactic areas are joined when one considers the stylistic options that proficient speakers and readers have available to them: these readers also know how and when to use which forms. Indeed, practitioners might consider integrating oral-to-written and written-to-oral activities into clinical and educational practice with a focus on which language style works in which situation. Westby (1985) describes a number of excellent activities for the facilitation of oral-to-literate exercises in the early and middle grades. Wallach (1985, 1988) also describes a series of steps she takes students through to help them appreciate communication style differences. For example, in one of her sports units, she has students move from conversational activities to television reporting, to radio reporting, and finally to sports writing. She guides students through discussions of the different ways they might "say the same thing" to different audiences in different contexts. She also has students compare spoken and written texts. Wallach and Miller (1988) outline many activities with accompanying lesson plans that facilitate structural awareness and provide students with models of literate language along both spoken and written dimensions. Gee (1988) suggests that children with oral or pragmatic language styles practice in groups with children who have already mastered syntactic modes. He gives the example of children sitting in a group trading baseball cards and says that the baseball card context provides a scenario in which children will talk about the cards, read what is on the cards, discuss why they are trading or keeping certain cards, and so forth. Gee (in press) says that the social practice and the script that goes with a particular practice pull language, literacy, and socialization closer together.

LITERACY AS A LIFELINE TO LEARNING NEW INFORMATION

Access to the written word enables people to do many things. They can escape to faraway countries, they can communicate with friends, they can organize their week, they can learn new words and concepts, and they can store some of the information of their culture. For children, "[literacy] marks the beginning of the ability to exist in a linguistically specified hypothetical world . . . and enables [them] . . . to live in the multifaceted world opened up by texts" (Wallach & Miller, 1988, p. 7). What would the world, particularly the world of western society, be without written text? What demands would be placed

on people's auditory systems? What would school be like if children had to process, store, retrieve, and recite all the information they were being given by their teachers without the benefit of notebooks, textbooks, computer printouts, and other written reminders?

As children move through the grades, being able to read becomes their lifeline to learning. By fourth grade, the curriculum is presented almost exclusively in written form. Students advance from learning to read to reading to learn in the middle grades (Bashir, 1988). Geography, social studies, science, and, more obviously, English literature are transmitted through books. By sixth and seventh grades, students have an additional challenge. They must manage a curriculum that is presented almost exclusively in expository style. Language-disabled students who also have reading problems have fewer options than nondisabled students. They have fewer places to turn when trying to absorb new content. In many cases, they turn to their already overloaded auditory systems when trying to absorb and retain information. Students without language problems have an immediate advantage over language- and reading-disabled students because nondisabled students have the written word, in addition to their intact spoken language systems, to facilitate further language development and learning. The availability of backup systems, where spoken language facilitates written language and written language facilitates spoken language, provides students with a strong base for learning and school achievement.

What other sources of information provide ideas for fostering literacy in students with and without language-learning disabilities? Are there additional ways to integrate oral and written intervention recommendations? Two overlapping concepts address these questions: the role of background knowledge and experience in the acquisition of literacy and the nature of structure and content interactions. Implications for intervention are drawn from the research with characteristic caution.

World knowledge and content schema

Ohlhausen and Roller (1988) have written that learning to read is "a complex interplay between prior knowledge, schooling, and text" (p. 70). The role of prior knowledge as it relates to both schooling and text is a concept receiving considerable attention today. In his book *Cultural Literacy*, Hirsch (1987) points out that being literate includes being knowledgeable about the events of one's culture. He says that informationally deprived people, even people who can read individual sentences and who can handle the vocabulary of a particular text, have difficulty making sense out of text when they lack background knowledge about a text's topic. Drawing from the results of his research with different groups of college students, Hirsch reports that students who had lim-

Informationally deprived people, even people who can read individual sentences and who can handle the vocabulary of a particular text, have difficulty making sense out of text when they lack background knowledge about a text's topic.

ited knowledge of the Civil War found selections about its generals, Grant and Lee, extremely difficult to understand. On the other hand, readers who knew about the historical events surrounding the Civil War and who had some idea about who its players were found the passages very easy to retain and absorb. The passage that follows from the classic article by Bransford and Johnson (1973) may be difficult to comprehend and retain for readers who have never seen or heard it, even though the sentence structures and vocabulary words are within readers' repertoires:

The procedure is actually quite simple. First you arrange the items in different piles. Of course one pile may be sufficient depending on how much there is to do. If you have to go somewhere else due to lack of facilities that is the next step; otherwise you are pretty well set. It is important not to overdo things. That is, it is better to do too few things at once than too many. (p. 400)

Adding the backgrounding title, *Washing Clothes*, should make the passage more comprehensible than it is without the title. Although limited in scope, the *Washing Clothes* passage provides a flavor of the multidimensional layers of literacy. Proficient readers decode text quickly and automatically, they use their knowledge of sentence structure and vocabulary, and they relate messages in the text to something they already know. Hirsch says that *knowing* relates to knowledge of the events of one's culture; others add that what readers know includes linguistic knowledge reflected in metaawareness of sounds, words, sentence structures, and structural cues within texts (van Kleeck & Schuele, 1987). Still others talk about *knowing* as monitoring oneself when reading

(Marzano, Hagerty, Valencia, & DiStefano, 1988).

Culture and value systems

Gee (1988) adds to what Hirsch, Bransford and Johnson, and others have said about the role of background information and experience in the acquisition of literacy. Gee (1988) says that readers' value systems affect what they glean from text. The idea that one's social and cultural values influence retention and comprehension may seem obvious. However, Gee (1988) believes that curriculum planners sometimes forget the obvious. Consider the following excerpt used by Gee (1988, p. 25).

The Alligator River Story

Once upon a time there was a woman named Abigail who was in love with a man named Gregory. Gregory lived on the shore of a river. The river which separated the two lovers was teeming with man-eating alligators. Abigail wanted to cross the river to be with Gregory. Unfortunately the bridge had been washed out. So she went to Sinbad, a river boat captain, to take her across. He said he would be glad to if she would consent to go to bed with him preceding the voyage.

"The Alligator River Story" continues to describe Abigail's plight. She asks her friend Ivan about the situation, and he chooses to remain uninvolved. With no one to turn to, Abigail accepts Sinbad's offer. Sinbad delivers Abigail to Gregory, who rejects her after she tells him about her bargain with Sinbad. Slug, another one of Abigail's friends, feels compassion for her, seeks out Gregory, and beats him up. Abigail is happy because Gregory has gotten what he deserves.

Gee (1988) asked three groups of high school students to read "The Alligator River Story": African American students, working-class white students, and upper-class white students. He then asked the groups to participate in a story retelling activity. Students reviewed the story and ranked characters from most offensive to least offensive. The students worked in small groups and voted on the responses they were going to give Gee about the story and its characters. Gee (1988) analyzed the responses of the students from a number of perspectives: how inferences were drawn, construction of social relations among story characters, moral lexicon, and language (including style and pronoun usage), among other variables.

Interesting differences surfaced among the groups. For example, the African American students made inferences based on the social world. They talked about how people should relate to one another in the broader sense and then tied the characters from the story to the world in general. The working-class white students made inferences by sticking to the text itself. They talked about the characters from the perspective of the story and the story plot. The upper-class white students related inferences to themselves. They talked about how their group decided on what was reasonable and nonreasonable behavior from their value systems.

Gee (1988) points out that word choice was also somewhat different among the groups. The African American students preferred words and phrases like *right/ wrong, should,* and *have to* when assessing characters' actions. The working-class white students used words like *felt as if* and *really didn't listen,* which focused on the psychological state and reasoning efforts of the characters. The upper-class white students used vocabulary like *from his point of view* and *we couldn't see any real good* to reflect psychological states of their characters and self-reaction.

Gee (1988) reiterates some of the points made earlier about oral and literate cultures. He says that the African American students in his study appeared to take a social approach to literacy, that is, text is part of society and interpretation of relations expressed in text connect to values within the society. According to Gee (1988) text is nonautonomous from society for the African American students. The working-class white students seemed to separate text from other aspects of their lives. The responses of the working-class white students reflected literal interpretations of the text. For them, text is autonomous. Upper-class white students related judgments about characters to their value systems and made verbal distinctions between themselves and the characters. Thus, the text is nonautonomous from self for the upper-class white students.

Study of structural variations across the groups also reinforced the differences between oral and literate cultures. For example, the African American students made the assumption that the listener (the teacher/researcher) already knew the story. Thus, they used pronouns initially in their explanations before clarifying referents (as might be done in oral exchanges between a speaker and listener who are familiar with each other and the topic). The white working-class students used the proper names first, followed by pronouns, in their discussions of the story (moving to a more formal or literate style). The upper-class white students rarely used pronouns

but chose proper names throughout their discussions (moving further away from oral modes). The following examples from Gee (1988) reflect differences between the pragmatic and syntactic modes:

Pragmatic mode:
> What an ass that guy was, you know, her boyfriend
> I should hope if I ever did that to you, you would shoot the guy
> He uses her and he says he loves her
> Sinbad never lies, you know what I mean?

Syntactic mode:
> Well, when I thought about it,
> I don't know, it seemed to me that Gregory should be the most offensive
> He showed no understanding for Abigail when she told him what she was forced to do
> He was so callous
> He was hypocritical, in the sense that he professed to love her he then acted like that

What can professionals do? They might consider developing language-reading programs that match more closely the linguistic, cultural, and social knowledge of students with and without language-learning disabilities, at least at the entry levels to literacy, with modifications of content and structure added as students advance. Certain types of discourse may be easier for some students to master before others (Gee, 1988). Gee (1988) notes that school reading curricula most frequently match the literal-autonomous model, reflected in the working-class white patterns described in the story. Curricula focus on the text and what the text says. Professionals might question this one-mode approach to curriculum development. As suggested in the previous section, children bring different kinds of background knowledge to text.

Intervention plans that encourage children to use background knowledge and to make inferences about what they are reading may be helpful if caution is exercised about judging right and wrong responses.

Blachowicz (1986) has developed many excellent suggestions for activating children's knowledge that combine interactional activities with metalinguistic and metacognitive activities. She uses brainstorming activities and group discussions about topics that encourage students to talk about what they know before they read. She also has children pick out words from geography, science, and history lessons that they know and do not know. Blachowicz guides students through a series of awareness activities whereby they rate themselves along a *can define, have seen the word somewhere*, and *need to know the word* continuum. She uses many other prediction activities that encourage students to talk about the text in relation to themselves as well as the text itself.

Wallach (1988) uses sports discourses to foster literacy in adolescent language-disabled students who have a keen interest in and knowledge of sports. In one activity, she has a group of students search for headlines from the sports section of newspapers and magazines. The headlines are used to encourage group discussion and demonstrate the role that prior knowledge

---

Intervention plans that encourage children to use background knowledge and to make inferences about what they are reading may be helpful if caution is exercised about judging right and wrong responses.

---

plays in comprehension. Wallach has students discuss the purpose of headlines. She asks the student group to outline the key points of an article from its headline. The students vote on the appropriateness and inappropriateness of guesses based on what the headline says and their knowledge of what really happened. Wallach guides students through discussions of old information (which they already knew) and new information (which appeared in the article but was previously unknown). Students have contributed headlines like "Magic Buries Celtics" (to recount the Los Angeles Lakers' defeat of the Boston Celtics, with Magic Johnson as the Lakers' star) and "Seoul Puts Best Foot Forward" (to describe the site of the 1988 Summer Olympics). Discussion of double meaning and metaphor is incorporated into the social context of the information-gathering sessions.

Many other excellent suggestions that combine oral and written activities and that encourage students to use background knowledge and experience appear in journals such as *Reading Research Quarterly, Reading Psychology, Journal of Reading*, and *Reading Teacher* and books by Irwin (1986), Kamhi and Catts (1989), and Wallach and Miller (1988).

Structure and content interactions revisited

Readers and listeners try to fit new information into the frame of reference, or schema, they already have. From Hirsch's (1987) point of view, new information has a better chance of being comprehended and retained when it is processed within a larger context or backdrop. The larger context or backdrop includes a tremendous amount of content, or world knowledge. In addition to content knowledge, proficient readers also use linguistic clues in the text to help them get and absorb critical points. "If the text is difficult, adults seem to attempt to use their structure schema . . . [to deduce what the author is trying to say]. If the text is well-structured . . . signaling appears to facilitate the ability of adults to activate and . . . focus on content strategy" (Ohlhausen & Roller, 1988, p. 86). If specific structural clues are absent, proficient readers try to make up a structure for the text by using their prior knowledge of the topic and its components (Meyer, 1984). Good fifth grade readers seem more sensitive to structural cues than poor fifth grade readers, and some language-learning–disabled students have more difficulty appreciating the conventions of the written word than their average-achieving age mates (Hahn, 1987; Scott, 1988b). Brannan, Bridge, and Winograd (1986) showed that even young readers are sensitive to story structure. They reorganized second grade basal readers and then tested children's comprehension and retention. For example, passage A represents a portion of a witch story from a basal reader:

In the grass was a little hill.
On the hill was a little house
In the little house was a little witch
On the little witch was a big hat.

Passage B is a portion of the rewritten version:

Setting: The little witch lived in a house on the hill.
　　　She had a big hat. The big hat was magic.

The content in the Brannan et al. (1986) study was held constant. Children read both versions, which were about a witch who lived in a house on a hill and used her magic hat to play with the animals near the pond. Passage B differed from passage A by virtue of its "storiness." Passage B was constructed using the Stein and Glenn (1979) story elements—setting, initiating event, internal response, attempt, consequence, and reaction. Brannan et al. (1986) found that the second grade readers in their study retained and comprehended more information from the story versions than from the basal readers. However, the children in their study were average readers who were familiar with the narrative genre. Results might differ if the study were done across cultures, as suggested by Gee (1988).

Ohlhausen and Roller (1988) used social studies stimuli to study content–structure interactions in middle and later elementary grades. The selections used in the original study were quite long and covered much information about a remote group of Pacific islands called Melanesia. The following passages are excerpts from the Melanesia passages:

1. Melanesia (content/structure version)

Melanesia is a relatively unknown country. In order to learn more about Melanesia, *we will describe both the physical and cultural geography of the country. We will first describe the physical geography of Melanesia. Specifically, we will focus on its location, then the land forms, and finally the climate. First, we will look at the location as an aspect of physical geography* [italics added]. Melanesia is an island located in the Pacific Ocean, northeast of Australia. The curving chains of islands stretches from New Guinea to the Fiji Islands. (p. 74)

2. Melanesia (content version)

Each tribe exchanged goods with other tribes such as food, animals, clay, and wooden bowls, woven mats, weapons, and even canoes. Religious ceremonies were often used to protect crops from harm or to increase their yields. Melanesia is a relatively unknown country. Some of the islands of Melanesia are large, single islands (New Britain and New Ireland), and some are made up of island groupings (The Solomon Islands and New Hebrides). Often villagers used magic to protect themselves from enemies or against villagers who failed to pay a debt or who broke a rule. (Ohlhausen & Roller, 1988, pp. 74–75)

Ohlhausen and Roller (1988) found that students below grade 7 performed better on comprehension activities when structural cues made content relations explicit. The first Melanesia passage was much easier for fifth grade students than the second passage. Seventh and ninth grade students, on the other hand, performed well on both passages. According to Ohlhausen and Roller, passage 1's content is expressed through explicit structure. The second passage appears to require more internal structuring on the part of the reader. Fifth grade students, according to Ohlhausen and Roller, are not as experienced as seventh and ninth grade students with social studies schema and expository text. They go on to say that seventh and ninth grade students have a distinct advantage over their younger peers, not because they read better, but because students in the later elementary grades study the characteristics of nations. Studying nations means studying their locations, landforms, climates, and so forth. Since they are familiar with the social studies schema, older students appear to have an easier time imposing structure on the content-

oriented selections like the second Melanesia passage than their younger schoolmates. According to Ohlhausen and Roller (1988), additional research will say more about prior knowledge, schooling, and text interactions. However, these findings show that structural sensitivity can facilitate the memory and retention for new and difficult content. Likewise, practice with content schema (like knowing the subtopics included in discussions about countries) can facilitate the processing of text that is organized poorly.

What can professionals do? They might help students recognize the distinctive structural patterns of the different discourse genres (Scott, 1988b). Westby (1985, 1988) indicates that exposing children to narratives may be a way to begin. She points out that narratives fall midway on the oral-to-literate continuum. Narratives are more formal than conversations but less formal than expository texts. Children can learn about idea units, or content schema, like physical states, physical events, internal states, goals, consequences, and so on through narratives. They can also learn how narrative structures differ from expository structures in the structure schema (Roller & Schreiner, 1985). Roller and Schreiner point out that children's sensitivity to text structure differences can be heightened by exposing them to familiar stories couched in expository structures. Piccolo (1987) provides many excellent examples of structural awareness for expository text. She shows how expository text training can improve students' organization and retention of curricular content. She also shows how content and structure training can be combined. For example, key words or phrases can be color-coded in

Children's sensitivity to text structure differences can be heightened by exposing them to familiar stories couched in expository structures.

reading texts to signal important information. Students can be asked to describe the writer's reason for writing in a particular style, and they can be asked to identify the kind of genre in which an idea has been presented (Wallach & Miller, 1988).

Armbruster, Anderson, and Ostertag (1987) also provide excellent suggestions for content and structure awareness activities. They point out that instruction in problem and solution structures, an organizational pattern commonly found in social studies textbooks, helps students organize their own writing summaries of what they have read. Professionals might consider providing some structural training before addressing summary and paraphrase, which is often required in the middle grades (Armbruster et al., 1987). Perera (1985) says that problem writers need explicit instructions in the ways in which speech and writing differ and the reasons why they differ. The idea that "almost 92% of school writing is done for the teacher as the sole audience, and that in half of all pieces of school writing, the students are being formally examined" creates a different communicative scenario than is created when one writes a spontaneous note to a friend or prepares a history essay for a statewide contest (Scott, 1988b, p. 79). Scott (1988b) reiterates Perera's notion by saying that students must understand the structural, content,

and pragmatic characteristics of different discourse genres. Many innovative suggestions are available currently. Scott (1988a, 1988b, 1989) should be consulted for indepth information about discourse genres and structure interactions in addition to the other sources referenced in this section.

KNOWING AND INTERPRETING THE RESEARCH

For professionals involved in the business of facilitating literacy in language-learning–disabled individuals, the greatest challenge is to remain both cautious and open-minded when interpreting and using research, test manuals, and intervention programs. The transition to literacy may be a difficult one for children for many reasons. An understanding of speech and print differences and the particular dilemmas related to decoding alphabetic systems can help professionals appreciate some of the difficulties encountered by young readers.

The discussion of discourse as a multilayered continuum, with unplanned and personal communication like chat at one end and impersonal and planned written language, such as speculation and argumentation on the other end, has also contributed much to the professional knowledgebase (Scott, 1988b). The age of pragmatics brought enlightenment about communication and a broadened view of children and their problems, but it is now evident that the principles and sequences gleaned from oral language development may apply to written language more indirectly than was previously thought. Indeed, whole-language approaches to reading, which encourage children to write like they talk and edit their own writing, become half-language approaches for children who have had little exposure to literate styles and who are less advanced metalinguistically (Bashir, 1988). Statements like "Phonics is an inappropriate approach to early reading," "Oral language activities should always precede written language work," and "Encourage children to write like they talk" reflect literal interpretations of complex concepts.

Understanding the supposedly simple headline "Magic Buries Pistons" requires a combination of many things—the ability to find English words in the written symbols quickly and effortlessly, an understanding of the spoken words represented by the symbols, an appreciation for metaphor, and a background knowledge of the events and people being described. Indeed, even skilled readers may be tempted to check their decoding and memory skills only to discover that the new information (Pistons) is connected to the old information, Magic Buries (Celtics), in a very special way for basketball fans from California.

REFERENCES

Allan, K.K. (1982). The development of young children's metalinguistic understanding of the word. *Journal of Experimental Child Psychology, 41*, 336–366.

Armbruster, B.B., Anderson, T.H., & Ostertag, J. (1987). Does text structure and summarizing instruction facilitate learning from expository text? *Reading Research Quarterly, 22*, 331–346.

Backman, J. (1983). The role of psycholinguistic competence in the acquisition of reading: A look at early readers. *Reading Research Quarterly, 18*, 466–479.

Bashir, A. (1988, June). *Language and literacy across the age and grade span: Clinical and educational implications.* Workshop presented at the Emerson College LLD Institute, Boston.

Blachman, B. (1984). Language analysis skills and early reading acquisition. In G.P. Wallach & K.G. Butler (Eds.), *Language learning disabilities in school-age children.* Baltimore, MD: Williams & Wilkins.

Blachman, B. (1989). Phonological awareness and word recognition: Assessment and intervention. In A.G. Kamhi & H.W. Catts (Eds.), *Reading disabilities: A developmental perspective.* Boston: College Hill/Little, Brown.

Blachowicz, C. (1986). Making connections: Alternatives to the vocabulary notebook. *Journal of Reading, 29*, 643–649.

Bradley, L., & Bryant, P.E. (1983). Categorizing sounds and learning to read: A causal connection. *Nature, 310*, 419–421.

Brannan, A.D., Bridge, C.A., & Winograd, P.N. (1986). The effects of structural variation on children's recall of basal reader stories. *Reading Research Quarterly, 21*, 91–104.

Bransford, J.D., & Johnson, M. (1973). Considerations of some problems in comprehension. In W. Chase (Ed.), *Visual information processing.* New York: Academic Press.

Catts, H.W. (1989, June). *Language basis of reading disabilities.* Workshop presented at the Emerson College LLD Institute, Boston.

Chall, J.S. (1983). *Stages of reading development.* New York: McGraw-Hill.

Fox, B., & Routh, D. (1975). Analyzing spoken language into words, syllables, and phonemes: A developmental study. *Journal of Psycholinguistic Research, 4*, 331–342.

Gee, J. (in press). Two styles of narrative construction and their linguistic and educational implications. *Discourse Processes.*

Gee, J. (1988, June). *Perspectives on literacy: Cultural and social diversity.* Workshop presented at the Emerson College LLD Institute, Boston.

German, D. (1987). Spontaneous language profiles in children with word finding problems. *Language, Speech, Hearing Services in Schools, 18*, 217–230.

Hahn, A.L. (1987). Developing a rationale for diagnosing and remediating strategic-text behaviors. *Reading Psychology, 8*, 83–92.

Hallie, K.K. (1988). The validity and reliability of phonemic awareness tests. *Reading Research Quarterly, 23*, 159–178.

Hirsch, E.D. (1987). *Cultural literacy: What every American needs to know.* Boston: Houghton-Mifflin.

Irwin, J. (1986). *Teaching Reading Comprehension*. Englewood Cliffs, NJ: Prentice-Hall.

Kail, R., & Leonard, L. (1986). Word-finding abilities of language-impaired children. *Applied Psycholinguistics, 5*, 37–49.

Kamhi, A.G., & Catts, H.W. (Eds). (1989). *Reading disabilities: A developmental perspective*. Boston: College Hill/Little, Brown.

Liberman, I. (1973). Segmentation of the spoken word and reading acquisition. *Bulletin of the Orton Society, 21*, 71–87.

Liberman, I.Y., Shankweiler, D., Camp, L., Blachman, B., & Werfelman, M. (1980). Steps toward literacy. In P. Levinson & C. Sloan (Eds.), *Auditory processing and language: Clinical and research perspectives*. New York: Grune & Stratton.

Marzano, R., Hagerty, P., Valencia, S., & DiStefano, P. (1988). *Reading diagnosis and instruction*. Englewood Cliffs, NJ: Prentice-Hall.

Meyer, B.J.E. (1984). Text dimensions and cognitive processing. In H. Mandel, N.L. Stein, & T. Trabasso (Eds.), *Learning and the comprehension of text*. Hillsdale, NJ: Erlbaum.

Miller, L. (1988, July). *Language competence and organization strategies: A framework for assessment and intervention*. Workshop presented at the Emerson College LLD Institute, Well, Holland.

Ohlhausen, M., & Roller, C. (1988). The operation of text structure and content schemata in isolation and interaction. *Reading Research Quarterly, 23*, 70–88.

Perera, K. (1985). "Do your corrections": How can children improve their writing? *Child Language Teaching and Therapy, 1*, 5–16.

Piccolo, A. (1987). Expository text structure. *The Reading Teacher, 5*, 838–847.

Roller, C.M., & Schreiner, R. (1985). The effects of narrative and expository organization instruction on sixth-grade children's comprehension of expository and narrative prose. *Reading Psychology, 6*, 27–42.

Rubin, H. (1986, August). *Linguistic awareness in relation to reading and spelling abilities*. Workshop presented at the Emerson College LLD Institute, San Diego, CA.

Scott, C.M. (1988a). A perspective on the evaluation of school children's narratives. *Language, Speech, and Hearing Services in Schools, 19*, 67–82.

Scott, C.M. (1988b). Spoken and written syntax. In M. Nippold (Ed.), *Later language development: Ages 9 through 19*. Boston: College Hill/Little, Brown.

Scott, C.M. (1989). Problem writers: Nature, assessment, and intervention. In A. Kamhi & H. Catts (Eds.), *Reading disabilities: A developmental language perspective*. Boston: Little, Brown/College Hill.

Stark, J., & Wallach, G.P. (1982). The path to a concept of language learning disabilities. In G.P. Wallach & K.G. Butler (Eds.), *Language disorders and learning disabilities*. Rockville, MD: Aspen Publishers.

Stein, N.L., & Glenn, C.G. (1979). An analysis of story comprehension in elementary school children. In R.O. Freedle (Ed.), *Advances in discourse processing: Vol. 2. New directions*. Norwood, NJ: Ablex.

Tunmer, W.E., Herman, M., & Nesdale, A.R. (1988). Metalinguistic ability and beginning reading. *Reading Research Quarterly, 23*, 134–158.

van Kleeck, A. (1984a). Metalinguistic skills: Cutting across spoken and written language and problem solving abilities. In G.P. Wallach & K.G. Butler (Eds.), *Language learning disabilities in school-age children*. Baltimore, MD: Williams & Wilkins.

van Kleeck, A. (1984b). Assessment and intervention: Does "meta" matter? In G.P. Wallach & K.G. Butler (Eds.), *Language learning disabilities in school-age children*. Baltimore, MD: Williams & Wilkins.

van Kleeck, A., & Schuele, C. (1987). Precursors to literacy: Normal development. *Topics in Language Disorders, 7*(2), 13–31.

Wallach, G.P. (1985). What do we really mean by verbal language proficiency? Higher level language learning and school performance. *Peabody Journal of Education, 62*(3), 44–60.

Wallach, G.P. (1988, July). *Prediction and inference strategies, word naming, and other meaningful connections*. Workshop presented at the Emerson College LLD Institute, Well, Holland.

Wallach, G.P. (1989). Current research as a map for language intervention in the school years. *Seminars in Speech and Language, 10*(5), 205–217.

Wallach, G.P., & Miller, L. (1988). *Language intervention and academic success*. Boston: College Hill/Little, Brown.

Warren-Leubecker, A. (1987). Competence and performance factors in word awareness and early reading. *Journal of Experimental Child Psychology, 43*, 62–80.

Westby, C. (1984). Development of narrative language abilities. In G.P. Wallach & K.G. Butler (Eds.), *Language learning disabilities in school-age children*. Baltimore, MD: Williams & Wilkins.

Westby, C. (1985). Learning to talk, talking to learn: Oral-literate language differences. In C. Simon (Ed.), *Communication skills and classroom success*. San Diego, CA: College Hill Press.

Westby, C. (1988, October). *Oral language and reading connections*. Paper presented at ASHA Weekend Workshop, Denver, CO.

Word-finding intervention for children and adolescents

Diane J. German, PhD
Professor
Holder of the Endowed Chair in Special
*   Education*
Department of Special Education
National-Louis University
Evanston, Illinois

PROBLEMS IN WORD FINDING have been observed in young children with known language disorders (Fried-Oken, 1984), in elementary and adolescent students with learning disabilities (German, 1984; Wiig & Semel, 1984), and in students with reading disorders (Wolf & Goodglass, 1986). Those definitions focused on the source describe word-finding difficulties as a disorder of either information storage or information retrieval. (See the article by Nippold in this issue.) Those definitions focused on its characteristics describe children with word-finding disorders as having difficulty retrieving specific words or producing discourse (or both) (German, 1991).

Difficulties in retrieval of specific words (e.g., character names, locations, dates, and specific facts from a story) can occur in single-word naming contexts or discourse (or both). Word finding problems in discourse (e.g., relating experiences or events) reveal a high incidence of word-finding behaviors in students' narratives (i.e., many repetitions, reformulations, substitutions, empty words, insertions, delays, and times fillers) (German, 1991). Other students

Top Lang Disord, 1992,13(1),33–50
© 1992 Aspen Publishers, Inc.

may have difficulty retrieving narrative schemata, resulting in low language productivity. These students then have problems making conversation since their discourse is so brief.

Given the negative impact of word-finding disorders on communication, it is important to provide language services to those students with word-finding difficulties. A diagnostic-remediation gap exists as implementation of intervention programs specific to word-finding difficulties has not kept pace with the recognition of this problem. Even though research investigators have reported a high incidence of word-finding difficulties in special needs populations and the standardized measures for word-finding assessment have been developed (German, 1989, 1990, 1991; see the article by Snyder and Godley in this issue), little guidance for word-finding programming has emerged in the literature. Thus, models to facilitate word-finding intervention are needed.

This article focuses on word-finding intervention for children and adolescents in a variety of contexts. First, efficacy studies and models for word-finding remediation are presented, followed by a three-fold model for word-finding intervention with general principles and specific objectives. Strategies to aid children's retrieval are highlighted, and guidelines for choosing a language curriculum and specific vocabulary are recommended.

EFFICACY STUDIES IN WORD-FINDING INTERVENTION

Efficacy studies focused on word-finding intervention in children are sparse. Those that have been conducted have contrasted elaboration with retrieval treatment procedures to enhance children's word-finding skills. In these investigations, elaboration treatment procedures provided children with a richer knowledge of the target word to aid their retrieval. In contrast, retrieval treatment approaches taught children to use phonemic, locative, and category retrieval cues to enhance their word-finding skills. Contrasting these elaboration and retrieval treatment procedures, McGregor and Leonard (1989) indicated that a word-finding treatment that combined both elaboration training and retrieval strategies was the most effective, as measured by increased accuracy on picture naming and higher recall scores in a repeated free recall task. The children they studied had both language-comprehension problems and word-finding difficulties. Similarly, Rubin, Rotella, and Schwartz (1988) reported improvement in picture-naming performance of third graders with age-appropriate language skills, after both elaborative and retrieval training (e.g., phonemic analysis, retrieval cuing, and manipulation of word segments).

Wing (1990) reported somewhat different results. She compared the effects of three treatment programs:

1. a semantic treatment to improve elaboration and organization of the semantic lexicon,
2. a phonological treatment to increase metalinguistic awareness of the phonological structure of words, and
3. a perceptual/imagery treatment that provided auditory and visual imagery cues.

Wing noted that subjects receiving the phonological and imagery treatments improved significantly in retrieving untrained targets, whereas the semantic treatment group made no significant improvement. Yet Beck, Perfetti, and McKeown (1982) reported that a treatment focused on establishing more elaborate semantic representations resulted in their subjects' improving on both receptive and expressive language tasks with trained and untrained words.

The results from these investigations indicate that specific intervention can improve word-finding skills in children. The findings are in conflict, however, regarding the appropriateness of elaborative versus retrieval approaches. In fact, some authors differ as to what they identify as representative of these remedial approaches. For example, rhyming techniques are referred to as elaboration training in one investigation (McGregor & Leonard, 1989) and as phonological treatment in another study (Wing, 1990). Similarly, category techniques used as semantic elaboration techniques in one investigation (Wing, 1990) are referred to as retrieval strategies in other investigations (McGregor & Leonard, 1989). Therefore readers need to be cautious in concluding that either elaborative or retrieval approaches are more appropriate for children with word-finding problems. Rather, it is possible that activities that provide students with information relative to the phonological and semantic specifications of words as well as strategies that enhance cues for retrieval may be beneficial in improving retrieval strength. (See also the article by Nippold in this issue.)

MODELS FOR WORD-FINDING INTERVENTION

Models for word-finding intervention in children are also sparse. Some authors have recommended that remediation models typically used with adults be applied to children (Wiig & Semel, 1980, 1984). Johnson and Myklebust (1967) have suggested, among other procedures, the facilitation of recall through word associations; word series; and visual, kinesthetic, and tactile cues.

Wiig and Becker-Caplan (1984) stress that word-finding intervention is complex, requiring juxtaposition of many variables and continuous program planning and revision. They suggest that clinicians consider students' age and diagnostic findings, as well as models of lexical storage, when planning intervention. They also recommend that clinicians determine whether students have storage or access and retrieval difficulties. They state that when there are significant delays in "concept formation and in semantic hierarchical classification" (p. 15), therapy objectives should focus on identification and elaboration of the semantic features of words. These could include grouping and categorization of words by class, contrasts of likenesses and differences of related words, and identification of the best exemplars of word categories. When a student needs help in accessing or retrieving target vocabulary, however, remediation should focus on identifying appropriate retrieval strategies, as well as on developing flexibility with these strategies. Such strategies could include accessing the motor schema and visual images associated with a target word or accessing scripts, semantic categories, and subcategories related to the target word. In contrast, for the student who exhibits word-finding difficulties in spontaneous language, they recommend that intervention focus on reducing dysfluency and revision patterns in discourse.

Finally, Segal and Wolf (in press) discuss a word-finding intervention plan directed toward increasing retrieval accuracy, fluency rate, and vocabulary elaboration among dyslexic children. Word games and language exercises (word association, verbal fluency, and rapid naming drills) are suggested to increase automaticity in retrieval rate. They recommend a child be taught to use, as needed, a pool of retrieval approaches, that is, phonological, visual, and semantic strategies. Examples include relating to words according to morphophonemic principles, definitions, personal experiences, and multiple meanings.

A WORD-FINDING INTERVENTION PROGRAM

German (1992) has developed a threefold model for word-finding intervention that considers not only word-finding remediation, but also self-advocacy instruction and compensatory programming. Built into German's Word Finding Intervention Program (WFIP) is a "real" life focus. That is, objectives set, materials used, and contexts practiced are relevant to everyday life of the student. Described next are the principles and selected objectives from the WFIP.

Intervention principles for the WFIP

Presented below are those pedagogical principles more general to the intervention program, followed by specific intervention principles for each component of the WFIP.

Principle 1—Determine the source of the word-finding problem: Difficulties in language comprehension or word retrieval

Before an intervention program in word-finding disorders is implemented it is important to try to determine the source of students' word-finding difficulties. As Nippold reports in this issue, every word in memory is thought to have both a storage strength (how well a word is learned) and a retrieval strength (how easily a word can be recalled) (Bjork & Bjork, 1992). Thus, two sources for word-finding disorders may be limitations in lexical storage and/or poor retrieval skills (Kail, Hale, Leonard, & Nippold, 1984).

On the basis of this work, hypotheses should be formulated relative to whether students have word-finding difficulties because (1) they do not have well established word meanings, which contributes to *weak storage strength*; or (2) they have word-finding problems on target words they understand, which suggests *weak retrieval strength*. To aid in this process, it is helpful to conceptualize these students as classified in one of three groups.

Group 1

The first group is represented by students with word-finding difficulties in the presence of good understanding of language (the classic definition of word-finding disorders in children and adults). This group has problems in retrieval strength or production. Children with this profile have been identified in the speech and language, learning disabilities, and reading literature. Lahey (1988) indicates that word-finding difficulties are a problem in form and Carrow-Woolfolk and Lynch (1982) indicate that they are a problem in formulation. Wiig and Semel

(1984) indicate that word-finding problems occur even when the words the children are trying to retrieve are familiar to them and easily recognized on picture vocabulary tasks. Johnson and Myklebust (1967) and Lerner (1988) also state that a word-finding difficulty is an expressive language disorder. In addition, results of investigations in the reading literature showed that it was not students' understanding of vocabulary that differentiated poor from good readers (Murphy, Pollatsek, & Well, 1988; Rubin & Liberman, 1983; Wolf & Goodglass, 1986) or learning disabled from normal learning children (German, 1979, 1984, 1985) but, rather, their word-retrieval skills.

Theoretically, students in Group 1 could manifest word-finding problems due to breakdowns at two different levels of retrieval. Research in normal memory processing is helpful in understanding the nature of these retrieval breakdowns. For example, Bjork and Bjork (1992) have identified two levels of retrieval, relative and absolute. The first step in retrieval occurs when "a given item must be discriminated from the other items associated to a given cue configuration which is a function of its strength relative to the strengths of the other cued items" (p. 60). This is identified as the "relative retrieval strength" (p. 60) of an item in memory. At the second step of retrieval the item "must be reconstructed once it is discriminated" (p. 43). Such reconstruction is a function of the "absolute retrieval strength" (p. 60) of an item in memory. Bjork and Bjork point out that such a two-step retrieval process is similar to the search-plus-recovery process in the Search of Associative Memory model of Raaijmakers and Shiffrin (1981).

Clinical observations appear to support

applications of this research to children and adolescents in this first group. For example, two different word-finding patterns, potentially representative of these levels of retrieval have been noted among these students. In the first pattern, the students indicate good target word comprehension, but manifest inconsistent word-finding facility on target words producing "in class" substitutions (barometer for compass, calculator for computer, Jefferson for Kennedy). This pattern may be more representative of a breakdown in the student's relative retrieval strength since it appears that his or her retrieval errors are the result of other words in the same category competing for selection. In fact, Bjork and Bjork (1992) indicate that the greatest challenge for accurate retrieval at the relative retrieval stage is the competition from items from the same semantic category. Therefore the superordinate, subordinate, and coordinate substitutions often observed in children with word-finding problems may be examples of this retrieval competition. Further, the observation that these students may retrieve the word correctly in other contexts as well as substitute a more abstract word (tool for drill) for the target word identifies them as a member of this category.

In the second pattern, students also know the meaning of the words they want to retrieve, but they experience difficulty because the phonological specifications of target words are not completely established for retrieval. Consider, for example, students who retrieve "cornelia" for cornucopia during a Thanksgiving presentation at school or "Themes of Geofrephy" for "Themes of Geography" in social studies class. They may know the meaning of these words on a multiple-choice test or on a picture identification task and have no difficulty repeating these words correctly on stimulation. If the phonological specifications of these target words are not well established, however, they may exhibit difficulty retrieving these multisyllabic words in spontaneous usage. This may represent a breakdown in absolute retrieval strength, revealing difficulty reconstructing the phonological schema for the target words.

Group 2

In contrast to Group 1, students in Group 2 have difficulty establishing the storage strength of words (Bjork & Bjork, 1992). (See also the article by Nippold in this issue.) These students have problems understanding language and manifest difficulties finding words they do not know or whose meanings may not be stable in long-term memory, reflecting underlying problems in language comprehension. They do not, however, show a high incidence of word-finding difficulties on words they understand. Group 2 students reveal word-finding problems stemming from "semantic problems that limit the richness of the knowledge one has stored about the word or access to this knowledge" (Smith, 1991, p. 200). Smith indicates that word-finding problems stemming from semantic difficulties include shallow word meanings, problems in reference shifting, and weak analytic and synthetic skills.

Group 3

Finally, students classified in Group 3 have difficulty establishing both the storage and retrieval strength of words (Bjork & Bjork, 1992). They have problems in understanding language and problems in retrieval of words whose meanings are

well established. As reported earlier, Kail et al. (1984) investigated language-impaired students with a composite receptive expressive/language score of 3 years 2 months below chronological age. These students demonstrated both word-finding difficulties on experimental recall tasks and were judged to have difficulties finding words due to poorly established representations in memory.

The literature cited above supports the presence of three groups of students with word-finding difficulty. Differentiating among these subgroups of students is one of the major challenges facing professionals working with language-impaired students. Although the relationship between language comprehension and production is not yet completely understood (Reed, 1986), identifying the underlying source of a student's word-finding difficulties before engaging in a language intervention program should be attempted. Intervention focused on improving lexical organization and storage is appropriate when there is evidence of significant delays in concept formation and in semantic hierarchical classification (Wiig & Becker-Caplan, 1984). Intervention of this nature is appropriate for students who manifest problems finding words due to unstable meanings in the lexicon or weak storage strength (i.e., students in Group 2) or for students who have underlying comprehension and word-retrieval difficulties (i.e., students in Group 3). Techniques of this nature would enhance the child's comprehension, but alone may not significantly improve his or her retrieval skills. Language intervention approaches that focus on both comprehension and production would be needed for these students (Johnson & Myklebust, 1967; Mann & Baer, 1971; Ruder & Smith,

1974). In fact, McGregor and Leonard (1989) report that their students (students who would be classified in Group 3) showed the greatest gains in word-finding skills when presented with a combination of elaboration and retrieval training.

Although this article focuses primarily on strategies for improving students' retrieval strength, activities for improving word knowledge and storage strength of target words are important for students who have difficulty establishing target word meanings (i.e., students in Groups 2 and 3). Wiig and Semel (1984) recommend several formats for such intervention. For increasing literal comprehension skills, they suggest using activities that contrast similarities and differences between the semantic components of target words (e.g., antonyms and synonyms), using open-ended sentences to teach the use of semantic and syntactic cues, and identifying phrases or clauses that violate "semantic referential context" (p. 207).

When teaching inferencing skills, Wallach and Miller (1988) recommend integrating oral and written language tasks. For example, strategies for drawing inferences from text might include having students relate real-life experiences to the content they are reading (Hansen & Pearson, 1983) and having students restate or rewrite text on the basis of modifications in the title, the location, and so forth (Wallach & Lee-Schachter, 1984).

Nippold (in this issue) indicates, however, that "word knowledge and storage strength alone will not ensure adequate word finding." She further states that "once a set of words has been learned . . . greater emphasis should be placed on retrieval activities" (p. 11). Therefore, for those students with word-finding disor-

ders in the presence of age-appropriate language comprehension (i.e., students in Group 1), intervention activities focused on improving retrieval skills of words the student understands would seem appropriate. The WFIP focuses primarily on intervention of this nature; it consists of activities designed to build students' retrieval strength, thus enhancing students' storage strength of target vocabulary. Such activities would also be appropriate for students in Group 3, when core vocabulary used consists of words the student understands.

Principle 2—Establish a broad-based program

Programming for children with word-finding problems must consider not only remediation, but also compensatory programming and self-advocacy instruction (German, 1992). The primary objective of the *remedial component* is to provide students with word-finding strategies and retrieval techniques that will facilitate retrieval in single-word naming contexts or in discourse. The major objective of *compensatory programming* is to modify the school and home environment, so that activities that put high demands on the student's oral retrieval can be reduced. Finally, the purpose of *self-advocacy instruction* is to help students develop adequate "executive control" of those functions related to their word-finding skills.

Principle 3—Ensure that word-finding profiles dictate intervention focus

A student's word-finding profile should determine the focus of remediation and compensatory programs. On the basis of the diagnosis, clinicians need to determine the nature of students' word-finding prob-

lems *across* retrieval contexts (i.e., retrieval problems with specific words or
discourse) and *within* retrieval contexts
(slow and fast namers versus accurate and
inaccurate namers in single-word naming
contexts; high and low language productivity versus high and low incidence of word-
finding behaviors in discourse), so that
appropriate intervention objectives can be
established. Once students' word-finding
strengths and weaknesses are determined,
an intervention program specific to the
student can be designed. Moreover, as
students' word-finding skills improve, modifications in the original intervention plans
need to be made.

Principle 4—Move from individual intervention to group work

The degree of structure used for language intervention will vary depending on
student needs and the school or clinic
setting. Lahey (1988) recommends that it
is the student's attention and learning
performance that determine the appropriate degree of structure for a particular
student. When the focus is on remediation, strategies for retrieval may need to be
presented initially in a one-to-one format.
Similarly, individual treatment may be
more appropriate initially for helping students differentiate between those situations that put the most and least stress on
their word-retrieval skills (self-advocacy
instruction). When students are focusing
on self-application of retrieval strategies in
sentences and in discourse, however, language lessons allowing for group interaction (in the clinic, classroom, school cafe-
teria, or playground) are preferable. This
model is consistent with intervention structure recommended for remediation of other
linguistic disorders (Reed, 1986).

Principle 5—Provide intervention in various settings

A variety of service delivery models
should be used when conducting intervention in word finding. Miller (1989) discusses five such models, all of which
would be appropriate at various times.

Whereas a traditional remediation format could be used for the identification
and introduction of appropriate retrieval
strategies and remedial techniques in a
clinical setting; subsequent sessions could
follow a more current format. For example, to facilitate conversations and dialogue, group work could take place in the
regular classroom during cooperative learning activities. In contrast, to meet objectives in compensatory programming, a
consultation–collaboration model (Miller,
1989) would facilitate modification of the
student's language environment.

The use of these different service delivery models may mean a modification in the
traditional role of the school clinician. As
Lahey (1988) indicates, the school clinician's role now requires adaptation to
current ideas about language intervention
in naturalistic contexts. She states, "One
cannot be isolated in a room apart from the
child's life . . . and expect them to learn
early content/form/use interactions that
will generalize to other aspects of their
lives" (p. 361). This is also the case for
many components of word-finding intervention.

Remediation components of the WFIP

The objectives for word-finding remediation will vary depending on whether the
student manifests difficulty generating discourse or retrieving specific words.

For students with word-finding problems in discourse, remediation should fo-

cus on activities that extinguish or modify inappropriate word-finding behaviors (repetitions, reformulations, substitutions, insertions, empty words, delays, and time fillers) or increase language productivity. Extinguishing or modifying inappropriate word-finding behaviors moves from self-identification of behaviors, to external modification of behaviors, to self-inhibition of behaviors. Wiig and Semel (1984) suggest that behavior-management techniques may be needed to help extinguish some distracting word-finding behaviors. They also suggest verbal elaboration activities, which focus on the ability to retrieve details in response to direct questions as well as verbal description of pictured objects and familiar events. German (1992) recommends self-instruction sequences to decrease the occurrence of inappropriate word-finding behaviors. For students with low productivity due to difficulties retrieving discourse components, German suggests that the use of guides to cue the discourse components is helpful. Such guides should be coupled with continual rehearsal of relevant discourse.

For students who have difficulty with specific words, the primary goal of remediation is to identify and teach retrieval strategies and remedial techniques that will aid a student's retrieval of single words or short phrases in both the convergent (single-word retrieval) and divergent (discourse) retrieval contexts. These strategies and techniques are applied only to words whose storage strength is well established. As indicated earlier, the focus is on elaboration of the target word's retrieval strength, which in turn will further enhance its storage strength.

The intervention principles related to remediation are described next.

Principle 1—Enhance students' retrieval strength of target words

Although students with word-finding difficulties may indicate that they comprehend the meanings of target words, they may not have adequate retrieval strength. Therefore, remediation needs to focus on the elaboration of retrieval strength. The goal is to increase retrieval accuracy and speed of target words. Remediation includes teaching retrieval cues, providing semantic attributes that differentiate target words, and establishing the phonological specification of multisyllabic target words.

Bjork and Bjork (1992) note that retrieval is cue dependent; "what we can and cannot recall at a given point in time appears to be governed by the cues that are available to us, where such "cues" may be environmental, interpersonal, emotional, or physical (body states) as well as ones that bear a direct associative relationship to the target item" (p. 36). Therefore, strategies that provide retrieval cues may help enhance the retrieval strength of target words by serving to differentiate them from other competing words in the cued set. Retrieval strategies that provide target word cues include attribute cuing (phonemic, graphemic, semantic, imagery, and gesture cuing) and associate cuing.

In addition, students are taught strategies to circumvent the word-finding block. Specifically, students are taught target word synonyms, category words, or multi-word word descriptions to be used in place of evasive target words. Finally, reflective pausing is recommended for those students who require more time to select and apply any of the above described strategies.

Other students may need techniques to

reinforce the phonological specification of difficult-to-retrieve target words. These include rehearsal only, rhythm plus rehearsal, segmenting plus rehearsal, and rapid naming. These remedial techniques increase retrieval strength of target words by increasing the frequency with which particular words have been retrieved (Bjork & Bjork, 1992). See Table 1 for a description of these strategies and techniques.

Principle 2—Identify retrieval strategies and remedial techniques appropriate for the student

The strategies and techniques used in word-finding intervention should facilitate students' retrieval. Clinicians and teachers should identify a combination of such strategies and techniques for a particular student. Random application of retrieval strategies or remedial techniques may

Table 1. Retrieval strategies and remedial techniques used in the remediation component of the Word Finding Intervention Program (WFIP) (German, 1992)

Retrieval strategies		Descriptions
Attribute cuing	Phonemic cuing	The initial sound, vowel nucleus, digraph, or syllable is used to cue the target word.
	Semantic cuing	The category name or function is used to cue the target word.
	Graphemic cuing	The graphic schema is used to cue the target word.
	Imagery cuing	A revisualization of the referent is used to cue the target word.
	Gesture cuing	The motor schema of the target word action is used to cue the target word.
Associate cuing (story for book)		An intermediate word is used to cue the target word.
Semantic alternates	Synonym/category substitutions	Semantic components (synonym or category words) are substituted for the target word.
	Multiword substitutions	Semantic components (functions or descriptions) are substituted for the target word.
Reflective pausing		Constructive use of pausing is used to reduce inaccurate competitive responses.

Remedial techniques		Descriptions
Stabilization of phonological specifications	Rehearsal	Students practice saying or writing the target words five times alone and then in five different sentences.
	Rhythm + rehearsal	Each syllable is marked with a tap during the above rehearsal of the target word.
	Segmenting + rehearsal	A line is drawn between each syllable during the above rehearsal of the target word.
Rapid naming		Students rapidly say names of and phrases with target words until their response time is reduced.

prove distracting to the student, who may then fail to learn and apply those strategies that are most helpful. This individual focus on word-finding remediation is consistent with remedial procedures recommended for other language disorders (Lahey, 1988; Reed, 1986). Ultimately, the strategy combinations that are the most successful in facilitating students' retrieval will be those that students continue to use. In summary, there are two guidelines clinicians initially can use to identify strategies potentially appropriate for a particular student: (1) the student's word-finding profile and (2) the nature and pattern of his or her target-word substitutions.

Student's Word-Finding Profile

As indicated in Principle 3, a clinician should consider a student's word-finding profile when individualizing each component of the WFIP. For example, retrieval strategies appropriate for an inaccurate namer could be drawn from the set of cuing or alternate semantic strategies or from the rehearsal techniques discussed earlier. These strategies provide retrieval cues, and highlight the phonemic specifications and semantic nature of target words, to improve retrieval accuracy. In contrast, retrieval strategies and remedial techniques for a slow namer could include semantic alternates and rapid naming (Wiig & Semel, 1984) to increase speed of retrieval.

Nature and Pattern of Student's Target Word Substitutions

The nature of a student's target word substitutions should also be considered when identifying the retrieval strategies or remedial techniques appropriate for a particular student. To determine the nature of target word substitutions, the examiner compares the substitutions with the target word. In this comparison the clinician determines what attributes of the target word are represented in the substitution and then categorizes naming errors on the basis of those attributes (German, 1989, 1990). For example, when students manifest phonemic substitutions—that is, substitute real words phonetically similar to the target word (e.g., cage, for page)—they have made a phonological encoding error (Levelt, Schriefers, Meyer, Pechmann, Vorberg, & Havinga, 1991). Here the clinician may want to provide the student with phonemic cuing strategies, such as the initial sound (p), vowel nucleus, digraph, or syllable, to help the student differentiate internally the target word (page) from competing words that have similar phonological attributes (e.g., cage). If the student's phonemic substitutions are only the initial sound or vowel nucleus (bi, bi, for binoculars) of the target word or similar sounding nonsense words (biniculus, for binoculars), however, a rehearsal technique to help stabilize the phonological specifications of target words should be used. Students who make semantic substitutions (saw for hammer, cane for crutch) reveal breakdown in lexical activation and selection (Levelt et al., 1991). The clinician then might provide functional cues ("pounding" for "hammer") or imagery cuing (visualizing a crutch, in contrast to a cane) to internally differentiate the target word from competing words in the same semantic category. For students who make semantic substitutions + self-corrections (cheek, no chin), clinicians may suggest that reflective pausing be used to help the student monitor and suppress the verbalization of competing coordinate words in his or her lexicon.

With the use of a somewhat different

approach, clinicians may want to teach the semantic-alternate strategy (e.g., providing students with additional semantic components of the target word, like synonyms, category words, or word descriptions, to use in place of target words that they are unable to retrieve). For example, this strategy could be used for those students who reveal a facility for retrieving a discourse script (e.g., I put it on my hamburger at lunch/for mustard). This semantic alternate strategy may help those students who often produce circumlocutions for target words circumvent a word-finding block without notice. Further, for the "no response" category, the clinician may want to design rapid-naming activities when the error is due to needing more time to respond, attribute cuing or rehearsal techniques if the student appears to be unable

to retrieve the phonological form, or semantic alternates if the student is unable to find the lexical match for the target word. (See Table 2 for a sample remedial lesson plan.)

Principle 3—Use relevant and thematic curriculum for word-finding remediation

The language curriculum for remediation should be based on relevant content and vocabulary drawn from the child's classroom curriculum, daily routines, recreational experiences, and home environment. Remedial lessons should be thematic with the vocabulary to be studied conceptually grouped. Vocabulary practice should consist of words drawn from three sources:

1. words that the student had difficulty retrieving

Table 2. Lesson plan for teaching application of the semantic alternate retrieval strategy used in the remediation component of the Word Finding Intervention Program (WFIP) (German, 1992)

LESSON: Semantic Alternates (Category Word Substituting)

Retrieval Context: Retrieval of specific words
Remedial Objective: Teach category word substituting for target words difficult to retrieve.
Retrieval Strategy/Remedial Technique Taught to Student: Substitute the category word for a target word that is difficult to retrieve.

Activities:
1. Indicate to the student that when he or she is having difficulty retrieving a word, it is appropriate to substitute the name of the category in which the target word would be classified.
2. With the student, identify five known and relevant words.
3. Reviewing the vocabulary list, explain that each of these words can be matched with the name of its category.
4. Have the student practice each word by verbalizing first the word and then the name of the category in which the target word is classified.
5. Have the student say a sentence for each target word, substituting the category name for the target word.
6. Have the student say each target word in three different sentences.
7. Have the student engage in a short discourse using the five words under study. (If students have difficulty, encourage them to switch to the name of the category in which the target word is classified.)
8. Repeat 1 through 7 for another set of five words.

Materials: Word lists, sentences, and discourse developed from student's word retrieval errors or content material from the classroom.

Source: Adapted from Word Finding Intervention Program (WFIP), German (1992). Used with permission of author.

2. vocabulary drawn from the student's classroom curriculum (reading, science, social studies content)
3. vocabulary drawn from home or recreational contexts

For example, lessons for elementary students could be focused on applying word-finding strategies to retrieval of art, reading, computer, science, or social studies vocabulary. Similarly, a remediation curriculum could be based on students' recreational interests. For example, for students interested in sports, football or basketball content could be the theme of word-retrieval lessons. This intervention principle is consistent with Reed's (1986) point that language content studied must be useful to the student receiving remediation.

Principle 4—Move from single word to discourse

The goal for the student with word-finding difficulties is to apply the retrieval strategies in meaningful discourse. Therefore only in initial remedial lessons in which word-finding strategies are introduced and applied do activities focus on the target vocabulary in isolation. In subsequent lessons, thematically related sentences containing that vocabulary should be developed and practiced. After this, scripts consisting of these sentences should be practiced as examples of discourse with this vocabulary.

Principle 5—Encourage ongoing rehearsal of vocabulary in isolation, sentences, and discourse

The literature on memory appears to support rehearsal to maintain retrieval strength and to enhance storage strength

of information. Bjork and Bjork (1992) indicate that the more frequently information is retrieved the more retrievable it becomes. They state, "As an overall generalization, the act of retrieving an item of information is considerably more potent in terms of facilitating its subsequent successful recall than is an additional study trial on that item" (p. 37). In addition, they indicate that the act of retrieving an item also increases that item's storage strength, which further enhances its retrieval strength.

Generalizing from this literature, it seems important that students practice and rehearse target vocabulary. Target word rehearsal in isolation should occur briefly in the beginning lessons only. It should then be followed by creating and practicing sentences with the target words and, finally, rehearsing brief narratives that contain the target vocabulary. This rehearsal should occur during the language lesson and at home. Since the research literature on memory indicates that with disuse there is a loss of access to the most recent items retrieved (Bjork & Bjork, 1992), vocabulary rehearsal should occur with both new and previously studied target vocabulary. Students should be encouraged to keep a list of such words in a notebook to use as a guide during rehearsal sessions. They should also be instructed to rehearse a planned discourse (e.g., participating in a dialogue at a basketball game) before engaging in that particular conversation.

Principle 6—Teach self-application of retrieval strategies and remedial techniques

For retrieval strategies and remedial techniques to be truly useful, students must learn to apply these aids for themselves when they are having word-finding difficulties. To facilitate self-application, cognitive-modification techniques such as self-monitoring and self-instruction are used. (A discussion of these techniques may be found in the section on self-advocacy instruction below, after Principle 7.)

Principle 7—Create carry-over activities to support generalization of strategies in the classroom and at home

At this point in remediation, students know how to apply their retrieval strategies. They now need to have experiences that will help with application of these strategies in classroom situations and at home. Two means by which this can be accomplished by the clinician are (1) to consult with classroom teachers and parents on how to monitor students' retrieval behavior in the classroom and at home and (2) to observe and instruct students in the classroom during situations in which they are required to participate in oral discussion. The role here of the clinician, classroom teacher, and parent is to serve as a visible reminder to students to apply the retrieval strategies appropriate for that language context.

Self-advocacy instruction

The purpose of self-advocacy instruction is to help students develop their executive system around their word-finding abilities. Instruction in this area is important if students are to be motivated to self-apply retrieval strategies and learn to negotiate necessary compensations in their learning environment (e.g., arrange for compensatory programming). As Ylvisaker and Szekeres (1989) indicate, "in the absence of adequate executive control, intervention that targets specific cognitive or communicative deficits is unlikely to have noteworthy generalizable effects" (p. 42).

The following components of executive functioning have been identified by these authors: "goal setting (based on an awareness of one's strengths and weaknesses), planning, self-directing and initiating, self-inhibiting, self-monitoring, self-evaluating, self-correcting, and flexible problem solving" (p. 35). The ability to carry out many of these executive functions is critical to experiencing success in word-finding remediation. These functions are thus considered in self-advocacy instruction.

In particular two cognitive-modification strategies are used to develop the executive functions necessary for self-monitoring, self-evaluating, and self-correcting. These are learning self-monitoring techniques to identify and record specific target behaviors and applying self-instruction sequences to modify target behaviors. Such strategies have been recommended for academic instruction with students who are learning disabled because they require the student to become actively involved in the teaching–learning process (Rooney & Hallahan, 1985). Activities that use self-monitoring help students become aware of their word-finding strengths and weaknesses. Self-instruction requires students to apply a sequence of self-verbalized directions to modify a specific behavior. Actively using self-instruction will help students modify or extinguish certain target behaviors as well as stabilize the self-application of retrieval strategies. As part of becoming aware of their strengths and weaknesses in oral retrieval, students are taught to identify settings (classroom, playground, home), speaking situations (group discussion, one-on-one interactions), and retrieval contexts (single word or discourse) that create the most difficulty in retrieval versus those that facilitate word retrieval. Once identified, intervention focuses on application of strategies to facilitate students' language in those contexts that are the most difficult. This includes both self-application of the retrieval strategies by the student and negotiating modification of the oral retrieval demands in the classroom with the teacher. Table 3 presents a sample lesson plan for self-advocacy programming.

Compensatory programming

Compensatory programming focuses on reducing the oral language demands placed on students at home, at school, and in recreation. The goal is to facilitate communication by temporarily circumventing students' weak retrieval areas. Modification of the language contexts facilitates students' ability to express their understanding of the content being discussed or studied. This is particularly important when trying to assess students' understanding of curricular content. For example, students with word-finding difficulties are often judged to have poor understanding when in reality they know, but are unable to express that knowledge. For these students modification of the school and home language environments needs to occur, so that they will not be judged as failing when they are actually learning. This may require modifying evaluation procedures and language formats used with these students.

Second, students with word-finding difficulties find it very frustrating to engage in a discourse with peers and adults. As Smith (1991) indicates, their word-finding difficulties can be a "lifelong source

Table 3. Lesson plan for teaching self-monitoring skills in the self-advocacy component of the Word Finding Intervention Program (WFIP) (German, 1992)

LESSON: Self-Advocacy Program

Self-Advocacy Objective: Teach student self-monitoring techniques for identification of target behaviors.
Strategy Taught to Student: Self-monitor his or her own retrieval behavior.

Activities:
1. Explain to students that they can observe their own behavior and record when and where they used specific behaviors.
2. Using a gesture behavior (raising arm or moving hand) while engaged in a discourse with the student, ask him or her to orally indicate each time you make that gesture.
3. For additional practice, choose a second behavior and ask the student this time to monitor his or her own use of that behavior. Have the student record each time he or she uses that behavior while engaged in a discourse with you.
4. Identify a gesture (target behavior) that the student typically does when he or she is having difficulty retrieving a target word. Ask the student to monitor his or her use of this target behavior at home or at school.
5. Ask the student to report his or her usage of this behavior at the next language session.

Materials: Student notebook: Self-monitoring worksheet

Source: Adapted from Word Finding Intervention Program (WFIP), German (1992). Used with permission of author.

of reading, learning and expressive difficulties" (p. 162). Their inability to express their knowledge often angers and frustrates them, causing them to withdraw from communicative contexts. When the language environment is restructured to compensate for their retrieval difficulties, however, students are more able to demonstrate their knowledge and experience a sense of achievement.

For students whose retrieval skills are better in discourse, instructional and home language environments should be modified to allow students to elaborate orally. For these students, use of convergent naming tasks, requiring the retrieval of specific facts, names, or dates at home or in school, should be minimized initially. Conversely, for those students who reveal better retrieval skills in single-word retrieval tasks, instructional, home, and recreational language environments should be restructured to minimize oral production. Oral or written frames that facilitate retrieval should be provided for those students with good convergent naming skills. For students who indicate word-finding difficulties in both language contexts, multiple-choice frames should initially be used.

For students who are slow and accurate namers, teachers should provide additional "wait time" when calling on them in class. Or, for those students who are fast and inaccurate namers, teachers should instruct students to reflect on their answers before giving a response. Finally, for the slow and inaccurate namer, the teacher should use the multiple-choice format. As students' word-finding skills improve, modifications should become less necessary.

Compensatory programming should be applied across curriculum areas. Demands for quick oral retrieval of answers should be reduced in

- language settings, such as school (e.g., classroom, playground) and non-school settings (e.g., home, recreation)
- language contexts, such as groups cooperative learning groups, play groups), and/or in individual language assignments (e.g., verbal reports)
- retrieval contexts identified as difficult by the student (single word vs. discourse).

This would include reducing retrieval demands in

- oral language activities (e.g., story telling, event relating, mathematics drills, oral discussion or oral quizzes),
- reading activities (e.g., oral reading, reading comprehension assessment through oral questioning), and
- written language activities (e.g., essays, spelling tests, examinations).

A summary of recommendations is provided in Table 4.

One material that aids children with word-finding disorders in the classroom is the advance organizer (Bloom, 1984). It consists of questions, word lists, and content materials that serve to cue students into certain aspects of forthcoming learning tasks before their implementation (Ausubel & Robinson, 1969). The organizer is helpful since it provides students with needed materials in advance which permits them to rehearse to facilitate their participation in class discussion. It also serves as a cue for retrieval during class discourse.

• • •

There is a high incidence of word-finding difficulties in children with special

Table 4. Modifications of classroom oral questioning activities used in the compensatory component of the Word Finding Intervention Program (WFIP) (German, 1992)

Word-finding profile	Content areas	Classroom activity	Recommended modifications for teacher	New materials
Difficulty retrieving specific words: inaccurate namer	All	Oral questioning	1. Use multiple-choice frames 2. Accept volunteer participation only 3. Provide target word cues (e.g., initial sound, syllable) 4. Use questions that require yes/no or true/false response	Advance organizer
Difficulty retrieving specific words: slow namer	All	Oral questioning	1. Prime student for questioning 2. Give student additional time to answer 3. Use multiple-choice frames 4. Use questions that require yes/no or true/false response	List of possible questions

Source: Adapted from Word Finding Intervention Program (WFIP), German (1992). Used with permission of author.

needs. It is not surprising that concern for this language difficulty is a central theme in programming for children with language and learning disorders. Although the implementation of intervention programs specific to this language difficulty has not kept pace with the recognition of this problem, early and direct intervention for students with word-finding difficulties is needed. The intervention recommendations presented here have been drawn from both child and adult psychological and neurological research, as well as my own clinical work with children. Although additional efficacy studies validating these procedures are necessary, clinicians are encouraged to use these intervention suggestions and document their findings. If students' word-finding disorders are not directly served, they may grow into adulthood with few strategies to aid them with their word-finding difficulties. In fact, Wiig and Becker-Caplan (1984) cautioned that "stress and increasing age may cause the language/learning-disabled speaker to lose control and flexibility in the use of productive lexical accessing strategies" (p. 16), a most undesirable outcome. It is, therefore, important that speech and language pathologists and other school personnel program directly for problems in word finding in children and adolescents.

REFERENCES

Ausubel, D., & Robinson, F. (1969). *School learning: An introduction to educational psychology.* Orlando, FL: Holt, Rinehart & Winston.

Beck, I.L., Perfetti, C.A., & McKeown, M.G. (1982). Effects of long-term vocabulary instruction of lexical access and reading comprehension. *Journal of Educational Psychology, 74,* 506–521.

Bjork, R., & Bjork, L. (1992). A new theory of disuse and an old theory of stimulus fluctuation. In A.F. Healy, S.M. Kosslyn, & R.M. Shiffrin (Eds.), *From learning processes to cognitive processes: Essays in honor of William K. Estes* (Vol. 2, pp. 35–67). Hillsdale, NJ: Erlbaum.

Bloom, B. (1984). The 2 sigma problem: The search for methods of group instruction as effective as one-to-one tutoring. *Educational Research, 13,* 4–16.

Carrow-Woolfolk, E., & Lynch, J.I. (1982). *An integrative*

approach to language disorders in children. San Diego, CA: Grune & Stratton.

Fried-Oken, M.B. (1984). *The development of naming skills in normal and language deficient children.* Unpublished doctoral dissertation, Boston University.

German, D.J. (1984). Diagnosis of word-finding disorders in children with learning disabilities. *Journal of Learning Disabilities, 17,* 353–358.

German, D.J. (1985). The use of specific semantic word categories in the diagnosis of dysnomic learning disabled children. *British Journal of Disorders of Communication, 20,* 143–154.

German, D.J. (1989). *National College of Education Test of Word Finding (TWF).* Allen, TX: DLM Teaching Resources.

German, D.J. (1990). *National College of Education Test of Adolescent/Adult Word Finding (TAWF).* Allen, TX: DLM Teaching Resources.

German, D.J. (1991). *Test of Word Finding in Discourse (TWFD).* Allen, TX: DLM Teaching Resources.

German, D.J. (1992). *Word finding intervention program (WFIP).* Unpublished manuscript.

German, D.J.N. (1979). Word-finding skills in children with learning disabilities. *Journal of Learning Disabilities, 12,* 176–181.

Hansen, J., & Pearson, P.D. (1983). An instructional study: Improving the inferential comprehension of good and poor fourth-graders. *Journal of Educational Psychology, 75,* 821–829.

Johnson, D., & Myklebust, H. (1967). *Learning disabilities: Educational principles and practices.* San Diego, CA: Grune & Stratton.

Kail, R., Hale, C.A., Leonard, L.B., & Nippold, M.A. (1984). Lexical storage and retrieval in language-impaired children. *Applied Psycholinguistics, 5,* 37–49.

Lahey, M. (1988). *Language disorders and language development.* New York, NY: Macmillan.

Lerner, J. (1988). *Learning disabilities: Theories, diagnosis, and teaching strategies.* Boston, MA: Houghton Mifflin.

Levelt, W.J.M., Schriefers, H., Meyer, A.S., Pechmann, T., Vorberg, D., & Havinga, J. (1991). The time course of lexical access in speech production: A study of picture naming. *Psychological Review, 98,* 122–142.

Mann, R.A., & Baer, D.M. (1971). The effects of receptive language training on articulation. *Journal of Applied Behavior Analysis, 4,* 291–298.

McGregor, K.K., & Leonard, L.B. (1989). Facilitating word-finding skills of language impaired children. *Journal of Speech and Hearing Disorders, 54,* 141–147.

Miller, L. (1989). Classroom-based language intervention. *Language, Speech, and Hearing Services in Schools, 20,* 153–169.

Murphy, L., Pollatsek, A., & Well, A. (1988). Developmen-tal dyslexia and word retrieval deficits. *Brain and Language, 35,* 1–23.

Raaijmakers, J.G.W., & Shiffrin, R.M. (1981). Search of associative memory. *Psychological Review, 88,* 93–134.

Reed, V. (1986). *An introduction to children with language disorders.* New York, NY: Macmillan.

Rooney, K.J., & Hallahan, D.P. (1985). Future directions for cognitive behavior modification research: The quest for cognitive change. *RASE–Remedial-and-Special-Education, 6,* 46–51.

Rubin, H., & Liberman, I. (1983). Exploring the oral and written language errors made by language disabled children. *Annals of Dyslexia, 33,* 110–120.

Rubin, H., Rotella, T., & Schwartz, L. (1988). The effect of phonological analysis training on naming performance. Unpublished manuscript.

Ruder, K.F., & Smith, M.D. (1974). Issues in language training. In R.L. Schielfelbusch, & L.L. Loyd (Eds.), *Language perspectives—Acquisition, retardation and intervention* (pp. 565–605). Baltimore, MD: University Park Press.

Segal, D., & Wolf, M. (in press). Automaticity, word-retrieval, and vocabulary development in reading disabled children. In L. Meltzer (Ed.), *Strategy assessment and instruction for students with learning disabilities: From theory to practice.* Boston, MA: Little, Brown.

Smith, C.R. (1991). *Learning disabilities: The interaction of learner, task, and setting.* Newton, MA: Allyn & Bacon.

Wallach, G., & Miller, L. (1988). *Language intervention and academic success.* Austin, TX: Pro-Ed.

Wallach, G.P., & Lee-Schachter. (1984). *Language activities for learning disabled students.* Boston, MA and Toronto, Canada: The Scarborough Board of Education.

Wiig, E.H., & Becker-Caplan, L. (1984). Linguistic retrieval strategies and word finding difficulties among children with language disabilities. *Topics in Language Disorders, 4,* 1–18.

Wiig, E.H., & Semel, E.M. (1980). *Language assessment and intervention for the learning disabled.* Columbus, OH: Charles E. Merrill.

Wiig, E.H., & Semel, E.M. (1984). *Language assessment and intervention for the learning disabled* (2nd ed.). Columbus, OH: Charles E. Merrill.

Wing, C.S. (1990). A preliminary investigation of generalization to untrained words following two treatments of children's word-finding problems. *Language, Speech, and Hearing Services in Schools, 21,* 151–156.

Wolf, M., & Goodglass, H. (1986). Dyslexia, dysnomia, and lexical retrieval: A longitudinal investigation. *Brain and Language, 28,* 154–168.

Ylvisaker, M., & Szekeres, S. (1989). Metacognitive and executive impairments in head-injured children and adults. *Topics in Language Disorders, 9,* 34–39.

Cognitive and academic instructional intervention for learning-disabled adolescents

Pearl L. Seidenberg, EdD
Associate Professor
Department of Special Education and Reading
Long Island University
Brookville, New York

TRADITIONALLY, research in the field of learning disabilities has focused on the younger school-aged student. In recent years, however, more attention has been devoted to the adolescent with learning problems. A considerable body of evidence suggests that learning disabilities are not transitory conditions that disappear after the elementary-school years. A number of studies have shown that problems in learning persist through adolescence and that many learning-disabled (LD) students are unable to cope effectively with the increasingly complex academic demands of secondary-school classrooms (Alley, Deshler, & Warner, 1979; Faford & Haubrich, 1981; Gottesman, 1979). Recent research findings have characterized the demands of secondary-school settings and identified the specific learning needs of LD adolescents (Deshler, Schumaker, & Lenz, 1984).

At the same time, the recent literature on metacognitive development has led to a

Top Lang Disord, 1988, 8(3), 56–71
© 1988 Aspen Publishers, Inc.

new understanding of the role of cognitive and language processes in learning. Effective learners are characterized as active processors, interpreters, and synthesizers of information who know how to use appropriate strategies to organize and monitor learning (Brown, 1978; Flavell, 1978). This metacognitive orientation has restructured clinicians' understanding of students with learning problems. The unitary, underlying-ability-deficit explanation (e.g., visual and auditory perceptual processing problems) of learning disabilities has been replaced by more complex notions (Forness, 1981), and the principles and procedures associated with the traditional learning-disability approach to instruction have been called into serious question (Arter & Jenkins, 1979; Larsen, Parker, & Hammill, 1982; Torgesen, 1979).

In contrast to an underlying-ability-deficit hypothesis, metacognitive research has focused attention on the importance of strategic activities for efficient learning. The learning-disabled student currently is viewed as someone who fails to spontaneously access or use task-appropriate cognitive strategies when they are needed (Brown, 1980; Sternberg & Wagner, 1982; Torgesen, 1977, 1982a). Although many learning-disabled students appear to lack the complex verbal processing and metacognitive strategies needed to meet the demands of academic settings (Bos & Filip, 1984; Wong & Wilson, 1984, Wong, 1985a), a number of intervention studies have shown that strategy instruction proves effective with these students (Brown & Palinscar, 1982, 1984; Gelzheiser, 1984; Pflaum & Pascarella, 1980; Wong & Jones, 1982).

In addition to maximizing the likelihood of improving the strategic processing of LD students through instruction and intervention, the research relating metacognitive development to academic learning has provided a conceptual framework for understanding the important factors that underlie academic performance requiring higher-order cognitive and language abilities (Baumann, 1984; Berkmire, 1985; Brown & Campione, 1979; Englert & Heibert, 1984; Williams, 1984).

The relevant research in the fields of learning disabilities and metacognition is reviewed and integrated here with the aim of establishing a conceptual base for the design of instructional interventions that can improve the learning effectiveness and academic performance of LD secondary-school students. Two major sources of information are examined: (1) the research that has focused on the learning needs of the LD adolescent, and (2) the research in metacognition that illustrates its relationship to academic learning. Implications are drawn for the improvement of instructional practices based on a metacognitive orientation.

ACADEMIC, ENVIRONMENTAL, AND INSTRUCTIONAL FACTORS

Academic deficits

While information pertaining to the academic deficits of secondary-school students with learning problems remains limited, some commonalities and some of the most enduring learning difficulties manifested by LD adolescents have been identified. An impressive body of work suggests that secondary-school LD students may be characterized as inactive learners

(Torgesen, 1982b), lacking in motivation (Adelman, 1978), exhibiting deficits in attention and automatization of functions (Sternberg & Wagner, 1982), underachieving in academic and cognitive skills (Deshler, Schumaker, & Lenz, 1984), and having poor ability to understand the varied academic demands of the secondary school (Deshler, Alley, & Carlson, 1980).

The one common characteristic found among adolescents with learning disabilities is a discrepancy between apparent ability to learn and actual academic achievement (Algozzine & Ysseldyke, 1983). This finding is not surprising in light of the federal criteria of a severe discrepancy between ability and achievement for identification of LD students (*Federal Register*, 1976). Most LD secondary-school students are reported to exhibit problems in a number of academic areas that appear to be the consequence of deficits in more complex cognitive and linguistic processing abilities. For example, many LD adolescents generally exhibit low performance in reading comprehension and composition skills even when they are compared with other low-achieving students (Warner, Schumaker, Alley, & Deshler, 1980). Also of interest is the finding that during adolescence, despite continued traditional basic skill remediation, growth in reading and writ-

---

The one common characteristic found among adolescents with learning disabilities is a discrepancy between apparent ability to learn and actual academic achievement.

---

ing reaches a plateau by the 10th grade, and achievement remains two to four years below grade-level expectancy (Deshler, Lowrey, & Alley, 1979).

A trait often cited as characteristic of LD adolescents is the inability to efficiently organize and retain information, which leads to poor test-taking and study skills (Alley, Deshler, & Warner, 1979; Lehtinan-Rogan, 1971). Also, many LD secondary-school students are reported to do poorly in note-taking, monitoring of written errors, skimming a reading passage and deriving the main points, integrating information from different sources, and listening comprehension (Carlson & Alley, 1981; Schumaker, Deshler, Alley, Warner, & Denton, 1984).

Environmental demands

An emerging issue in the field of learning disabilities is the relationship between the setting in which the individual must function and his or her disability. Therefore, the impact and demands of the classroom learning environment on the LD student need to be better understood. A number of researchers have provided information about the complex demands placed on LD students by secondary-school classroom settings.

Studies of secondary-school settings have found that the predominant classroom format used by secondary-school teachers comprises seatwork and lecture followed by some class discussion. There is little student–teacher interaction, and minimal feedback is given to students. Teachers provide few advance organizers for students that might help them listen or take notes more effectively and only infrequently check for students' understanding of instructions or content. Students are required to work independently on assignments requiring reading and writing skills.

In general, teachers expect students to have acquired the skills to function independently in a number of areas such as volunteering answers, requesting assistance, locating the correct page(s), and budgeting time without continuous monitoring. The findings indicate that to be successful in academic settings, LD students need to have a number of complex cognitive and linguistic competencies (e.g., listening, note-taking, attending, and problem-solving skills) to effectively manage the information-processing demands of the classroom (Moran, 1980; Schumaker, Warner, Deshler, & Alley, 1980; Schumaker & Deshler, 1984; Zigmond, 1978).

Instructional interventions

Findings from current research appear to document the need for instructional interventions for LD adolescents that go beyond the traditional tutorial approach for the remediation of basic skills (e.g., reading and writing) or the acquisition of subject content. The finding that LD students reach a plateau in basic skill development in the secondary grades and the general lack of data with regard to the effectiveness of the tutorial approach have brought into question the appropriateness of this approach in providing the support needed by LD students to cope with the demands of a secondary-school curriculum. While the tutorial approach may help students pass required courses, it does not appear to adequately support long-term achievement gains, nor does it help

students learn to attempt and complete tasks on their own (Schumaker, Deshler, Alley, & Warner, 1983).

Similarly, there are limitations to the compensatory approach, which attempts to modify or change the formats of instruction and/or instructional materials (e.g., taped texts, taped lectures) to facilitate the LD student's acquisition of content material. The assumption that changing the method of instruction or modifying instructional materials would affect learning has been challenged (Schumaker, Deshler, Alley, & Warner, 1983). Also, the changes required in the overall educational delivery system to implement effective compensatory procedures are cumbersome and require the cooperative efforts of administrative and instructional staff (Hartwell, Wiseman, & Van Reusen, 1979). Finally, the compensatory approach shifts the responsibility and focus for change from the student to the system and does not provide LD students with the competencies they need to cope effectively and independently with the demands of a secondary-school instructional program (Deshler & Graham, 1980).

Recently, interest has emerged in the training of task-specific cognitive strategies. A strategic processing approach to intervention has been proposed that goes beyond the traditional approaches outlined earlier. The findings of a number of intervention studies have been reported that appear to validate the effectiveness of this approach in improving the LD secondary-school student's performance on a variety of tasks. The rationale underlying the strategic processing approach is derived from a metacognitive orientation that has focused on the importance of strategic activities for learning (Brown, 1978). The learning-disabled student is viewed as someone who fails to deploy cognitive resources effectively. A number of research studies have indicated that many LD students do not spontaneously access or use task-specific cognitive strategies when they are needed (Brown, 1980; Seidenberg & Bernstein, 1986; Torgesen, 1982b; Wong, 1985b).

At the same time, a number of intervention studies have shown that when LD secondary students are taught a task-specific cognitive strategy, many can and do use the strategy effectively (Wong & Jones, 1982; Gelzheiser, 1984; Schumaker, Deshler, Alley, Warner, & Denton, 1984). Based on a metacognitive approach, a systematic instructional methodology leading to the acquisition and use of learning strategies by LD secondary-school students has been proposed. The major instructional goals are activation and engagement of the learner and direct training in the selection and use of task-specific performance strategies (Schumaker, Deshler, Alley, Warner, & Denton, 1984).

A number of training studies have demonstrated that the acquisition and use of task-specific learning strategies enabled LD secondary-school students to perform a variety of academic tasks (e.g., comprehension of text materials, monitoring of written errors, test-taking, and paraphrasing of text information) more effectively (Deshler, Alley, Warner, & Schumaker, 1981; Lee & Alley, 1981; Schumaker, Deshler, Alley, & Warner, 1983).

Furthermore, research on metacogni-tive development has led to a reconceptualization of factors that underlie academic performance requiring more complex linguistic and cognitive abilities. The next section defines metacognition and identifies some of the important metacognitive content variables that should be incorporated in instructional interventions for LD secondary-school students.

METACOGNITION AND LEARNING

Metacognition plays a vital role in learning (Wong, 1985a). The term, as used by cognitive psychologists, refers to both the knowledge and the control individuals have over their own thinking and learning. Successful learners engage in a variety of strategic behaviors that influence learning. These strategic behaviors, for example, include such things as the learner being able to determine the goal of the learning activity, his or her personal strengths and weaknesses, effective strategies to complete the learning activity, and evaluation of the implementation of the strategies (Palinscar, 1986). Metacognition in learning also involves regulation of and control over the coordination of these complex interactive factors (Brown, 1978; Dansereau, 1984; Flavell, 1978).

An important body of work on the development of metacognition has focused on the interaction of these strategic behaviors and learning from text. A metacognitive orientation to learning from text involves the learner's knowledge and control of four factors and an understanding of how these interact to produce learning. The four factors are the learner's knowledge of

1. the features of text;
2. the nature of the task;
3. the activities or strategies that need to be engaged in; and
4. his or her own learning characteristics.

Features of text

Research has identified a number of textual features that influence learning, including topic familiarity, vocabulary, clarity (i.e., style, structure, coherence), and syntax. Metacognitive research has focused on structure—the logical organization of the reading material—and found that structure influences learning even when the learner is not aware of the effects. Moreover, learning is maximized when the learner is aware of the text features and is able to consciously use these features. Conscious abilities concerning text features that have been identified as salient in learning are

- the ability to identify important idea units,
- the ability to identify organizational patterns,
- the ability to identify different levels of importance of ideas, and
- the ability to evaluate textual consis-

Metacognitive research has focused on structure—the logical organization of the reading material—and found that structure influences learning even when the learner is not aware of the effects.

tency and coherence (Baumann, 1984; Bridge, Belmore, Moskow, Cohen, & Matthews, 1984; Brown & Smiley, 1978; Englert & Hiebert, 1984; Owings, Peterson, Bransford, Morris, & Stein, 1980; Williams, 1984). Several training studies have shown that students can be taught to identify and use text structures to facilitate learning. By using techniques such as making advance organizers, searching for embedded headings, and recognizing organizational patterns, high school and college students have been trained to identify and use common expository text structures as an aid to learning (Dansereau, 1984; Richgels, McGee, Lomax, & Sheard, 1987; McGee, 1982; Pehrsson & Denner, this issue).

Nature of the task

In learning from text, the reader may have many different purposes or tasks, depending on the kinds of cognitive demands that are made. The learner must be aware of the processing and retrieval demands of the task and be able to adapt reading and studying accordingly. For example, the processes involved in locating specific information in a text differ greatly from those required to write a summary or take a test. Students' ability to skim for relevant information and their ability to read for studying (e.g., selection of suitable retrieval cues) have been examined. While developmental differences occur in the acquisition of these abilities, the findings have also indicated that good readers are more aware of processing and retrieval demands of different tasks and are better able to adapt their reading strategies to meet these demands (Brown & Campione, 1979; Kabasigawa, Ransom, & Holland, 1980; Myers & Paris, 1978; Winograd, 1984).

Activities or strategies

Metacognition also involves knowledge of what to do to repair comprehension breakdowns and to enhance storage and retrieval of information. A number of studies have looked at comprehension monitoring and repair strategies as well as study strategies. Comprehension monitoring and repair strategies are dependent on the purpose set for reading. They include storing the comprehension failure in memory with the expectation that the forward text will bring clarification; rereading the prior text; scanning the forward text; and consulting an outside source.

The strategic activities that have received the most attention are knowledge of text structure (e.g., recognition of the logical organization of text and use of advance organizers, embedded headings, self-questioning) and repair strategies such as "lookbacks" (i.e., looking back or rereading relevant sections of previously read tests). Here again, older children are more aware of these strategies and use them more effectively than younger children. Also, good readers are better than poor readers in comprehension monitoring and in repairing comprehension failures (Alessi, Anderson, & Goetz, 1979; Brown, Smiley, & Lawton, 1978; Garner & Reis, 1981; Owings, Petersen, Bransford, Morris, & Stein, 1980; Paris & Meyers, 1981).

It has been proposed that while these strategies are necessary conditions for resolving general comprehension failures, they are not sufficient for resolving specific comprehension failures for inconsistencies in text (e.g., contextual anomalies or ambiguities that result from anaphoric usage, metaphoric meanings, analogies, idioms). While students need to recognize text features and be able to use general repair strategies such as lookbacks, they also need to recognize specific comprehension breakdowns and know how to access and use specific strategies (e.g., engaging in comparative behaviors, matching equivalence of meaning among linguistic elements, generating and matching semantic attributes) for repair of comprehension failures that are a consequence of textual inconsistencies or ambiguities (Seidenberg & Bernstein, in press).

Another important area for learning is study strategies, which include underlining, self-questioning, note-taking, outlining, semantic mapping, and summarizing. Studies have found that successful training includes instruction addressing students' metacognitive awareness of text and task factors as well as information about when, where, and how a strategy should be used. (Andre & Anderson, 1978–1979; Brown & Palincsar, 1982; Palincsar & Brown, 1983; Rinehart, Stahl, & Erickson, 1986; Taylor & Beach, 1982; Wong, 1979).

Learner characteristics

Another important factor for efficient learning from text is the learner's awareness of his or her own characteristics (e.g., memory limitations, prior knowledge, motivational factors), how these characteristics affect learning, and how the learner should modify reading and studying activities based on his or her awareness of these factors.

One learner characteristic that has been studied is the awareness and ability to use prior knowledge. This concept is also consistent with the notions proposed in schema theory (Pearson & Spiro, 1980; Seidenberg, 1982). According to Rumelhart (1980), schemata—the building blocks of cognitive activity—are hypothetical knowledge structures that are similar to concepts but more inclusive. According to schema theory, learning is directly related to schema availability (e.g., prior knowledge), the ability to select schema, and the maintenance of schema. The findings of a number of studies have consistently indicated that the activation and the extent of background knowledge used during reading and studying differentiates good and poor readers (Berkmire, 1985; Bransford, Stein, Shelton, & Owings, 1980; Sullivan, 1978).

Another learner characteristic that has been examined is effectance motivation (e.g., the learner's causal attributions concerning successes and failures) and its relationship to performance behaviors and achievement outcomes. LD secondary-school students have been characterized as lacking in motivation, and this has been conceptualized in terms of causal attributions. It has been suggested that LD students' passive approach to learning is the result of their tendency not to link performance outcomes to their own efforts or abilities (Butkowsky & Willows, 1980; Dudley-Marling, Snider, & Tarver, 1982; Licht, Kistner, Ozkaragoz, Shapiro, & Clausen, 1985). It has also been proposed

that there is an explicit link between causal attributions and metacognitive development (Harter, 1982; Winograd & Niquette, this issue).

To the extent that students with learning problems are less aware of the identifiable causal factors affecting their task performance, they will be less likely to exploit these factors (e.g., accessing and/or using a strategy) and more likely to approach a task in a passive manner.

A substantial body of research evidence indicates that motivational deficits are correlates of reading problems and interfere with the development of effective strategic reading behaviors (Butkowsky & Willows, 1980; Diener & Dweck, 1980; Fowler & Peterson, 1981; Heibert, Winograd, & Danner, 1984; Johnston & Winograd, 1985; Licht, 1984; Pearl, 1982; Torgesen & Licht, 1983). A number of researchers who have examined the effects of attribution retraining on reading performance have concluded that when attribution retraining is combined with instruction in specific strategies it is most likely to result in improvements (e.g., increased effort and confidence) that will be maintained over time. In other words, it has been suggested that the retraining of attributions is more effective if it is provided within a strategic learning instructional context than if it is decontextualized (Borkowski, Peck, Reid, & Kurtz, 1983; Hallahan & Sapona, 1984; Pflaum & Pascarella, 1982).

IMPLICATIONS FOR INSTRUCTIONAL INTERVENTION

It is essential for practitioners who work with adolescent students with learning problems to enlarge the scope of their instructional practices. The research that has identified the specific learning needs of the LD adolescent, together with the research illustrating the relationship between metacognitive activities and academic learning, provides a conceptual base for the design of instruction that focuses on both the content that must be learned and on the cognitive strategies that promote efficient learning.

The major practical implications of the literature describing the specific learning needs of LD secondary-school students are that many of these students exhibit deficits in reading, writing, and studying strategies, and that these students can be taught specific cognitive strategies that will improve their academic performance. Teaching LD students to identify and use strategies that promote, monitor, and evaluate learning has a positive effect on learning outcomes. The training studies have demonstrated that LD secondary-school students can be successfully taught task-specific cognitive strategies that they subsequently are able to apply to academic materials used in regular classroom settings and enhance academic achievement as a result (Pflaum & Pascarella, 1980; Schumaker, Deshler, Alley, Warner, & Denton, 1984; Wong & Jones, 1982).

This body of work has also suggested that, in the design of instructional interventions for LD secondary-school students that encourages active processing of information, motivational factors must be considered. Motivated students are more persistent and more likely to expend the effort required to access, monitor, and evaluate strategic activities (Butkowsky & Willows, 1980). Because of the apparent

Motivated students are more persistent and more likely to expend the effort required to access, monitor, and evaluate strategic activities.

connection between motivational orientation and metacognitive development, LD students should be taught not only the cognitive strategies needed to improve task performance but also how they can control task performance and achievement outcomes through their own efforts and abilities (Harter, 1982; Licht, 1984; Winograd & Niquette, this issue).

The research on the role of metacognition in learning has identified the features of successful instructional interventions for complex academic tasks requiring strategic processing. These features include:

- heightening the learner's awareness of the task demands;
- instructing the learner in appropriate strategies to facilitate successful task completion;
- explicitly modeling the use of the strategies;
- providing guided practice and feedback regarding the application of the strategies; and
- providing instruction for generalized use of the strategies.

The box entitled "Procedure for Teaching a Cognitive Strategy for a Complex Academic Task" provides an example of an instructional sequence for teaching strategic processing skills.

Recent intervention studies with LD secondary-school students that focused on the acquisition and use of strategic pro-

**Procedure for Teaching a Cognitive Strategy
for a Complex Academic Task**

Step 1.   Introduction of strategy and performance review
The teacher explains the strategy (e.g., summarizing an expository paragraph) and students and teacher review the students'
current level of performance (e.g., pretest results).

Step 2.   Relevance of the strategy
The teacher explains why the strategy should be learned, and
students and teacher generate examples of strategy application
(e.g., note-taking from a text or classroom lecture depends on
good summarization skills).

Step 3.   Strategy description
The teacher describes how to use the strategy and provides the
students with a "help sheet" listing the steps (e.g., (a) find the
main idea and underline it, (b) replace a list of items with a
single word or phrase, (c) leave out unnecessary information, (d)
leave out repeated information, (e) write your summary, (f) reread and revise summary).

Step 4.   Model the strategy
The teacher models the use of the strategy (e.g., summarizes a
paragraph, demonstrating aloud the thinking process underlying
the separate steps). The teacher and students, as a group, model
and rehearse the use of the strategy.

Step 5.   Practice in controlled materials
The students apply the strategy to controlled practice materials
while the teacher provides prompts and corrective feedback as
necessary.

Step 6.   Evaluation
The students and teacher collect data and evaluate the students'
performance on the controlled practice materials.

Step 7.   Practice in text materials
The students apply the strategy to textbook materials used in
regular content area classrooms.

Note. Adapted from *Instructor's Guide: Integrated Reading-Writing Strategies Curriculum* by
P. L. Seidenberg, 1987, Greenvale, NY: Long Island University. Adapted with permission.

cesses and included the features outlined here have shown the effectiveness of metacognitive instruction for the enhancement of memory skills (Gelzheiser, 1984), comprehension monitoring (Pflaum & Pascarella, 1980; Wong & Jones, 1982), general reading comprehension abilities (Brown & Palincsar, 1982; Palincsar & Brown, 1984, 1986; Schumak-er, Deshler, Alley, Warner, & Denton, 1984), and spelling skills (Gerber, 1983, 1986; Wong, 1986). The following descriptions of the instructional procedures used in three recent intervention studies designed to increase text comprehension further illustrate the key features of a metacognitive approach to strategic learning.

Deshler and his colleagues have based their intervention model on a learning-strategies approach that is designed to teach LD adolescent students how to learn rather than to teach specific content (Deshler, Alley, Warner, & Schumaker, 1981; Deshler, Schumaker, & Lenz, 1984; Ellis & Lenz, 1987; Ellis, Lenz, & Sabornie, 1987; Schumaker, Deshler, Alley, Warner, & Denton, 1984). For example, it has been proposed that students should be taught techniques for organizing text material that must be memorized for a social studies test rather than teaching them the actual social studies content. An example of an intervention program designed to teach a specific learning strategy is Multipass, which was developed to enhance students' abilities to acquire information from text material.

Schumaker, Deshler, Alley, Warner, and Denton (1984) investigated the use of the Multipass strategy with junior high and high school students who were identified as learning disabled. Initially, they evaluated the students' approach to reading materials. Following this evaluation, they discussed with the students their lack of a strategic approach to studying from text. Then the teacher outlined and modeled the following steps: (a) survey the text chapter for the purpose of understanding the chapter organization and the main ideas, (b) read the questions at the end of the chapter to figure out which facts are important, and (c) reread the chapter to determine the important content and generate key questions. Initially, practice in controlled materials written at an appropriate instructional reading level was provided, followed by practice in grade-level materials with teacher feedback. Results indicated that, although none of the students used this strategy before instruction, following instruction each student could apply the strategy in ability-level textbooks as well as textbooks used in regular classrooms. Also, after they had learned the strategy, their grades on tests covering regular class text material improved markedly.

Wong and Jones (1982), working with junior high school students in the eighth and ninth grades, examined the effects of teaching LD students how to generate questions to enhance comprehension monitoring. The first stage of their instructional procedure involved teaching LD students how to identify the main ideas in text material until the students, over three consecutive days, were able to do so with 80% accuracy. In the second stage, subjects in the experimental group were taught the following steps through modeling and corrective feedback: (a) find and underline the main idea(s), (b) develop a question about the main idea(s), (c) learn the answer to the question, and (d) review the questions and answers to be sure information is understood. The LD students in the control group read the same text material to evaluate the writing for clarity and coherence. The results of the intervention program indicated that the procedures were effective for the LD experimental students, who were able to identify more main-idea units, answer more comprehensive questions correctly, and recall more relevant information than the LD control students.

In a series of intervention studies (Brown & Palincsar, 1982; Palincsar & Brown, 1984, 1986), the effects of an instructional program labeled "reciprocal teaching" were investigated. This program involved a structured dialogue between teacher and students and included instruction in four strategies (summarizing, question generating, clarifying, and predicting) and focused on the comprehension of expository text. Interventions with LD junior high school students took place over a period of 20 consecutive school days. The program was based, in part, on Vygotsky's (1978) theory of the internalization of self-guiding speech into thought and on the concept of mediated or scaffolded learning that is central to many naturally occurring teaching situations (e.g., the acquisition of language by young children) in which the adult mediates the environment to the student by framing, selecting, focusing, and elaborating experiences to produce new learning (Bruner, 1978; Feuerstein, 1980).

At first, the teacher initiated and modeled the strategies during instruction, providing guidance and encouragement to the students to participate at whatever level they could. With each subsequent day of instruction, by coaching and providing feedback, the teacher transferred more responsibility to the students. Provision was also made for daily group review of the strategies (e.g., what strategies they were learning, why they were learning them, and when they would be helpful). The results of the reciprocal teaching program indicated that with guided practice the students were able to maintain independent use of the strategies and showed significant improvement on criterion tests of reading comprehension, as well as improvement in classroom performance. Five of the six students participating in the original study reached skill levels similar to those of their normally achieving counterparts. In a follow-up study using groups of students instructed by their regular remedial teachers, the results were essentially replicated.

Although each of these intervention approaches represents a somewhat different theoretical orientation, emphasis, and application, they have a number of features in common. They all have shown that cognitive functions can be modified. Secondary-school LD students can be taught to approach learning more strategically through intervention procedures designed to provide an organized sequence of activities that have been found to promote optimal learning for academic tasks. They also have shown that the use of task-specific cognitive strategies can be generalized to improve classroom performance.

•   •   •

Metacognitive research in text processing has suggested that active learning from text involves a dynamic, interactive repertoire of activities that foster the development of comprehension abilities as well as salient metacognitive comprehension-monitoring strategies. Students must be taught to consider the four factors involved in learning from text and how these factors interact to influence learning outcomes (Brown, Campione, & Day, 1981). Specifically, students must be taught to recognize text features that influence comprehension and recall of information (e.g., the organization of text structure) and to recognize the processing and retrieval demands of a task so that they can adapt reading and studying to meet these demands (e.g., students must recognize that it is necessary to prepare differently for an essay examination than for a multiple-choice test).

General comprehension strategies (e.g., self-monitoring, drawing inferences, resolving contextual ambiguities) and specific study strategies (e.g., paraphrasing, summarizing, note-taking), as well as factors related to learner characteristics (e.g., motivational factors, and integration of prior knowledge with text information), should be addressed in instructional intervention programs designed for LD secondary-school students.

Many students with learning problems continue to be constrained by ill-defined or ineffective instructional programs that

may be as disabling as their cognitive or linguistic deficits. A metacognitive orientation, by defining both the content and the cognitive processes that will promote independent learning, provides a conceptual base on which to build instructional interventions for LD secondary-school students. Interventions based on a metacognitive orientation that address LD learners' reading and writing deficits and incorporate a teaching methodology that promotes strategic learning appear to hold the most promise for enabling LD students to become more successful learners. The development of such comprehensive intervention programs is a special challenge for practitioners who work with secondary-school students with learning handicaps.

REFERENCES

Adelman, H.S. (1978). The concept of intrinsic motivation: Implications for practice and research related to learning disabilities. *Learning Disability Quarterly, 1,* 43–54.

Alley, G.R., Deshler, D.D., & Warner, M.M. (1979). Identification of learning disabled adolescents. *Learning Disability Quarterly, 2,* 76–83.

Alessi, S.M., Anderson, T.H., & Goetz, E.T. (1979). An investigation of lookbacks during studying. *Discourse Processes, 2,* 197–212.

Algozzine, B., & Ysseldyke, J. (1983). Learning disabilities as a subset of school failure: The over sophistication of a concept. *Exceptional Children, 50,* 242–246.

Andre, M.E., & Anderson, R.I. (1978–1979). Effects of inconsistent information on text processing. *Reading Research Quarterly, 14,* 605–625.

Arter, J.A., & Jenkins, J.R. (1979). Differential diagnosis-prescriptive teaching: A clinical appraisal. *Review of Education Research, 49,* 517–555.

Baumann, J. (1984). The effectiveness of a direct instruction paradigm for teaching main idea comprehension. *Reading Research Quarterly, 20,* 93–115.

Berkmire, D.P. (1985). Text processing: The influence of text structure, background knowledge, and purpose. *Reading Research Quarterly, 20,* 314–326.

Borkowski, G.G., Peck, V.A., Reid, M., & Kurtz, B.E. (1983). Impulsivity and strategy transfer: Metamemory as mediator. *Child Development, 54,* 459–473.

Bos, C.S., & Filip, D. (1984). Comprehension monitoring in learning disabled and average students. *Journal of Learning Disabilities, 7,* 229–233.

Bransford, J.D., Stein, B.S., Shelton, T.S., & Owings, R.A. (1980). Cognition and adaptation: The importance of learning to learn. In J. Harvey (Ed.), *Cognition, social behavior and the environment.* Hillsdale, NJ: Erlbaum.

Bridge, C.A., Belmore, S.M., Moskow, S.P., Cohen, S.S., & Matthews, P.D. (1984). Topicalization and memory for main ideas in prose. *Journal of Reading Behavior, 20,* 314–326.

Brown, A.L. (1978). Knowing when, where and how to remember, a problem of meta-cognition. In R. Glaser (Ed.), *Advances in instructional psychology.* Hillsdale, NJ: Erlbaum.

Brown, A.L. (1980). Metacognitive development and reading. In R.J. Spiro, B.C. Bruce, & W.F. Brewer (Eds.), *Theoretical issues in reading comprehension.* Hillsdale, NJ: Erlbaum.

Brown A.L., & Campione, J.C. (1979). The effects of knowledge and experience on the formation of retrieval plans for studying from texts. In M.M. Grueneberg, P.E. Morris, & R.N. Sykes (Eds.), *Practical aspects of memory*. London: Academic Press.

Brown, A.L., Campione, J.C., & Day, J.D. (1981). Learning to learn: On training students to learn from texts. *Educational Researcher, 10,* 14–21.

Brown, A.L., & Palincsar, A.S. (1982). *Inducing strategic learning from texts by means of informed, self-control training* (Technical Report No. 262). Urbana, IL: University of Illinois, Center for the Study of Reading.

Brown, A.L., & Smiley, S.S. (1978). The development of strategies for studying texts. *Child Development, 49,* 1079–1088.

Brown, A.L., Smiley, S.S., & Lawton, S.C. (1978). The effects of experience on the selection of suitable retrieval cues for studying texts. *Child Development, 49,* 829–835.

Bruner, J. (1978). The role of dialogue in language acquisition. In A. Sinclair, R.J. Jaroella, & J.M. Levelt (Eds.), *The child's conception of language*. Berlin: Springer-Verlag.

Butkowsky, I.S., & Willows, D.M. (1980). Cognitive-motivational characteristics of children varying in reading ability: Evidence for learned helplessness in poor readers. *Journal of Educational Psychology, 72,* 408–422.

Carlson, T.G., & Alley, G.R. (1981). *Performance and competence of learning disabled and high-achieving high school students on essential cognitive skills* (Technical Report No. 53). Lawrence, KS: University of Kansas, Institute for Research in Learning Disabilities.

Dansereau, D.F. (1984). Learning strategy research. In S. Chapman, J. Segal, & R. Glaser (Eds.), *Thinking and learning skills* (Vol. 2). Hillsdale, NJ: Erlbaum.

Deshler, D.D., Alley, G.R., & Carlson, S.A. (1980). Learning strategies: An approach to mainstreaming secondary students with learning disabilities. *Education Unlimited, 2,* 6–11.

Deshler, D.D., Alley, G.R., Warner, M.M., & Schumaker, J.B. (1981). Instructional practices for promoting skill acquisition and generalization in severely learning disabled adolescents. *Learning Disability Quarterly, 4,* 415–421.

Deshler, D.D., & Graham, S. (1980). Tape recording educational materials for secondary handicapped students. *Teaching Exceptional Children, 12,* 52–54.

Deshler, D.D., Lowrey, N., & Alley, G.R. (1979). Programming alternatives for learning disabled adolescents. *Academic Therapy, 14,* 54–63.

Deshler, D.D., Schumaker, J.B., & Lenz, B.K. (1984). Academic and cognitive interventions for LD adolescents: Part I. *Journal of Learning Disabilities, 17,* 108–117.

Diener, C.I., & Dweck, C.S. (1980). An analysis of learned helplessness: Continuous change in performance, strategy and achievement cognitions following failure. *Journal of Personality and Social Psychology, 39,* 940–952.

Dudley-Marling, C.C., Snider, V., & Tarver, S.G. (1982). Locus of control and learning disabilities: A review and discussion. *Perceptual and Motor Skills, 54,* 503–514.

Englert, C.S., & Heibert, E.H. (1984). Children's developing awareness of text structures in expository materials. *Journal of Educational Psychology, 76,* 65–74.

Ellis, E.S., & Lenz, B.K. (1987). A component analysis of effective learning strategies for LD students. *Learning Disabilities Focus, 2,* 94–107.

Ellis, E.S., Lenz, K.B., & Sabornie, E.J. (1987). Generalization and adaptation of learning strategies to natural environments. Part 1: Critical agents. *Remedial and Special Education, 8,* 6–20.

Faford, M.B., & Haubrich, P.A. (1981). Vocational and social adjustment of learning disabled adults: A follow-up study. *Learning Disability Quarterly, 4,* 122–130.

Federal Register. (1976, November). Washington, DC: Department of Health, Education and Welfare.

Feuerstein, R. (1980). *Instrumental enrichment*. Baltimore, MD: University Park Press.

Flavell, J.H. (1978). Metacognitive development. In J.M. Scandura & C.J. Brainerd (Eds.), *Structural process theories of human behavior*. Hillsdale, NJ: Erlbaum.

Forness, S.R. (1981). Concepts of learning and behavior disorders: Implications for research and practice. *Exceptional Children, 48,* 56–64.

Fowler, J.W., & Peterson, P.L. (1981). Increasing reading persistence and altering attributional style of learned helpless students. *Journal of Educational Psychology, 73,* 251–260.

Garner, R., & Reis, R. (1981). Monitoring and resolving comprehension obstacles. *Reading Research Quarterly, 16,* 569–582.

Gelzheiser, L.M. (1984). Generalization from categorical memory tasks to prose by learning disabled adolescents. *Journal of Educational Psychology, 76,* 1126–1138.

Gerber, M.M. (1983). Learning disabilities and cognitive strategies. *Journal of Learning Disabilities, 16,* 255–260.

Gerber, M.M. (1986). Generalization of spelling strategies by LD students as a result of contingent imitation/modeling and mastery criteria. *Journal of Learning Disabilities, 19,* 530–537.

Gottesman, R.L. (1979). Follow-up of learning disabled children. *Learning Disability Quarterly, 2,* 60–69.

Hallahan, D.P., & Sapona, R. (1984). Self-monitoring of attention with learning-disabled children: Past practice and current issues. *Annual Review of Learning Disabilities, 2,* 97–101.

Harter, S. (1982). A developmental perspective on some parameters of self-regulation in children. In P. Koraly &

F.H. Kanfer (Eds.), *Self-management and behavior change: From theory to practice.* New York: Pergamon.

Hartwell, L.K., Wiseman, D.E., & Van Reusen, A. (1979). Modifying course content for mildly handicapped students at the secondary level. *Teaching Exceptional Children, 12,* 28–32.

Heibert, E.H., Winograd, P.N., & Danner, F.W. (1984). Children's attributions of failure and success for different aspects of reading. *Journal of Educational Psychology, 76,* 1139–1148.

Johnston, P.H., & Winograd, P.N. (1985). Passive failure in reading. *Journal of Reading Behavior, 4,* 279–301.

Kabasigawa, Ransom C.C., & Holland, C.J. (1980). Children's knowledge about summing. *Alberta Journal of Educational Research, 26,* 169–182.

Larsen, S.C., Parker, R.M., & Hammill, D.D. (1982). Effectiveness of psycholinguistic training. *Exceptional Children, 49,* 60–66.

Lee, P., & Alley, G.R. (1981). *Training junior high school students to use a test-taking strategy* (Research Report No. 38). Lawrence; KS: University of Kansas, Institute of Research in Learning Disabilities.

Lehtinan-Rogan, L.E. (1971). How do we teach him? In E. Schoss (Ed.), *The educator's enigma.* San Rafael, CA: Academy Therapy Publications.

Licht, B.G. (1984). Cognitive-motivational factors that contribute to the achievement of learning-disabled children. *Annual Review of Learning Disabilities, 2,* 119–126.

Licht, B., Kistner, J., Ozkaragoz, T., Shapiro, S., & Clausen, L. (1985). Causal attributions of learning disabled children: Individual differences and their implications for persistence. *Journal of Educational Psychology, 77,* 208–216.

McGee, L.M. (1982). Awareness of text structure: Effects on children's recall of expository text. *Reading Research Quarterly, 17,* 581–590.

Moran, M.R. (1980). *An investigation of the demands on oral language skills of learning disabled students in secondary classrooms* (Research Report No. 1). Lawrence, KS: University of Kansas, Institute for Research in Learning Disabilities.

Myers, M., & Paris, S.G. (1978). Children's metacognitive knowledge about reading. *Journal of Educational Psychology, 72,* 250–256.

Owings, R.A., Peterson, G.C., Bransford, J.D., Morris, C.D., & Stein, B.S. (1980). Spontaneous monitoring and regulation of learning. *Journal of Educational Psychology, 74,* 250–256.

Palincsar, A.S. (1986). Metacognitive strategy instruction. *Exceptional Children, 53,* 118–124.

Palincsar, A.S., & Brown, A.L. (1983). *Reciprocal teaching of comprehension-monitoring activities* (Technical Report No. 269). Champaign, IL: University of Illinois, Center for the Study of Reading.

Palincsar, A.S., & Brown, A.L. (1984). Reciprocal teaching of comprehension fostering and comprehension monitoring activities. *Cognition and Instruction, 1,* 117–175.

Palincsar, A.S., & Brown, A.L. (1986). Interactive teaching to promote independent learning from text. *The Reading Teacher, 39,* 771–777.

Paris, S.G., & Meyers, M. (1981). Comprehension monitoring, memory and study strategies of good and poor readers. *Journal of Reading Behavior, 13,* 7–22.

Pearl, R. (1982). Children's attributions for success and failure: A replication with a labeled learning disabled sample. *Learning Disability Quarterly, 5,* 173–176.

Pearson, P.D., & Spiro, R.J. (1980). Toward a theory of reading comprehension instruction. *Topics in Language Disorders, 1* (1), 71–88.

Pflaum, S.W., & Pascarella, E.T. (1980). Interactive effects of prior reading achievement and training in context on the reading of learning disabled children. *Reading Research Quarterly, 16,* 138–158.

Pflaum, S.W., & Pascarella, E.T. (1982). Attribution retraining for learning disabled students: Some thoughts on the practical implications of the evidence. *Learning Disability Quarterly, 5,* 422–426.

Richgels, D.G., McGee, L.M., Lomax, R.G., & Sheard, C. (1987). Awareness of four text structures: Effects of expository text. *Reading Research Quarterly, 22,* 177–196.

Rinehart, S.D., Stahl, S.A., & Erickson, L.G. (1986). Some effects of summarization training on reading and studying. *Reading Research Quarterly, 12,* 422–438.

Rumelhart, D.E. (1980). Schemata: The building blocks of cognition. In R.J. Spiro, B.C. Bruce, & W.F. Bremer (Eds.), *Theoretical issues in reading comprehension.* Hillsdale, NJ: Erlbaum.

Schumaker, J.B., Deshler, D.D., Alley, G.R., & Warner, M.M. (1983). Toward the development of an intervention model for learning disabled adolescents. *Exceptional Education Quarterly, 4,* 45–74.

Schumaker, J.B., & Deshler, D.D. (1984). Setting demand variables: A major factor in program planning for the LD adolescent. *Topics in Language Disorders, 4*(2), 22–40.

Schumaker, J., Deshler, D., Alley, G., Warner, M., & Denton, P. (1984). Multipass. A learning strategy for improving reading comprehension. *Learning Disability Quarterly, 5,* 295–304.

Schumaker, J.B., Warner, M.M., Deshler, D.D., & Alley, G.R. (1980). *An epidemiological study of learning disabled adolescents in secondary schools* (Research

Report No. 12). Lawrence, KS: University of Kansas, Institute for Research in Learning Disabilities.

Seidenberg, P.L. (1982). Implications of schemata theory for learning disabled readers. *Journal of Learning Disabilities, 15*, 352–354.

Seidenberg, P.L., & Bernstein, D.K. (1986). The comprehension of similes and metaphors by learning disabled and non-learning disabled children. *Language, Speech, and Hearing Services in the Schools, 17*, 219–229.

Seidenberg, P.L., & Bernstein, D.K. (in press). Metaphor comprehension and performance on metaphor-related language tasks: A comparison of good and poor readers. *Remedial and Special Education.*

Sternberg, R.J., & Wagner, R.K. (1982). Automatization failure in learning disabilities. *Topics in Learning and Learning Disabilities, 2*(2), 1–11.

Sullivan, J. (1978). Comparing strategies of good and poor comprehenders. *Journal of Reading, 21*, 710–715.

Taylor, B.M., & Beach, R.W. (1982). The effects of text structure instruction on middle-grade students' comprehension and production of expository text. *Reading Research Quarterly, 19*, 134–146.

Torgesen, J.K. (1977). The role of nonspecific factors in the task performance of learning disabled children. *Journal of Learning Disabilities, 12*, 514–521.

Torgesen, J.K. (1979). What shall we do with psychological processes? *Journal of Learning Disabilities, 12*, 514–521.

Torgesen, J.K. (1982a). The study of short-term memory in learning disabled children. In K. Gadow & I. Bialer (Eds.), *Advances in learning and behavioral disabilities* (Vol. 1). Greenwich, CT: JAI Press.

Torgesen, J.K. (1982b). The learning disabled child as an inactive learner: Educational implications. *Topics in Learning and Learning Disabilities, 2*(2), 45–52.

Torgesen, J.K., & Licht, B.G. (1983). The learning disabled child as an inactive learner: Retrospect and prospects. In J.D. McKinney & L. Feagans (Eds.),

Current topics in learning disabilities (Vol. 1). Norwood, NJ: Ablex.

Vygotsky, L.S. (1978). *Mind in society: The development of higher psychological processes.* Cambridge, MA: Harvard University Press.

Warner, M.M., Schumaker, J.B., Alley, G.R., & Deshler, D.D. (1980). Learning disabled adolescents in the public schools. *Exceptional Education Quarterly, 1*, 27–36.

Williams, J.P. (1984). Categorization, macrostructure, and finding the main idea. *Journal of Educational Psychology, 76*, 874–879.

Winograd, P. (1984). Strategic difficulties in summarizing texts. *Reading Research Quarterly, 21*, 404–425.

Wong, B.Y.L. (1979). Increasing retention of main ideas through questioning strategies. *Learning Disabilities Quarterly, 2*, 42–47.

Wong, B.Y.L. (1985a). Metacognition and learning disabilities. In T.G. Weller, D. Forrest, & E. Mackinnon (Eds.), *Metacognition, cognition and human performance.* New York: Academic Press.

Wong, B.Y.L. (1985b). Self-questioning instructional research. *Review of Educational Research, 55*, 227–268.

Wong, B.Y.L. (1986). A cognitive approach to teaching spelling. *Exceptional Children, 53*, 169–173.

Wong, B.Y.L., & Jones, W. (1982). Increasing metacomprehension in learning disabled and normally achieving students through self-questioning training. *Learning Disability Quarterly, 5*, 228–246.

Wong, B.Y.L., & Wilson, M. (1984). Investigating awareness of and teaching passage organization in learning disabled children. *Journal of Learning Disabilities, 17*, 477–482.

Zigmond, N. (1978). A prototype of comprehensive services for secondary students with learning disabilities. *Learning Disability Quarterly, 1*, 39–49.

Improving composition skills of inefficient learners with self-instructional strategy training

Steve Graham, EdD
Associate Professor

Karen R. Harris, EdD
Assistant Professor
Department of Special Education
University of Maryland
College Park, Maryland

WRITING IS A particularly complex and difficult task. The writer must master the dialectical properties of written English; the stylistic requirements of the various forms of written discourse; and the mechanics of handwriting, punctuation, and spelling (Bereiter & Scardamalia, 1982; Graham, 1982). Skillful writing also requires the ability to monitor and regulate the composing process. A variety of cognitive activities, including planning, translating, reviewing, and revising, must be managed and orchestrated, and the writer must be able to switch attention between these functions and a variety of mechanical and substantive concerns (Scardamalia & Bereiter, 1986). These activities require the writer to automatize a vast array of skills so that he or she can execute them with little conscious attention and focus attention on a number of ongoing and competing tasks without any serious lapses or interference (Bereiter & Scardamalia, 1982).

For writers who demonstrate disabili-

Top Lang Disord, 1987, 7(4), 66–77
©1987 Aspen Publishers, Inc.

ties, the composing process can be especially challenging. However, the writing of inefficient learners, including adolescents and young adults with reading and language disorders, can be improved by teaching them appropriate composition strategies and self-management routines that they can use independently. The writing behavior of many of these learners suggests that they use inefficient writing strategies and that they can profit from instruction aimed at improving strategic performance. Inefficient writers can, for instance, be taught strategies for maintaining active task involvement and productivity, activating a search of appropriate memory stores for writing content, facilitating advance planning, and editing and revising texts.

We have developed self-instructional strategy-training procedures for teaching composition skills to inefficient learners. These strategies can be used to supplement existing, effective procedures in order to improve writing skills and the quality of students' written language.

SELF-INSTRUCTIONAL STRATEGY TRAINING

The development of our self-instructional strategy-training approach was based on three important sources: (1) Meichenbaum's (1977) development of cognitive–behavior modification (CBM) training; (2) the concept of self-control training developed by Brown and her colleagues (Brown, Campione, & Day, 1981; Brown & Palincsar, 1982); and (3) the development and validation of the learning strategies model for severely learning disabled adolescents by researchers at the Univer-

sity of Kansas Institute for Research in Learning Disabilities (Deshler, Alley, Warner, & Schumaker, 1981; Schumaker, Deshler, Alley, & Warner, 1983). These three approaches share many characteristics; most important, each emphasizes teaching inefficient learners to use task-specific and metacognitive (self-regulation) strategies.

The CBM approach to strategy training emphasizes interactive learning between teacher and student, and responsibility for recruiting, applying, and monitoring strategies is eventually placed on the student. To develop effective use of strategies by inefficient learners, sound instructional procedures, such as initial teacher direction and modeling, active learner involvement, graduated difficulty, feedback, reinforcement, maintenance of an academic focus, and individualization, are incorporated into training.

Based on these principles and a model of normal development of self-regulation, Meichenbaum (1976, 1977) developed a strategy-training procedure referred to as *self-instructional training*. Self-instructional training is individually tailored to the student's cognitive and language capabilities, and it views the student as an active collaborator (Harris, 1985). Four basic steps are followed in self-instructional training:

1. The teacher models relevant task-specific and metacognitive strategies aloud while performing the task.
2. The student performs the task using the same or similar self-instructions given aloud, assisted at first by the teacher and then alone.
3. Overt guidance and verbalizations are slowly faded.

4. The student performs the task independently, presumably guided by covert (internal) self-instructions.

Four basic types of statements are modeled and developed to assist the student in comprehending the task, producing appropriate strategies, and using these strategies and verbalizations to mediate behavior: (a) problem definition, (b) task-appropriate and metacognitive strategies, (c) self-reinforcement, and (d) self-evaluation (including coping and error correcting).

Meichenbaum's (1977) self-instructional training provided the basis for the development and proliferation of strategy-training techniques for language-disordered and other handicapped students. Emphasis on the development of strategic and self-regulatory behaviors appears particularly appropriate for students who exhibit such characteristics as impulsivity, low productivity, an external locus of control, deficits in the production and effective application of strategies they are capable of using, and an ineffective linguistic control system (i.e., difficulty in establishing correspondence between saying and doing or in using verbalizations to guide behavior).

As Pressley and Levin (in press) noted, strategy researchers have only begun the task of creating and empirically validating interventions. However, a substantial amount of research indicates that strategy-training interventions can be highly effective across a variety of academic areas and populations. In fact, strategy-training procedures frequently enable mildly to moderately handicapped students to perform as well as their nonhandicapped peers (Harris, 1982, 1985, 1986a; Pressley & Levin, in press; Wong, 1985).

The components necessary for effective strategy training in different areas and for different populations are being rigorously researched. Brown and her colleagues (Brown et al., 1981; Brown & Palincsar, 1982) suggested that an ideal training package for students with learning problems would include skills training (including task-appropriate strategies), metacognitive training (instruction in the self-regulation of those strategies), and instruction in the significance of such activities. This approach has been labeled self-control training. Thus, our strategy-training procedures for the development of composition skills (which are based on a self-instructional training model) have incorporated additional self-regulation components, including self-determined criteria (goal setting), self-assessment, and self-reinforcement. Furthermore, the strategy-acquisition steps developed by Deshler and his colleagues (Deshler et al., 1981; Schumaker et al., 1983) to provide students with the knowledge, motivation, and practice needed to apply a skill or strategy have also been incorporated into our training procedures.

EFFECTIVENESS OF SELF-INSTRUCTIONAL STRATEGY TRAINING

Research conducted with a variety of inefficient and normal learners at different age levels has provided initial evidence that self-instructional strategy-training procedures can have a positive effect on writing performance. One area of interest to strategy researchers is the use of self-instructional procedures to increase writing output. Ballard and Glynn (1975) reported that a combination of self-assessment and self-recording had little or no effect on the narrative-writing productivity of normal third-grade students. The addition of self-determined and self-administered reinforcement, however, resulted in an increase in the students' number of sentences, number of different action words, and number of different describing words, as well as in higher quality ratings by independent judges.

In a series of experiments conducted by Hull (1981), self-monitoring plus goal setting was found to be effective in increasing the amount and frequency of journal writing done by college freshmen in both a traditional introductory writing course and a remedial writing course. Furthermore, Seabaugh and Schumaker (1981) concluded that a self-regulation package that included behavioral contracting, self-recording, self-monitoring, and self-reinforcement resulted in an increase in the number of writing assignments completed by both learning-disabled and normally achieving high school students.

Investigators at the University of Kansas Institute for Research in Learning Disabilities have developed composition strategies designed to improve the writing performance of adolescents with reading and other academic problems (Schumaker et al., 1983). Two of the strategies, one for sentence writing and one for paragraph writing, teach students to independently use a series of steps for generating a variety of types of sentences and paragraphs. The theme-writing strategy includes a heuristic for organizing and writing a five-paragraph theme. The error-monitoring strategy is a self-directed management procedure for detecting and correcting

errors of capitalization, punctuation, spelling, and overall appearance. Although not all of these strategies have been adequately validated, preliminary evidence on their effectiveness for improving the writing performance of learning-disabled adolescents is promising (Schumaker, Deshler, Alley, Warner, Clark, & Nolan, 1982).

We have also been involved in conducting a series of studies aimed at developing and validating various composition strategies with both early adolescents and elementary school students. The heuristics and self-regulatory procedures used in these studies were based on the principles presented in the previous section. In the first investigation (Harris & Graham, 1985), sixth-grade learning-disabled students with deficiencies in writing were taught to manage and regulate a five-step compositional strategy designed to increase diversity of vocabulary and the quality of their written stories. The self-instructional strategy-training program resulted in an increase in the number of different action words (verbs), number of different action helpers (adverbs), and number of different describing words (adjectives) in narratives written by these students. Moreover, the total number of words written increased, and quality ratings of the students' stories improved. Generalization from the training setting to the special education classroom was obtained, and the students' performance gains were maintained in follow-up probes.

In the second study (Graham & Harris, 1986), fifth- and sixth-grade learning-disabled students were taught self-instructional procedures designed to facilitate advance planning and promote the generation of elements commonly found in short stories (i.e., introduction of the main chracter, description of time and locale, goals and goal-directed behaviors, outcome, and reaction to consequences). Learning-disabled students generally have difficulties in these areas (Graham & MacArthur, 1987a; MacArthur & Graham, in press). Following the students' training in the use of a story grammar strategy and five steps for story writing, the number and variety of story elements they used increased, and these gains were maintained and generalized to the students' special education classroom. In addition, stories written immediately following training were judged to be superior to compositions written prior to training. Students also became more confident of their ability to write a "good" story, and, more important, strategy-trained learning-disabled students were as adept as normally achieving students in incorporating story grammar elements into their compositions.

A third study (Graham & MacArthur, 1987b) involved teaching fifth- and sixth-grade learning-disabled students a strategy for revising essays that were composed on the word processor. The strategy included a series of self-directed prompts for revising:

1. Read your essay.
2. Find the sentence that tells what you believe—is it clear?
3. Add two reasons why you believe it.
4. Scan each sentence (Does it make *sense?* Is it *connected* to your belief? Can you *add* more? *Note* errors.).
5. Make changes on the computer.
6. Reread your essay and make final changes.

Following training in the use of the revision strategy, learning-disabled students made two to five times as many revisions, and their final essays were approximately twice as long. More important, however, revised essays improved in terms of overall quality. We are currently conducting a fourth study to examine the effectiveness of a prewriting strategy for improving opinion essays written by learning-disabled students.

DESIGNING SELF-INSTRUCTIONAL STRATEGY TRAINING

Self-instructional strategy-training procedures can be applied to a variety of composition tasks and skills. However, the components and procedures illustrated here are not meant to be followed in a cookbook fashion. The selection and tailoring of components and procedures for self-instructional strategy training should be done in an individualized, flexible, and collaborative manner. Thus, the development of a new composition-strategy training intervention for language-impaired students begins with thorough task and learner analyses (Harris, 1982). These analyses are critical in determining the goals of training, selecting training tasks, and establishing the sequence of learning activities to reach the goals. Strategy and self-regulation components appropriate to the learners, tasks, and goals are then carefully selected. The introduction, acquisition, and evaluation of selected pre-skills, composition strategies, and metacognitive (self-regulatory) strategies are then designed and implemented. Evaluation of affective, behavioral, and cognitive effects takes place both throughout and after training.

Learner analysis

Characteristics of the learner that may interact with task and training requirements should be carefully considered. These may include age and maturity, cognitive capacity and capabilities (including memory and information-processing abilities), language development, learning style, tolerance for frustration, attitudes and expectancies, private speech, and initial knowledge state and strategy use. For example, students with limited cognitive capacity, younger students, and those with severe language deficiencies may require more extensive pretraining, more explicit training procedures and components (e.g., shaping, prompts, feedback), smaller training steps, or simpler strategies.

For the student with language deficits, the learner analysis must include careful consideration of the learner's receptive and expressive vocabulary, style and manner of speaking, and idiosyncratic preferences. Both the student's overall language ability level and the specific language skills (i.e., vocabulary words, concepts, etc.) necessary to master the composition strategy to be taught must be determined in order to model and develop effective self-instructions. For example, a student who cannot handle the vocabulary or complexity of a self-instruction such as

---

For the student with language deficits, the learner analysis must include careful consideration of the learner's receptive and expressive vocabulary, style and manner of speaking, and idiosyncratic preferences.

"the first thing I need to do is to decide on the main characters for my story" can be taught to use a self-instruction such as "OK, Step 1, who is my story about?". If the term *adjectives* is not appropriate for the student's vocabulary level or if learner analysis indicates that previous experiences have resulted in negative attitudes concerning the ability to understand and use such words, the phrase *describing words* can be used instead.

Task analysis

In conjunction with a careful and thorough analysis of the learner, considerable thought and attention must be given to the selection and development of the various tasks to be mastered. Instructional goals and expected outcomes must be specified in advance. Furthermore, the skills and processes targeted for instruction must be important enough to effect a reasonable change in the quality of the student's writing performance.

Once the goals of instruction are clearly determined, the strategies necessary for successful performance must be developed. We (Graham & Harris, 1986) taught students a mnemonic device that was used as a cue for generating a series of self-directed questions designed to stimulate the production of writing content for specific story elements that provided the raw material for the subsequent compositions. In addition, preskills not already in the learner's repertoire that needed to be mastered in order to learn and use the strategy were determined. Prior to teaching this strategy, we found that it was necessary to teach students labels for each of the narrative elements. Finally, the metacognitive skills that the learner needed to successfully regulate the newly learned strategy were identified. These may include, but are not limited to, self-assessment, self-reinforcement, and self-determined performance criteria.

One way to determine the skills, strategies, and cognitions (private speech, images, expectancies, etc.) necessary for successful performance of a particular task is to observe and question experts (adults or students) who are performing the task. These individuals can also be asked to report the skills, strategies, and cognitions that they employ. Moreover, those who perform poorly on the task can be observed and interviewed in order to speculate on what leads to poor performance. Cognitions and self-instruction involved in comprehending the task, the production of appropriate strategies, and the self-regulation of these strategies should all be considered (Harris, 1982).

Component development

Following the task analysis, the strategy and self-regulation components as well as the various training tasks must be developed. We have found the following steps helpful in designing specific strategies:

1. Compose a strategy that consists of a small enough number of components to be easily mastered. The exact number of components depends on the student's ability and the complexity of the task.
2. Provide students with either a mnemonic or a label for the various steps or components. For example, Graham and MacArthur (in press) used the mnemonic "SCAN" to help students remember the four steps to the following sentence-revising strategy:

(a) Does it make *sense?*, (b) Is it *connected* to my belief?, (c) Can I *add* more?, and (d) *Note errors.*
3. Take advantage of the student's existing self-management and writing skills by extending and refining strategies already in the student's repertoire.
4. Develop strategies that can be scaled upward or downward in complexity so that they can be modified according to the student's level of performance. For instance, the SCAN strategy could be extended by teaching students an additional strategy for noting errors.

Development, implementation, and evaluation

At the completion of the learner and task analyses, the preskills, composition strategies, and self-regulatory strategies necessary for the development of the targeted composition skill have been determined. Training components can now be tailored in accordance with the cognitive and language characteristics of the learners in order to utilize existing strengths and develop positive, adaptive characteristics.

Steps for introducing and integrating the components

The seven basic steps designed to introduce and integrate the selected components are presented next. Detailed descriptions of the actual use of these steps in training learning-disabled students to use a prewriting strategy for enriching and increasing vocabulary diversity can be found in Harris and Graham (1985).

Use of these steps in the teaching of creative writing is illustrated in Graham and Harris (1986).

Step 1: Pretraining

In Step 1, pretraining, training must be matched with the cognitive and language competencies of the trainees (Harris, 1982; Wong, 1985). Thus, any preskills that are necessary for learning and using the composition strategy to be taught but are not already in the learner's repertoire should be trained to mastery at this point. For example, pretraining in our vocabulary enrichment study involved instruction in the meaning and identification of action words, action helpers, and describing words. (Steps 1–7 were followed for action words first, instruction then began again at Step 1 for action helpers, and describing words were taught last.) Mastery of these concepts was necessary before Step 2 could be initiated. A simple procedure for generating a list of appropriate words ("look at a picture and list action words it makes you think of") was also taught at this point. This step was then used as part of the composition strategy taught in Step 3.

Students with language deficits may need further pretraining. This training might include vocabulary training as well as the generation and practice of self-instructions to be used in later steps. Such self-instructions may be related to either task requirements or cognitive or affective characteristics of the learner. For example, a student with a low tolerance for frustration might decide to say to himself, "Remember, getting angry makes me do poor work," or, as one of our younger students put it, "mad makes me do bad."

The student can practice using such self-instructions to help control frustration in a variety of situations as part of pretraining; these instructions can then later be incorporated into the composition-strategy training. In addition, for students whose language problems prohibit the use of overt self-instructions, alternative procedures, such as pictorial cue cards, tape-recorded self-instructions, or written self-statements, can be introduced at this point (Harris, 1982).

Step 2: Review Current Performance Levels

In Step 2, the instructor and student examine baseline data on the targeted composition skill. Negative or ineffective self-statements (e.g., "I'm no good at this," or "I hate this") and strategies the student has been producing might also be discussed. Instructor and student then discuss the goal and significance of training. This step enables the student to identify personal strengths and weaknesses, make a commitment to training, and establish motivation for change. It should be conducted in a positive, collaborative manner.

Step 3: Describe the Composition Strategy

In Step 3, composition strategy (e.g., recursive steps in prewriting or revision) is described and discussed. An understanding of the strategy is developed, and advantages of the strategy are made clear (Case, 1978; Meichenbaum, 1976).

Step 4: Model the Composition Strategy and Self-instructions

In Step 4, the instructor models the composition strategy and types of self-instructions while composing. Prompts (if any) that the student will be encouraged to use in later steps should be present. The model's performance should be matched with the student's verbal style and language ability level. The model should be natural (and enthusiastic) and should use self-statements with appropriate phrasing and inflection. After modeling the strategy, the instructor should discuss with the student the importance of the things people say to themselves while they work, and the instructor and student should identify together the types of self-instructions the teacher used (e.g., problem definition, use of strategy components, self-reinforcement). The instructor should then ask the student to generate and record his or her own self-instructions of these types and any others that he or she feels will be useful; these instructions will be used in later steps. The instructor and the student can also discuss the strategy steps and components and collaboratively decide if any changes are needed to make the procedure more efficient or effective.

Step 5: Mastery of the Composition Strategy

In Step 5, the student is required to memorize the steps in the composition strategy. Once the strategy is memorized, students can paraphrase as long as meaning remains intact. Students are required to memorize examples of each type of self-statement identified in Step 4 (in their own words).

Step 6: Controlled Practice of Strategy Steps and Self-instructions

In Step 6, we typically introduce any self-regulation components that we have determined to be appropriate. For example, students in our vocabulary enrich-

ment study (Harris & Graham, 1985) were taught to set criteria, self-assess, and self-record. These components were included to support motivation as well as generalization and maintenance of the learned strategy. The student then practices the strategy and self-instructions while performing the writing task. Interaction with and guidance from the instructor, as well as physical prompts (charts, etc.) are used as necessary. Guidance and prompts are faded over practice sessions until the student can perform independently. Initial goals are determined cooperatively, and graphic, self-recorded data are collected throughout this step (Harris, 1986b).

Step 7: Independent Performance

In Step 7, the student is instructed to use the strategy independently. Transition to covert (internal) self-instructions is encouraged. Self-regulation procedures are continued and monitored by the instructor, but can be gradually faded.

Generalization and maintenance components

Educators and speech–language pathologists are typically concerned with both the maintenance of a learned skill and its generalization across tasks (e.g., from narrative writing to persuasive writing) and settings (from the resource or training setting to the regular classroom). Harris (1982) reviewed 15 suggestions for obtaining maintenance and generalization; many of these are embedded in our seven training steps. Schumaker et al. (1983) discussed additional training steps that can be undertaken if generalization or maintenance is not achieved at the termination of strategy training. These steps include instructor and student analysis of opportunities for, and actual student use of, the strategy in the regular classroom; a behavioral contract between the instructor and student involving self-regulation of strategy use in the regular classroom; and a cooperative planning procedure developed by the special education teacher, the speech–language pathologist, and the regular classroom teacher.

Evaluation

Evaluation of strategy and skill development takes place throughout training, at the culmination of training, and in generalization and maintenance conditions. It is also important to continue assessing actual strategy use once students are performing independently; students are likely to modify the original strategies according to their perceived usefulness or cost–benefit ratio (Wong, 1985). A strategy may be subverted, becoming less effective than it was, or students may modify strategies in ways that make them more useful, powerful, or parsimonious.

Self-instructional strategy-training techniques stress the importance of affective and cognitive change and outcomes in addition to behavioral change and skill development. Certain training compo-

---

Self-instructional strategy-training techniques stress the importance of affective and cognitive change and outcomes in addition to behavioral change and skill development.

---

nents (e.g., self-statements, self-regulation components) may be aimed at producing desirable cognitive and affective changes for a particular student (this should be determined during the learner analysis). Assessment of these changes or outcomes is important and can be conducted through the use of such procedures as questionnaires, scales, interviews, observation, thought listing, and other self-report techniques (Harris, 1985).

Research has indicated that change can be targeted and achieved for important cognitive and affective learner characteristics, such as tolerance for frustration, persistence, organization, locus of control, self-efficacy, attributions, expectancies, attitudes, and emotions (Harris, 1985; Pearl, 1985; Wong, 1985). Sufficient time for training effects to appear must be allotted, as some changes may take time to manifest (Harris, 1985; Wong, 1985). Finally, student and instructor satisfaction with the strategies and training procedures should be evaluated.

GUIDELINES AND OBSERVATIONS

A few final guidelines and observations concerning training should be considered. The training steps and the content of each step are not inflexible; training steps and their content should be matched with the learner, tasks, and goals. For example, there may be no need for Step 1 in some cases, and training may begin at Step 2; or Steps 1 and 2 may be reversed. For some writing tasks (e.g., narrative writing), strategy steps can be used in a recursive manner; students may double back, reordering or repeating strategy steps, as they write. Certain components, such as the self-regulation procedures, can be presented at any of several steps.

Progression through the training steps and termination of training should be mastery or criterion based rather than time based, and booster sessions should be planned (Harris, 1982; Meichenbaum, 1983). Obviously, educators and speech–language pathologists will frequently need to develop composition strategies of their own and should take great care to determine whether a composition strategy they have devised is effective. Well-intentioned individuals may unwittingly teach strategies that do not work well (Pressley & Levin, in press).

Training can be facilitated when it is desired by the student and when the instructor has a favorable relationship with the student and an enthusiastic attitude. Difficulties and failures should be anticipated and subsumed into the training program (Meichenbaum, 1983). If students resist the use of overt self-instruction or find it embarrassing, training and practice can be done in isolation, or the student can be allowed to whisper or speak into a microphone. The student should also understand that "thinking out loud" is required only during training and that "thinking to yourself " (or "in your head") is the eventual goal.

Furthermore, training can be done successfully either individually or with small groups (Graham & Harris, 1986; Harris, 1982; Kendall, 1982). If small groups are used, self-instructions should continue to be individualized, and the guidelines presented in this article should be carefully considered.

Research continues on the components necessary for the acquisition, maintenance, and generalization of strategic behavior. It is likely that effective components differ depending on learner and task characteristics. Thus, those who design self-instructional strategy training must use a commonsense approach and monitor the results of current research.

REFERENCES

Ballard, K., & Glynn, T. (1975). Behavioral self-management in story writing with elementary school children. *Journal of Applied Behavior Analysis, 8,* 387–398.

Bereiter, C., & Scardamalia, M. (1982). From conversation to composition: The role of instruction in a development process. In R. Glaser (Ed.), *Advances in instructional psychology* (Vol. 2, pp. 1–64). Hillsdale, NJ: Erlbaum.

Brown, A.L., Campione, J.C., & Day, J.D. (1981). Learning to learn: On training students to learn from texts. *Educational Researcher, 10*(2), 14–21.

Brown, A.L., & Palincsar, A.S. (1982). Inducing strategic learning from texts by means of informed, self-control training. *Topics in Learning and Learning Disabilities, 2*(1), 1–17.

Case, R.A. (1978). A developmentally based theory and technology of instruction. *Review of Educational Research, 48,* 439–463.

Deshler, D.D., Alley, G.R., Warner, M.M., & Schumaker, J.B. (1981). Instructional practices for promoting skill acquisition and generalization in severely learning disabled adolescents. *Learning Disability Quarterly, 4,* 415–421.

Graham, S. (1982). Composition research and practice: A unified approach. *Focus on Exceptional Children, 14*(8), 1–16.

Graham, S., & Harris, K. (1986, April). *Improving learning disabled students' compositions via story grammars: A component analysis of self-control strategy training.* Paper presented at the Annual Meeting of the American Educational Research Association, San Francisco.

Graham, S., & MacArthur, C. (1987a). Written language of the handicapped. In C. Reynolds & L. Mann (Eds.), *Encyclopedia of special education* (pp. 1678–1681). New York: Wiley.

Graham, S., & MacArthur, C. (1987b). [Improving learning disabled students' skills at revising essays produced on a word processor: Self-instructional strategy training]. Unpublished raw data.

Harris, K.R. (1982). Cognitive behavior modification: Application with exceptional students. *Focus on Exceptional Children, 15*(2), 1–16.

Harris, K.R. (1985). Conceptual, methodological, and clinical issues in cognitive–behavioral assessment. *Journal of Abnormal Child Psychology, 13*, 373–390.

Harris, K.R. (1986a). The effects of cognitive–behavior modification on private speech and task performance during problem solving among learning disabled and normally achieving children. *Journal of Abnormal Child Psychology, 14*, 63–67.

Harris, K.R. (1986b). Self-monitoring of attentional behavior vs. self-monitoring of productivity: Effects on on-task behavior and academic response rate among learning disabled children. *Journal of Applied Behavior Analysis, 19*, 235–247.

Harris, K.R., & Graham, S. (1985). Improving learning disabled students' composition skills: Self-control strategy training. *Learning Disability Quarterly, 8*, 27–36.

Hull, G. (1981). Effects of self-management strategies on journal writing by college freshmen. *Research in the Teaching of English, 15*, 135–148.

Kendall, P.C. (1982). Individual versus group cognitive–behavioral self-control training: 1 year follow-up. *Behavior Therapy, 13*, 241–247.

MacArthur, C., & Graham, S. (in press). Learning disabled students' composing under three methods of text production: Handwriting, word processing, and dictation, *Journal of Special Education.*

Meichenbaum, D. (1976). Cognitive factors as determinants of learning disabilities: A cognitive–functional approach. In R. Knights & D. Bakker (Eds.), *The neuropsychology of learning disorders: Theoretical approaches* (pp. 423–442). Baltimore, MD: University Park Press.

Meichenbaum, D. (1977). *Cognitive behavior modification: An integrative approach.* New York: Plenum Press.

Meichenbaum, D. (1983). Teaching thinking: A cognitive–behavioral approach. In *Interdisciplinary voices in learning disabilities and remedial education* (pp. 1–28). Austin, TX: Pro-Ed.

Pearl, R. (1985). Cognitive–behavioral interventions for increasing motivation. *Journal of Abnormal Child Psychology, 13*, 443–454.

Pressley, M., & Levin, J.R. (in press). Elaborative learning strategies for the inefficient learner. In S.J. Ceci (Ed.), *Handbook of cognitive, social, and neuropsychological aspects of learning disabilities.* Hillsdale, NJ: Erlbaum.

Scardamalia, M., & Bereiter, C. (1986). Written composition. In M. Wittrock (Ed.), *Handbook of research on teaching* (3rd ed., pp. 778–803). New York: MacMillan.

Schumaker, J., Deshler, D., Alley, G., Warner, M., Clark, F., & Nolan, S. (1982) Error monitoring: A learning strategy for improving adolescent performance. In W.M. Cruickshank & J.W. Lerner (Eds.), *Best of ACLD* (Vol. 3, pp. 170–183). Syracuse, NY: Syracuse University Press.

Schumaker, J., Deshler, D., Alley, G., & Warner, M. (1983). Toward the development of an intervention model for learning disabled adolescents: The University of Kansas Institute. *Exceptional Educational Quarterly, 4*(1), 45–74.

Seabaugh, G., & Schumaker, J. (1981). *The effects of self-regulation training on the academic productivity of LD and NLD adolescents* (Research Report No. 37). Lawrence, KS: University of Kansas Institute for Research in Learning Disabilities.

Wong, B.Y.L. (1985). Issues in cognitive–behavioral interventions in academic skill areas. *Journal of Abnormal Child Psychology, 13*, 425–442.

Language and literacy: Participating in the conversation

Barbara Hoskins, PhD
Language/Learning Disabilities
Consultant
Pasadena, California

REDEFINING language as a social-interactive process has had important implications for those developing intervention programs for individuals with language disorders (Bates, 1976). Two issues that have had a major impact on the roles of language specialists have emerged.

First, the goal of intervention has shifted. No longer is it seen as appropriate to teach language as isolated skills. Instead, there is growing support for the notion that the end goal of language intervention should be effective conversational interaction (Larson & McKinley, 1985; Prutting, 1983). Achieving this goal requires focusing on the wide range of social, cognitive, conceptual, and linguistic skills needed for conversation and developing ways of facilitating use of these skills in the context of conversation (Blank & Marquis, 1987; Howe, 1981).

Second, it has become evident that oral language competence is inexorably linked to written language (Horowitz & Samuels, 1987; Olson, Torrance, & Hildyard, 1985).

Top Lang Disord, 1990,10(2),46–62
© 1990 Aspen Publishers, Inc.

As communicators, humans express themselves, in language, in a range of mediums. Although spoken and written language are distinct systems, they interact in intricate ways in each language learner. Disorders in oral language comprehension, auditory analysis, memory, and oral formulation interfere with performance in reading, spelling, and writing (Menyuk, 1983; Sawyer, 1985). As children move through the grades, written language disorders are often seen as the primary residual manifestations of what was initially an oral language disorder (Bashir, Kuban, Kleinman, & Scavuzzo, 1983; Bashir, Wiig, & Abrams, 1987; Wiig, 1984).

As a function of the new perspective on language, language specialists have begun to redefine their roles (Marvin, 1987). Many speech–language specialists are choosing to work with groups rather than in individual sessions so that they can facilitate effective conversational interaction (Bedrosian, 1985; Hoskins, 1987). Others are working as consultants with other educators to teach language skills needed for effective performance in the classroom (Comkowycz, Ehren, & Hayes, 1987). Catts and Kahmi (1986) point out that speech–language pathologists are playing "an integral role in the identification, assessment, and remediation of children with reading disorders" (p. 329). Increasingly, speech–language pathologists are acting as facilitators of communication in classrooms, in psychiatric hospitals, and even in courtroom settings. These new roles demand a richer, more inclusive recognition of the nature of language and increased understanding of the relationship between language and literacy.

This article (a) offers a framework for language intervention focusing on conversational interaction, (b) suggests some parallels between oral conversations and the development of literacy, and (c) offers guidelines for acting as facilitators in the development of language and literacy.

CONVERSATION AS THE CONTEXT FOR LANGUAGE LEARNING

Language is learned in the context of conversational interaction. Work by researchers such as Bates (1979), Halliday (1975), Howe (1981), Moerk (1977), and Snow (1977) has carefully delineated the nature of these interactions and has demonstrated that conversational interaction is the basis for learning oral language throughout the life span. This article explores the notion that not only oral language but also written language is learned in the context of conversation.

The major challenge for those working with individuals with language disorders is to design therapeutic contexts in which such interactive language learning will occur. In 1984, Snow, Midkiff-Borunda, Small, and Proctor provided an overview of the dilemma this design problem presents for clinicians. In reviewing the paradigmatic shift from behaviorism through psycholinguistics to sociolinguistics, they suggested that language specialists had not yet resolved how to integrate work on the various aspects of language into an integrated whole. Clinicians express this concern when they say that there is too much to focus on and that there is no consistent framework within which to work.

Snow et al. (1984) point out that one important guideline in designing intervention is the recognition that "all language is pragmatically based and that the social use of language gives rise to both the form (syntax) and meaning (content) expressed" (p. 78). The focus of intervention then shifts from sentence to conversational turn. They point to the need to establish contexts for real communication "in which partners share a topic of interest, imitations are meaningful, and meaning is continually negotiated" (p. 80). They suggest a shift of therapeutic practice toward an interactive style that facilitates natural language learning.

Recent work on written language has illustrated that reading and writing are social-interactive phenomena. There is a growing interest in how readers and writers interact as listeners and speakers in the medium of text (Horowitz & Samuels, 1987; Olson, Torrance, & Hildyard, 1985). Although some of the conventions for communicating in the written mode are different from those of spoken conversations, the principles for facilitating oral conversations may be used in developing more effective interactions in the written mode.

With a focus on reading as a social-interactive process, challenges similar to those confronting professionals working in the field of oral language arise. How does one teach the specific skills needed to be an effective reader, maintaining a focus on reading as a meaningful interactive process? To address this issue, a framework for oral language intervention will be examined and implications for an interactive approach to literacy explored.

A FRAMEWORK FOR FACILITATING CONVERSATIONAL INTERACTION

The approach to intervention described here was designed to be used to facilitate conversational interaction in language-learning disabled adolescents. It has been implemented and adapted for use with children, adults, and adolescents with a range of language disorders (Hoskins, 1988). This framework is based on the notion that language is learned in the context of conversational interaction (Wells, 1981). Intervention procedures are designed for work in small groups, so that conversation among peers can be facilitated. Sessions are organized so that participants learn a range of language skills needed to become effective conversational partners. (For a complete description of the program and its implementation strategies, see Hoskins, 1987.)

According to the conversations model, interacting in conversation involves negotiating a set of conversational moves: Introducing a topic, Maintaining a topic, Introducing a topic in an elaborated form, Extending a topic, Changing a topic, Requesting clarification, and Responding to requests for clarification (Hoskins, 1987). To make these moves appropriately, the speaker draws on a range of linguistic–conceptual and social–cognitive skills fundamental to effective conversational interaction.

Using the conversations framework for language intervention, the facilitator works with groups of participants to develop specific interactive abilities. Sessions are designed to focus on each of the seven conversational moves listed above. A series of sessions is held on introducing a topic, followed by a series of sessions on maintaining a topic. Sessions include guided conversations as well as activities to build foundation skills that are needed to use conversational moves effectively. In working on introducing a topic, for example, it may be noted that participants have difficulty using appropriate nonverbal communication to engage others in an interaction. As part of the series of sessions on introducing a topic, activities are planned to develop competence in nonverbal communication as a foundation skill for conversation.

In the conversational interaction approach, foundation skills are not taught as prerequisites to conversation, but rather are learned as needed in developing effective conversational abilities. The interface between skill building and conversation is observed in natural language learning: for example, a new term may be heard when listening to an explanation; a way to formulate questions may be noted as one observes another in conversation; and a young child practices skills in play situations and then uses the skills in other conversations (Weir, 1962). Thus, the cycle starts with conversation. As the child engages in inter-

---

In the conversational interaction approach, foundation skills are not taught as prerequisites to conversation, but rather are learned as needed in developing effective conversational abilities.

---

action, new skills are developed. These skills are then available for use in the next conversation.

Conversation group sessions consist of three parts: discussion, guided conversations, and activities to build foundation skills. During the discussion, the facilitator acts as a moderator, setting a context for the session. The facilitator greets the participants, states the purpose of the session, and engages the participants in a discussion regarding their experiences with the conversational move that will be the focal point of that session. When working on introducing a topic, for example, participants may discuss examples of times when they had difficulty knowing how to start a conversation.

The facilitator elicits topics from the group that can serve as bases for guided conversations. During these conversations, the participants are guided to develop competence in using a particular conversational move (e.g., introducing a topic). The facilitator assists by providing prompts and cues so that the participants experience effective interaction.

During guided conversations or as a result of a formal evaluation, the facilitator identifies specific foundation skills needed to build conversational competence. Activities are planned to build these skills. These activities can be selected from a range of curricular materials designed to build linguistic–conceptual and social–cognitive skills (e.g., vocabulary, syntax, turntaking, nonverbal communication skills). They may be the same activities that have been used in the past in language intervention programs; however, here they are taught in the context of developing conversational competence.

IMPLICATIONS FOR A MODEL OF WRITTEN LANGUAGE

Written language has recently been depicted as a social-interactive process similar in many ways to oral language (Horowitz & Samuels, 1987). Nystrand (1987) points out that although there is not the same kind of turntaking in written discourse as in spoken discourse, turntaking is not the essential aspect of the interaction. "Turntaking is the way conversants *accomplish* interaction, but the interaction of interest is what the turntaking accomplishes, namely *an exchange of meaning or transformation of shared knowledge*" (p. 206). He goes on to point out that "when writers do certain things and readers do certain other things, the result is the unique interaction of lucid, comprehensible text. This is why writing is no less interactive in either principle or practice than speech" (p. 207).

As with oral discourse, written discourse can be seen as an interactive process requiring a specific set of moves and a set of foundation skills. Reading can be seen as listening or engaging in a conversation with an author. Writing, on the other hand, can be described as interaction with a nonpresent audience. Although many of the foundation skills for oral language are needed for effective written language, reading and writing involve a different set of foundation skills as well as different conversational moves.

In his analysis of the differences between speaking and writing, Chafe (1985)

notes that "Written language is not a brand-new kind of language, but a kind that was founded on the resources of spoken language and that has in the meantime developed certain expanded possibilities" (p. 107). He points out that "Writing is in fact free of the constraints imposed by the limited temporal and informational capacity of focal consciousness; we have time to let our attention roam over a large amount of information and devote itself to a more deliberate organization of linguistic resources" (p. 107).

Because writing is a medium in which people can communicate with a nonpresent partner, it requires a unique set of skills. In their research on dinner table conversations, formal lectures, and written samples of letters and academic prose, Chafe and Danielewicz (1987) demonstrate that writing usually incorporates more complex sentence structure, more varied vocabulary, and different indicators of personal involvement than does spoken discourse.

In reviewing the foundation skills, it can be seen that written discourse involves additional linguistic–conceptual skills, different social–cognitive skills, and different conversational moves. In the linguistic–conceptual domain, an individual learning to read and spell must develop a level of phonological awareness appropriate to print (van Kleeck & Schuele, 1987). Moreover, print literacy involves mastery of a more extensive vocabulary and more complex sentence structure (Chafe, 1985). Memory and retrieval skills may be used differently in reading and writing (Israel, 1984). Lastly, mastery of reading and writing involves developing competence in using the discourse structure of narrative and expository text (Wallach & Miller, 1988).

The pragmatics of print literacy are also different. Since reading and writing usually involve communicating with a nonpresent partner, it is necessary to establish mutual focus in the text. Tannen (1985) points out that although written language is often described as decontextualized, the context is usually made more explicit in writing than in speaking. In writing, it is usually not possible to predict the background or beliefs of an audience; therefore, there is less room for presupposition. Nonverbal aspects of communication are expressed in handwriting or print rather than in vocal patterns. Pauses and intonation are indicated by punctuation. Stylistic variation is restricted in writing, since this is a mode of communication designed to communicate across time and space.

People develop foundation skills for language by participating in oral and literate discourses. By participating in primitive conversations, early foundation skills for oral language develop (Snow, 1977). Bruner (1975) points out that young children engage in mutual focus and joint activity with their caretakers and, during these interactions, begin to distinguish objects, actions, and agents that are the bases for lexicogrammatical speech. In his observations of 6- and 7-month-old children, Bruner reports "the most evident thing to be observed was the ubiquitousness of the mother's interpretations of the child's actions, almost inevitably taking the form of inferring the baby's intentions or other directive states" (p. 12). He points to the role of the adult as a facilitator in the language learning process. "The process is, of course, made possible by the presence of an interpreting adult who operates not so much as a corrector or reinforcer, but rather as a provider, an expander and idealizer of utterances while interacting with the child" (p. 17).

In his 1985 work, Bruner further describes the context in which language learning occurs. He notes that "language acquisition 'begins' before the child utters his first lexicogrammatical speech. It begins when mother and infant create a predictable format of interaction that can serve as a microcosm for communicating and for constituting a shared reality" (p. 31). Similarly, by being read to and by watching others read and write, children learn how to interact in the medium of written language (van Kleeck & Schuele, 1987). Moreover, by continuing to read and to write, language competence is extended. Although both normal and language-disordered children may need considerable instruction to develop specific foundation skills for reading and writing, the initial stage of literacy involves introducing them to interactions in text (Chall, 1983).

It should be noted that foundation skills

Although both normal and language-disordered children may need considerable instruction in order to develop specific foundation skills for reading and writing, the initial stage of literacy involves introducing them to interactions in text.

for mastering print are not prerequisites to literacy, but rather develop in part as a function of literate interactions. Increases in vocabulary, use of embedded phrases, and an understanding of the structure of stories and expository text are developed for the most part through reading. Chall (1983) notes "when Goethe was very old, someone asked him when he had learned to read. He reportedly answered that although he had spent a lifetime learning, he was still learning" (p. 4).

The interactive moves in written language differ somewhat from those in spoken conversation. In speaking, conversations start with introducing a topic. In writing, an author similarly chooses a topic of interest and introduces it to the reader. The topic is then developed, following the discourse structure of narrative or expository text. Lastly, the author may conclude or summarize the text. Reading begins with choosing a text. Readers may then skim texts or engage in thorough reading, depending on their purposes and levels of expertise. They may reread and take notes for future reference. Finally, they may choose other texts, thereby continuing their conversations.

Although written and oral language systems differ in some ways, the general framework for examining the relation between foundation skills and conversational interaction is of value for those interested in designing intervention from a social-interactive perspective. In this model, both oral and written language are seen as media for social interaction. A distinction is drawn between the foundation skills needed for interaction and conversational moves. Foundation skills for both spoken and written language are learned as means

to participate more effectively in spoken or written interactions.

FACILITATING LITERACY

As with oral language, when reading is taught by focusing on foundation skills in isolation, the essential purpose (i.e., interaction) is often overshadowed by concern with form (Bloom, 1978). Children who have difficulty with phonemic analysis, therefore, think that reading is essentially "sounding out the words." Although they may ultimately learn to decode relying primarily on other strategies, they may harbor the belief well into adulthood that they are not really reading unless they master phonics.

When a particular skill is taught within a context, what is taught is not only the skill itself but also its uses within that context. When reading is taught as an analytic process, children may make the assumption that reading is primarily "sound games." Similarly, if they are taught that reading is a linear process of gathering information (i.e., getting the right answer), they may find reading a tedious, slow process in which they are always in danger of "missing something."

When reading is taught as a conversation, a mode of interaction is also taught. When one enters a conversation with an author, one may enter with an expectation that there may be an opportunity—an opportunity to hear a story, an opportunity to learn about birds, an opportunity to explore together. When one does not recognize a word, there are a number of ways to "guess": guessing based on the context, recognizing the word as a whole, examining the structural components of the word, or following phonics rules to "sound it out" (Goodman & Goodman, 1977). Although beginning readers may use the latter strategy frequently, more proficient readers only rarely resort to this strategy. Instead, they recognize a large number of words by sight, guess based on the context, or use structural analysis to gain recognition (Chall, 1983).

The conversation that occurs in the medium of reading begins with a move to engage. One may have a question, an interest, an assignment. The conversation is initiated against a backdrop of already known information, questions, or assumptions. As the reader engages, he or she will need a set of foundation skills in order to interact effectively in the medium of text. These may include decoding skills as well as strategies for comprehension. Decoding skills include whole-word recognition, use of contextual cues, morphological analysis, and phonic analysis. Skills that facilitate comprehension include developing vocabulary, understanding complex syntax, recognizing the structure of narrative and expository text, and learning to assess the author's perspective.

This list is not meant to be exhaustive, but it may serve to illustrate the point that teaching reading as conversation may include teaching a set of specific skills. In this approach to facilitating literacy, however, these skills are not to be taught as prerequisite skills, but rather are taught as foundation skills for the primary task— which is engaging in the conversation.

Readers may learn to interact with texts in a variety of ways. They may learn to select texts for different purposes, much as we might select friends, teachers, social events, or classes. They may also select different strategies for interacting with different texts, such as skimming, reading thoroughly, rereading, or selecting passages that are of particular interest.

Proficient readers often demonstrate a conversational orientation to texts. They use texts to interact with authors and to construct knowledge for themselves (Chall, 1983). Students who have difficulty learning to read, however, rarely gain glimpses of this. Teaching traditionally starts by teaching foundation skills. Students who have difficulty with these skills may spend an inordinate amount of time building decoding skills and may have no opportunity to discover more about what it is to interact in the medium of text.

Teaching reading as a set of prerequisite skills is reminiscent of the ways in which oral language skills have been taught in the past. That is, specific skills were taught as part of a developmental sequence. Following mastery of a set of skills, the client or student was expected to "generalize." Unfortunately, students had not learned how to use these newfound skills in the context of conversation and often had difficulty communicating in everyday situations.

Presenting strategies for decoding and for comprehension as foundation skills allows students to develop a conversational orientation to reading. Teaching becomes a process of facilitation. The facilitator introduces the students to reading as a mode of communication in which they can find out about things that are of concern to them. Strategies are introduced to assist students in understanding how meaning is communicated through the medium of text. Students or participants may find that certain strategies are more useful to them than others, depending on their levels of expertise and their strengths and weaknesses as learners. Some may not, for example, initially be able to use phonics well. Many language-disordered children find building whole-word recognition a more usable initial strategy for accessing meaning from print. To some extent, strategies may be learned as participants read and are read to. Other skills will have to be taught in structured activities and further developed in the process of reading.

The approach to facilitating literacy suggested here is consistent with what has been observed in highly interactive classroom situations. Dudley-Marling and Rhodes (1987) provide an insightful comparison of two classrooms that demonstrates the contrast between an interactive approach and a more traditional approach to literacy. In classroom A in the Dudley-Marling and Rhodes (1987) study, the teacher read to the students and encouraged them to read to her as well as to each other. The teacher's feedback and comments during both reading and writing activities focused on meaning rather than form. Spelling and punctuation were taught after students had learned to communicate with a variety of audiences, for a range of purposes. Reading and writing were frequently within the classroom as a means of communication. In classroom B, children worked primarily on "individualized assignments designed to promote practice of written language forms such as word recognition, letter–sound correspondences, spelling, handwriting, and, occasionally, capitalization and punctuation" (pp. 48–49).

The teacher in this classroom focused her attention on form rather than meaning or use. The basal reader that was used featured rhyming words with a limited set of sound–letter relations. The teacher corrected most mispronunciations during reading. Written assignments were primarily corrected for spelling, punctuation, and handwriting. No comment was made to students on the content of their writing. Dudley-Marling and Rhodes (1987) point out that the two classrooms observed in their study taught the students "very different lessons about literacy" (p. 49). They suggested that classroom A taught them that "the use and meaning of written language, like oral language, depends upon the context of use" (p. 50). In classroom B, it was demonstrated that "written language is a matter of getting the forms right" (pp. 49–50).

Clearly, language form is important in developing language competence. Most language-disordered children do not develop adequate skills without specific instruction in foundation skills. It has been demonstrated in oral language intervention, however, that language-disordered children often do not transfer skills taught out of context to use of these skills in conversational interaction. The framework proposed here offers a means of

It has been demonstrated in oral language intervention that language-disordered children often do not use skills taught out of context in conversational interaction.

integrating work on a set of foundation skills in the context of conversational interaction.

GUIDELINES FOR ACTING AS A FACILITATOR

The process of facilitation differs from traditional teaching in several interesting ways. In what is termed traditional "teacher talk" (Mehan, 1979), the teacher controls the lesson by determining what is to be learned and the sequence in which it is to be learned. The teacher takes the central role in the process. The learner is viewed as a passive recipient of information, rather than one who constructs meaning. In facilitation, the locus of control shifts to the learner. Learning is based on the student's questions or concerns. The facilitator acts as a guide, providing a framework for the learning process, highlighting regularities, and planning activities in which the learner can develop competence.

The following three principles serve as guidelines in facilitating oral language conversation groups. These same principles are relevant in facilitating print literacy: (a) intervention is based on the participant's communication; (b) language is learned in interaction; and (c) the facilitator acts as a metalinguistic guide.

Intervention is based on the participant's communication

In facilitating conversations in spoken or written language, the focus is on the participant's interaction with the text or with a listener. Readers may read for a variety of purposes and make different

interpretations over several readings. Meaning is generated by readers, based on their backgrounds, interests, or concerns.

This is consistent with Williams's (1988) work, in which she points out that there is no main idea in the text. Instead, she explains, readers bring a range of backgrounds, concerns, and purposes to the interaction. They may, therefore, at different times, see different main points as salient.

In working with conversation groups, as well as in teaching reading or writing, one is facilitating the process of communication. The specific aspects of form may be seen as secondary to the primary goal: to communicate with another. Therefore, the content of the conversation is based on the participants' interests or concerns.

In conversation groups, topics are elicited from the group. In reading, students learn to select text based on their questions, interests, or concerns. For writing or for oral conversations, students can learn to brainstorm a set of topics, to choose one of interest, and then to elaborate on relevant aspects of the topic to include in the text.

Once a topic is selected, the facilitator may assist the group in exploring different aspects of the topic. Pehrsson and Denner (1988, 1989) suggest using semantic organizers or schemata to generate meaningful relationships among concepts for reading or writing. These schemata can similarly be used to explore relationships among topics for conversation. Pehrsson and Denner (1988) suggest drawing or organizing topics in a cluster around a central topic or sketching out a sequential series of episodes. For the most part, the cluster format is most useful for organizing expository text, whereas episodic structure is used most commonly for narratives. Brainstorming topics related in a cluster or organizing topics in an episodic schema can also prepare participants to tell a story as part of a conversation, to maintain a topic, or to extend from one topic to another logically related topic in conversation.

Throughout guided conversations, participants are assisted in communicating what they have to say. They are not corrected by the facilitator or by other participants. The facilitator may assist in the delivery of the message by postscript modeling (Duchan & Weitzner-Lin, 1987). Using the postscript modeling strategy, the facilitator follows the communicator's message with a corrected version but does not interfere with the communication or ask that his or her model be repeated. The facilitator may note that participants need work on specific foundation skills and plan activities to build these skills. Similarly, if participants are misinformed, they are not corrected in the midst of the conversation. Rather, they are allowed to complete their communications with the other participants. The facilitator's role is to assist in that communication.

Similarly, in writing, communication is primary. Participants are assisted in generating topics, using brainstorming as described earlier. They may be taught foundation skills to organize a story or expository text. They are encouraged to formulate their communications using a mode that is accessible to them. This may be by using pencil and paper, by typing into a computer, or by dictating to another and later copying the text. Writing is initially read to interpret the intended communication. Suggestions can then be made to assist the writer to communicate more effectively with a nonpresent listener or reader.

Language is learned in interaction

One of the basic assumptions of the approach described above is that language is the means by which we interact. It is therefore learned in the process of interaction. In his work on discourse comprehension, Kintsch (1988) contends that texts are understood through a construction–integration process in which participants integrate what they read with their available networks of knowledge. In conversation, both listener and speaker are active participants in this process. Listeners are not passive "receivers" of information, but rather construct meaning based on an interaction between what they hear and their backgrounds or experiences.

The constructive process that Kintsch (1988) talks about requires that the reader, or listener, makes predictions, anticipates outcomes, and searches actively for related patterns. In conversations, we have the experience that someone is listening when we recognize signs of these interactive processes—head nods, eye gaze, brief acknowledgments. On the other hand, we may note that although someone is sitting quietly across from us, no active listening is going on. In these cases we may make a judgment that no communication is taking place.

In oral language conversation groups, interaction is elicited by posing questions to engage the participants in the interaction. In setting up the group, the facilitator discusses the purpose of the session and asks questions to prompt participants to explore how the session might be of value to them. Topics are then elicited from the participants. As they enter into the conversation, the facilitator suggests particular skills to focus on during the guided conversation. Throughout the conversation, the facilitator provides prompts and cues so that the participants experience success.

Similar procedures may be used to facilitate interaction in reading. Using question probes as a preset for reading, during the reading process, and as a follow-up to reading sets a context for interaction (Flores & Graves, 1986). Initially, students can be guided in exploring their interests or concerns. These concerns can provide a basis for choosing a text. Once a text is chosen, a preparatory set for interaction can be developed by asking students the following *prereading* questions:

- What do you think this will be about?
- What do you already know about this?
- What questions can you ask?

During reading, students are asked to attend to the major distinctions posed in the text. For expository text, it may be suggested that they read the study questions at the end of a chapter or skim the text, focusing on major headings (Risko & Alvarez, 1986). When reading a story, questions can be posed based on the structure of a story or story grammar (Stein & Glenn, 1979; Wallach & Miller, 1988).

The following can serve as a guide *during the reading of narratives:*

For expository text, it may be suggested that students read the study questions at the end of a chapter or skim the text, focusing on major headings.

- Who is it about? Where did it happen?
- What happened?
- What was the reaction?
- What did they try to do then?
- What happened then?
- What was the ending?

The above questions can also be used to guide the reconstruction of a narrative or to facilitate the construction of a story in writing. Flores and Graves (1986) suggest that students be encouraged to read a text several times. They may notice that they make different interpretations each time. Rereading can be used to demonstrate that there is no "getting the information in the text." Rather, each person may come away from the interaction with something different, and, moreover, the same person may construct different meanings from the same text at different points in time.

After reading, *follow-up* questions can stimulate further action:

- What did you see that you did not see before?
- What do you see is possible?
- What else would you like to know?

Reading a text, writing, and oral conversation are all opportunities for interaction and for developing competence. In each of these interactions, foundation skills may be developed to bring to the next interaction.

The facilitator acts as a metalinguistic guide

The facilitator may assist in developing conversational competence by both highlighting the regularities in the language and by offering opportunities to practice specific foundation skills. In conversation groups, the facilitator structures guided conversations and designs activities to practice foundation skills.

During guided conversations, the facilitator does not play a central role, but rather moderates or coaches. As a moderator, he or she directs the participants' attention to relevant conversational moves and reviews aspects of the conversation to assist them in observing effective patterns of interaction. As a coach, the facilitator provides prompts or cues to encourage successful interaction.

As the facilitator observes the need for specific foundation skills, activities can be planned to develop or practice them. Activities can be designed that are both interactive and functional. Interactive activities are those in which participants communicate to one another. They may ask each other questions or give directions, for example. Activities that are functional are those in which something happens as a result of the communication, for example, someone follows an instruction or responds to the question. Thus, foundation skills are also learned within an interactive context.

In facilitating the development of literacy in children, adults often act as metalinguistic guides. Van Kleeck and Schuele (1987) point out that children are introduced to books as sources of interaction within their homes as well as in other social situations. Between 2 and 4 years of age many normal children are guided to recognize relationships between words and print. Van Kleeck and Schuele point out that children develop an awareness that words are arbitrary distinctions and may, therefore, be used in a variety of ways. Furthermore, they begin to recognize word boundaries in the ongoing flow of speech. Lastly, they develop a phonological aware-

ness that allows them to see words as comprising sounds that can be modified to change the meanings of words, and they begin to recognize the relations between sounds and symbols. These distinctions about language become evident to most normal children as a function of participating in a literate culture.

Schuele and van Kleeck (1987) suggest introducing language-disordered children to literacy at the preschool level. They point out the need for them to participate in verbal exchanges about written material. This includes reading stories together, retelling stories, and asking and answering questions about stories. They underline the importance of introducing language-disordered children to the functions of written language by reading signs and labels, using recipes, following written directions, and writing and receiving letters.

Moore (1988) provides an overview of research on an approach to facilitating literacy termed "reciprocal teaching" (Brown & Palincsar, 1985; Palincsar & Brown, 1984). This is an interactive teaching technique in which a teacher works with a small group of students to facilitate reading comprehension. The teacher initially models a set of strategies for interacting with text: predicting, questioning, clarifying, and summarizing. The teacher begins by leading the group to read a text and use these strategies to analyze the text in a small group discussion. The teacher/facilitator then turns over responsibility for leading the discussion to the participants in the group. Moore (1988) reports that the research on reciprocal teaching with students across grade and ability levels demonstrates that "through active involvement in real reading contexts, strategies can and do make a difference to comprehension" (p. 6).

Palincsar and Brown's work on reciprocal teaching points to the similarities in facilitating interaction in spoken and written discourse (Palincsar & Brown, 1984). In reciprocal teaching, spoken and written discourse are interwoven. Oral discussion sets a context for reading and allows for clarification and interaction with others who are reading the text. Reading becomes another medium in which learning and interaction occur.

Similarly, in the conversational approach to literacy proposed here, reading and writing are taught as a process of facilitation. The facilitator guides the participants to use written language to interact and also teaches specific foundation skills needed to be effective in those interactions. Rather than introducing the reading process as a set of skills to be developed, the first move in facilitating literacy involves assisting students in identifying their interests and concerns. Students are guided to explore and choose texts for a variety of reasons: to be entertained, to answer questions, to learn how to do things. They are encouraged to engage in the reading process by addressing the prereading questions outlined in the previous section.

As language-disordered children begin to interact with texts, they are assisted in building foundation skills needed to understand the relationship between meaning and text. This can be achieved by assisting them in building a repertoire of words they recognize as whole units. They may also benefit from learning to gain meaning from verbal and nonverbal contextual cues. In addition, they can be assisted in building skills in segmenting words into sylla-

bles. Lastly, they may need particular assistance developing phonological awareness. These skills are introduced as alternative strategies for engaging in meaningful interactions in the medium of text.

Facilitation of literacy as described here is not done in a linear way. Instead, the learner is introduced to the discourse and is assisted in developing effective interactions. A range of strategies may be offered to allow the learner to interact effectively. The choice and sequence of strategies to be learned will depend on the individual learner's strengths and weaknesses.

The approach to facilitating language and literacy presented here is an outgrowth of the current perspective on language as a social-interactive phenomenon. New developments in the study of language learning have led to the current thesis that language is not learned as an analytic, linear process, but rather as a process of participating in a discourse. This shift in perspective brings with it a new view of not only spoken language, but also of written language. Although these two mediums of interaction differ, the basic principles of language learning hold true for both. Continuing to examine the implications of an interactive view of language may be of value for professionals working with language-disordered individuals as they design new intervention practices and explore the implications of their roles as facilitators of language learning.

CONTINUING THE CONVERSATION

Good conversations leave one with further questions to pursue. With that in mind, the following questions and preliminary reflections are offered.

> *Continuing to examine the implications of an interactive view of language may be of value for professionals working with language-disordered individuals as they design new intervention practices.*

What does it mean to become literate? Hirsch (1987) suggests that to be literate is to participate in one's culture. Flores and Graves (1986) take this one step further to suggest that to become literate is to participate in the discourses that comprise a culture. The process of education can, then, be seen as a process of introducing others to these discourses. Some of these discourses may be seen as the fields of biology, physics, history, or mathematics. They exist as an intricate web of both spoken and written conversations.

What does it mean to facilitate others in the process of becoming literate? To facilitate becoming literate is to introduce students to the conversations that exist and to invite them to participate actively. Initially, this means introducing them to the opportunities in oral and written conversations. Following that, a range of skills can be taught as strategies to negotiate those interactions.

Clearly, most children need more than simply to be introduced to the opportunity. They must also be taught the skills needed to participate. As Bruner (1985) points out, in the development of oral language, these skills are learned as part of an interactive "dance" between child and caretaker or facilitator. Although this "introduction to the dance" happens naturally for the normal language learner, what can be learned about these interactive patterns that can assist language specialists in acting as facilitators for those with language disorders? How can the facilitator structure the learning situation so that the predictable formats of both spoken and written discourse become part of the child's interactive schema?

• • •

How does participating in a discourse through listening, speaking, or writing influence the development of one's sense of self? We continue to develop ourselves as communicators whenever we read something new, whenever we sit down to write, and whenever we engage in conversation. Maturana and Varela (1987) suggest that we continue to invent ourselves constantly in language. We not only are continuously learning language, but, in our interactions in language, we are constantly developing the narratives that comprise who we are, how we think of ourselves, and how we present ourselves to others.

In the study of language learning, we, as language specialists, have learned much about language, about learning, and about ourselves as facilitators of learning. As we continue to explore the language-learning process, we are certain to find valuable parallels as well as intriguing differences in the development of oral language, reading, and writing. We are beginning to establish a comprehensive frame of reference for the development of language and literacy. Our explorations should leave us better equipped to be effective facilitators in the teaching and learning process.

REFERENCES

Bashir, A., Kuban, K., Kleinman, S., & Scavuzzo, A. (1983). Issues in language disorders: Considerations of cause, maintenance, and change. In J. Miller, D. Yoder, & R. Schieflebusch (Eds.), *ASHA Report No. 12.* Rockville, MD: American Speech–Language–Hearing Association.

Bashir, A., Wiig, E., & Abrams, J. (1987). Language disorders in childhood and adolescence: Implications for learning and socialization. *Pediatric Annals, 16*(2), 145–156.

Bates, E. (1976). *Language and context.* New York: Academic Press.

Bates, E. (1979). *The emergence of symbols: Cognition and communication in infancy.* New York: Academic Press.

Bedrosian, J.L. (1985). An approach to developing conversational competence. In D.N. Newberry Ripich & F.M. Spinelli (Eds.), *School discourse problems.* San Diego, CA: College Hill Press.

Blank, M., & Marquis, M.A. (1987). *Directing discourse.* Tucson, AZ: Communication Skill Builders.

Bloom, L. (1978). The integration of form, content, and use in language development. In J.K. Kavanagh & W. Strange (Eds.), *Speech and language in the laboratory, school and clinic.* Cambridge, MA: MIT Press.

Brown, A., & Palincsar, A. (1985). *Reciprocal teaching of comprehension strategies: A natural history of one programme for enhancing learning* (Tech. Rep. No. 334). Urbana, IL: University of Illinois Center for the Study of Reading.

Bruner, J. (1975). The ontogenesis of speech acts. *Journal of Child Language, 2,* 1–19.

Bruner, J. (1985). The role of interaction formats in language acquisition, In J.P. Forgas (Ed.), *Language and social situations.* New York: Springer-Verlag.

Catts, H.W., & Kahmi, A.G. (1986). The linguistic basis of reading disorders: Implications for the speech-language pathologist. *Language, Speech, and Hearing Services in Schools, 17,* 329–341.

Chafe, W. (1985). Linguistic differences produced by differences between speaking and writing. In D.R. Olson, N. Torrance, & S. Hildyard (Eds.), *Literacy, language, and learning.* New York: Cambridge University Press.

Chafe, W., & Danielewicz, J. (1987). Properties of spoken and written language. In R. Horowitz & S.J. Samuels (Eds.), *Comprehending oral and written language.* San Diego, CA: Academic Press.

Chall, J. (1983). *Stages of reading development.* New York: McGraw-Hill.

Comkowycz, S.M., Ehren, B.J., & Hayes, N.H. (1987). Meeting classroom needs of language disordered stu-

dents in middle and junior high schools: A program model. *Journal of Childhood Communication Disorders, 11*(1), 199–208.

Duchan, J.F., & Weitzner-Lin, B. (1987). Nurturant-naturalistic intervention for language-impaired children: Implications for planning lessons and tracking progress. *Asha, 29*(7), 45–49.

Dudley-Marling, C.C., & Rhodes, L.K. (1987). Pragmatics and literacy. *Language, Speech, and Hearing Services in Schools, 18,* 41–52.

Flores, F., & Graves, M. (1986). *Reading a Text.* Unpublished manuscript.

Goodman, K.S., Goodman, Y.M. (1977). Learning about psycholinguistic processes by analyzing oral reading. *Harvard Educational Review, 47*(3), 317–333.

Halliday, M.A.K. (1975). *Learning how to mean.* London: Edward Arnold.

Hirsch, E.D. (1987). *Cultural literacy: What every American needs to know.* Boston: Houghton Mifflin.

Horowitz, R., & Samuels, J.S. (1987). *Comprehending oral and written language.* San Diego, CA: Academic Press.

Hoskins, B. (1987). *Conversations: Language intervention for adolescents.* Allen, TX: DLM/Teaching Resources.

Hoskins, B. (1988, November). *Facilitating conversational interaction in adolescents: An effectiveness study.* Paper presented at the annual convention of the American Speech–Language–Hearing Association, Boston.

Howe, C. (1981). *Acquiring language in a conversational context.* New York: Academic Press.

Israel, L. (1984). Word knowledge and word retrieval: Phonological and semantic strategies. In G.P. Wallach & K.G. Butler (Eds.), *Language learning disabilities in school-age children.* Baltimore: Williams & Wilkins.

Kintsch, W. (1988). The role of knowledge in discourse comprehension: A construction-integration model. *Psychological Review, 95*(2), 163–182.

Larson, V.L., & McKinley, N.I. (1985). General intervention principles with language impaired adolescents. *Topics in Language Disorders, 5*(3), 70–77.

Marvin, C.A. (1987). Consultation services: Changing roles for SLPs. *Journal of Childhood Communication Disorders, 11*(1), 1–15.

Maturana, H.R., Varela, F.J. (1987). *The tree of knowledge.* Boston: New Science Library, Shambhala Publications.

Mehan, H. (1979). *Learning lessons.* Boston: Harvard University Press.

Menyuk, P. (1983). Language development and reading. In T.M. Gallagher & C.A. Prutting (Eds.), *Pragmatic assessment and intervention issues in language*. San Diego, CA: College Hill Press.

Moerk, E.L. (1977). *Pragmatic and semantic aspects of early language development*. Baltimore: University Park Press.

Moore, P.J. (1988). Reciprocal teaching and reading comprehension: A review. *Journal of Research in Reading, 11*(1), 3–14.

Nystrand, M. (1987). The role of context in written communication. In R. Horowitz & J.S. Samuels (Eds.), *Comprehending oral and written language*. San Diego, CA: Academic Press.

Olson, D.R., Torrance, N., & Hildyard, A. (1985). *Literacy, language, and learning*. New York: Cambridge University Press.

Palincsar, A., & Brown, A. (1984). Reciprocal teaching of comprehension fostering and monitoring activities. *Cognition and Instruction, 1*, 117–175.

Pehrsson, R.S., & Denner, P.R. (1988). Semantic organizers: Implications for reading and writing. *Topics in Language Disorders, 8*(3), 24–37.

Pehrsson, R.S., & Denner, P.R. (1989). *Semantic organizers, a study strategy for special needs learners*. Rockville, MD: Aspen Publishers.

Prutting, C. (1983). Scientific inquiry and communicative disorders: An emerging paradigm across six decades. In T.M. Gallagher & C.A. Prutting (Eds.), *Pragmatic assessment and intervention issues in language*. San Diego, CA: College Hill Press.

Risko, V.S., & Alvarez, M.C. (1986). An investigation of poor readers' use of a thematic strategy to comprehend text. *Reading Research Quarterly, 21*, 298–315.

Sawyer, D.J. (1985). Language problems observed in poor readers. In C.S. Simon (Ed.), *Communication skills and classroom success*. San Diego, CA: College Hill Press.

Schuele, C.M., & van Kleeck, A. (1987). Precursors to literacy: Assessment and intervention. *Topics in Language Disorders, 7*(2), 32–44.

Snow, C., Midkiff-Borunda, S., Small, A., & Proctor, A. (1984). Therapy as social interaction: Analyzing the contexts for language remediation. *Topics in Language Disorders, 4*(4), 72–85.

Snow, C.E. (1977). The development of conversations between mothers and babies. *Journal of Child Language, 4*, 1–22.

Stein, N.L., & Glenn, C.G. (1979). An analysis of story comprehension in elementary school children. In R.O. Freedle (Ed.), *New directions in discourse processing*. Hillsdale, NJ: Erlbaum.

Tannen, D. (1985). Relative focus on involvement in oral and written discourses. In D.R. Olson, N. Torrance, & A. Hildyard (Eds.), *Literacy, language, and learning*. New York: Cambridge University Press.

van Kleeck, A., & Schuele, C.M. (1987). Precursors to literacy: Normal development. *Topics in Language Disorders, 7*(2), 13–31.

Wallach, G.P., & Miller, L. (1988). *Language intervention and academic success*. San Diego, CA: College Hill Press.

Weir, R. (1962). *Language in the crib*. The Hague, Holland: Mouton.

Wells, G. (1981). *Learning through interaction*. New York: Cambridge University Press.

Wiig, E.H. (1984). Language disabilities in adolescents: A question of cognitive strategies. *Topics in Language Disorders, 4*, 51–58.

Williams, J.P. (1988). Identifying main ideas: A basic aspect of reading comprehension. *Topics in Language Disorders, 8*(3), 1–13.

Enhancing communication in adolescents with autism

Catherine Lord, PhD
Associate Professor
Department of Pediatrics
University of Alberta and Glenrose
  Rehabilitation Hospital
Edmonton, Alberta, Canada

FOR YOUNGSTERS with autism, as for other children, adolescence represents a time in which there are often marked shifts in interests, expectations, and problems, as well as continued development of skills acquired in childhood. Because the range of communication skills of autistic adolescents is broad, it is necessary to link specific strategies of intervention to particular levels of skill. The focus of this article, therefore, is on autistic adolescents who are verbal, with mild or no general mental retardation, who are in their mid- to late teens. This is in contrast to earlier articles that dealt with programs for adolescents with more limited language and cognitive abilities (Lord & O'Neill, 1983; Watson & Lord, 1982; Watson, Schaffer, Lord, & Schopler, 1988). The criterion here is not so much IQ as the youngsters' participation at some level of independence in the academic mainstream.

Top Lang Disord, 1988, 9(1), 72–81
© 1988 Aspen Publishers, Inc.

COMMUNICATION ISSUES
ARISING DURING ADOLESCENCE

By adolescence, a substantial proportion of autistic youngsters regularly use language to express their needs and to comprehend basic instructions. Cantwell, Baker, and Rutter (1978) found that high-functioning autistic subjects of older school age and early adolescence did not differ in the complexity of their syntax from IQ-matched children with severe receptive delays. However, many functional communication difficulties remained in the autistic group. Similar findings have been reported for other populations of autistic adolescents.

Some of the more obvious abnormalities associated with autism, such as immediate echolalia, are often outgrown by adolescence. However, difficulties in pragmatics almost always continue (Baltaxe, 1977; Lord et al. (in press); Simmons & Baltaxe, 1975). Few autistic adolescents or adults can hold a reciprocal conversation; some are very uncomfortable talking at all except to express their needs; others may engage in long monologues, repeatedly ask the same questions, or talk to themselves (Rumsey, Rapoport, & Sceery, 1985). Intonation and rhythm remain notably odd (Baltaxe & Simmons, 1983), while grammar and use of words may be unusual or stereotyped (Lord & O'Neill, 1983).

Pragmatic aspects of language become especially significant at adolescence because the youngsters often become more interested in interacting with people outside the family. By this age, family members may have become so accustomed to each others' idiosyncratic ways of communicating that pragmatics are virtually transparent. However, when the adolescent has to deal with strangers or peers, *how* communications are made once again become as important as *what* the communications are. This interest in being with peers, and, even more so, experience in social situations outside the home, are areas of individual difference within a group of high-functioning autistic teenagers. Though few autistic persons have "real" friends (in the sense of true intimacy as well as shared activities) (LeCouteur et al., in press), some attend regular schools and some participate in a variety of community activities. Others may have very limited interactions even with siblings (O'Neill & Lord, 1982). The widening of social goals and individual differences in experience and motivation have definite implications for communication goals for adolescents.

Social needs for communication may also expand as relationships within the family change. Autistic adolescents may show the same desire for independence as their peers, but even more inconsistently than other teenagers. How much independence they can have is affected by their judgment and skills and also by family patterns of protectiveness, activities, or encouragement. These patterns are often related to the adolescents' functional communication skills.

It can be difficult for older autistic youngsters to find age-appropriate activities that interest them. Parents may be too tired after years of keeping their child busy to maintain intense schedules of planned activities with an adolescent. The possibility of using language as a leisure activity (e.g., reading, writing) also has implications for communication planning.

Similarly, at school, autistic adolescents may find themselves with no appropriate placement. Academically oriented programs may be too abstract or difficult, while vocational programs often assume relatively good social skills and specific interests, such as in mechanics or clerical work that are not relevant to many autistic youngsters. An autistic teenager who has some academic skills (e.g., who can read at a fourth or fifth grade level or higher; who can do some basic arithmetic), but who needs practice in applying these skills to functional, vocational, and leisure activities may be difficult to place in regular academic or vocational classes. Individualized planning, with communication and language needs as an important component, is critical.

To summarize, three changes associated with increasing independence and development have been identified as reasons for shifting communication goals as youngsters with autism enter adolescence. These include a widening of social interests and horizons, a need for age-appropriate leisure activities, and identification of requisite communication skills for greater independence and vocational planning.

RECENT CHANGES IN APPROACHES TO COMMUNICATION

Recent shifts in the emphases of communication programs have made many professionals better prepared to address the practical communication needs of adolescents with autism than in previous years (Lord & O'Neill, 1983). Communication is now almost automatically considered in the contexts in which it occurs—in terms of what the adolescent needs to learn, and how, when, and where he or she will use these skills. Programs specifically aimed at generalizing behaviors across contexts are now readily available to teachers and clinicians, though it would be interesting to see how much they are really used. Social aspects of language are routinely considered, as are the possible communicative roles of many specific behaviors, such as echolalia (Prizant & Wetherby, 1985).

In the last five years, greater attention has been paid to the role of nonverbal skills in communication (Mundy, Sigman, Ungerer, & Sherman, 1986). Especially with younger children, there has also been greater emphasis on peers in improving the social interactions of autistic children (Odom & Strain, 1986). A related approach from a different perspective has been activity-oriented groups designed to improve functional communication (Mesibov, 1984; Williams, in press).

Yet there is still much about communication in autistic persons that is not well understood. Relatively little is known about language comprehension, except that it often remains surprisingly poor even in adolescence (Lord & O'Neill, 1983; Cantwell, Baker, & Rutter, 1978). The relationship between nonverbal communication and language has barely been addressed, though there is suggestive evidence that the coordination of vocal and nonverbal behaviors may be a particular area of deficit (Lord, 1984; Magill & Lord, in press). The interface between cognition and social development has been an area of great interest, but the exact nature of this relationship is far from clear (Baron-Cohen, Leslie, & Frith, 1986; Hobson, 1986). Little is known about secondary effects of unfamiliarity, varying cognitive demands, and lack of social experience or knowledge on communication (Lord & Garfin, 1986; Lord & Magill, 1988). Finally, while IQ and language ability have been identified as factors in prognosis, little is known about what factors relate to "positive" outcome within a population of

While IQ and language ability have been identified as factors in prognosis, little is known about what factors relate to "positive" outcome within a population of relatively high-functioning, verbal adolescents and adults.

relatively high-functioning, verbal adolescents and adults (Bartak & Rutter, 1976). Although some information is available about developmental changes in specific aspects of communication, what these characteristics have to do with how well individual youngsters do as adolescents or adults is not known.

In fact, to date, positive outcome seems to have been defined principally by the lack of certain very negative features, such as institutionalization, complete social isolation, or the need for constant supervision and/or intensive psychiatric treatment (Lotter, 1974a, 1974b; Rutter, Greenfeld, & Lockyer, 1967). What are reasonable, positive expectations for an autistic adolescent with near-normal or

normal nonverbal intelligence? Clearly these questions have to be answered on individual bases as they relate to the needs of the individual student, the benefits and disadvantages of the available programs, and the aspect of communication considered (e.g., expressing oneself, understanding others). One must ask about both the amount and the success of communication by autistic youngsters in different residential and academic settings. As professionals, we must resist the temptation to accept simple answers to complex questions. For example, it may be an achievement for all concerned that an autistic adolescent boy attends regular high school classes, but if he has little or no spontaneous positive interaction with his classmates, then clearly, there is work to be done.

IDENTIFYING GOALS, RESOURCES, AND STRATEGIES FOR COMMUNICATION BY AUTISTIC ADOLESCENTS

Below is an attempt to identify positive goals for outcome, both overall and for communication, defined in terms of language, social, and cognitive needs of autistic individuals. Examples of specific objectives and associated treatment approaches are given for each goal.

Goal 1: To participate in age-appropriate social relationships outside the family

While it is difficult to select reasonable positive objectives from among all the communicative behaviors carried out by normally developing adolescents, several are suggested here out of many possible choices. Both research and clinical experience indicate that the following are feasible ideas with potential for immediate effects on social interaction, and that these behaviors are important aspects of interactions among normally developing adolescents or are obvious deficits in the behavioral repertoires of adolescents with autism.

Rituals

Rituals are communicative behaviors that are gradually modified into socially acceptable, conventional patterns of greetings or conversation openers. When such a ritual occurs, it is easier for the recipient to infer communicative intent (Lord & Magill, 1988; Prizant & Wetherby, 1985) than when the behavior pattern is less predictable. Along the same line, rituals typically involve predictable behaviors from both parties, so that they provide an autistic adolescent who is socially unsure with both a way of beginning an interaction and a way of evoking a predictable response from the other person. Rituals of greeting, parting, introducing oneself, asking for help, asking for clarification, and entering conversations can all be memorized, practiced, and used in many circumstances. Thus, rituals provide a concrete way for even a relatively socially unskilled person to enter an interaction and to structure it so that it is more comprehensible and predictable.

Conversely, a recent series of observational studies of social behavior among normally developing, behavior-disordered, and autistic peers in integrated social groups suggests that it is the normally developing children who violated the expected rituals, or at the least, modified them depending on many subtle cues (Lord & Magill, 1988; Magill & Lord, in press). Thus, providing autistic adolescents with a well-rehearsed greeting ritual does not necessarily make them "normal," but, nevertheless, may help them communicate more appropriately and effectively. At a minimum, rituals are a worthwhile approach to communication because they provide an entry point to interaction (Prizant & Wetherby, 1985).

Rituals can also provide positive alternatives to unusual behaviors sometimes produced by autistic individuals. These unusual behaviors can prevent communicative attempts from resulting in interactions, because a recipient does not know how to respond or even know that an initiation has been attempted (Lord & Magill, 1988; Magill, 1986). It is therefore suggested that in an interaction, the focus must be not only in teaching the ritual (e.g., when you see someone whom you like, stop walking, look right at them, and say "Hello"), but also to teach autistic youngsters to attend, at least at some level, to how the ritual fits in with the behavior of the other person (e.g., make sure that the other person is looking at you before you talk; do not insist on shaking hands with a young child or someone whose hands are full).

Identifying topics

Research with normally developing children has indicated that one of the most successful entry behaviors of children joining groups is simply to join in with whatever the group is doing (Dodge, Coie, & Brakke, 1982). In a way, this behavior is the opposite of a ritual, because it is completely context dependent. Recent studies of how children converse in groups have indicated that this joining in is a complex developmental process that is acquired gradually in the school years and teens (Dorval & Eckerman, 1984). One of the most complicated components is identifying the topic of the conversation, since often ongoing group topics are implicit, rather than identified clearly. For example, the statement "my grandmother and I saw a grizzly bear last weekend in the mountains" could be a contribution to discussions of last weekend, trips to the mountains, frightening experiences, grandparents, nearly extinct animals, or an implicit reference to an earlier conversation about storms.

Topics of conversation are relevant issues for autistic youngsters for several reasons. Adolescents with autism may have a particularly difficult time identifying implicit topics in ongoing conversations because they are unable to follow the nonverbal, as well as verbal cues, that modulate the direction of talk (Lord & Magill, 1988; Rutter, 1985). They also may not have the unstated knowledge shared by other participants about facts underlying specific statements (e.g., that grizzly bears are nearly extinct) or even if they have the knowledge (e.g., that it was raining last weekend), they may not realize that it is relevant to this instance (Lord, 1984; Tager-Flusberg, 1981). Autistic children and adolescents often choose somewhat unusual topics about which to speak or have difficulty shifting topics from one area to another when they are leading the conversation (Baltaxe, 1977; Rumsey, Rapoport, & Sceery, 1985).

As with the rituals, intervention can take the form of overtly structuring a rather unstructured process by teaching the autistic adolescent both self-prompts and ways of cuing the other person that help is needed. Providing clear guidelines that one must not talk, but *listen* for a while and *then* identify the topic when joining a conversation may be a start. Autistic adolescents and adults have also been taught to confirm the topic (e.g., "Are you talking about summer vacations?") or to check the appropriateness of one they might suggest (e.g., "Do you like to talk about elevations?") (Mesibov, 1984; Williams, in press). Although this process may seem artificial, in many ways it is just exaggerating and formalizing the communications that normally take the form of sighs, shifts in eye gaze, and changes in intonation patterns.

Practicing conversations may not solve the problem, but at least gives the adolescent a chance to build up some skill at identifying and following topics (McGee, Krantz, & McClannahan, 1984). Thus, selection of topics that are both age and culturally appropriate and of some interest to the autistic person can be helpful. Extending vocabulary programs from earlier years to include words and contexts chosen to meet current needs can address the autistic person's need for more knowl-

---

Extending vocabulary programs from earlier years to include words and contexts chosen to meet current needs can address the autistic person's need for more knowledge to back up his or her participation in conversation.

edge to back up his or her participation in conversation. It may be particularly useful to select terms and topics important to other teenagers.

Goal 2: The ability to use language to pursue one's interests

A second goal is to help adolescents use language to learn, develop their own interests, and participate as independently and fully as possible in everyday experiences. While this goal overlaps with the previous one, since there are social aspects to almost all experiences, the emphasis here is on learning and carrying out activities for their own sake. Reading (especially decoding) is an area of strength for some autistic adolescents (Cobrinik, 1974; Frith & Snowling, 1983) as is spelling (Rumsey, Rapoport, & Sceery, 1985).

Reading and spelling are modes of language that do not require *immediate* social interaction and so provide potential leisure activities that do not demand complicated plans or social pressure. In addition, reading and writing provide ways of acquiring new knowledge that, as discussed earlier, may lead to greater ability to participate in society.

Developing interests through reading and writing

A difficulty often encountered is that the autistic person's ability to decode far exceeds his or her comprehension of written or oral language, especially connected discourse, such as stories or essays. A person who can decode at a 12-year-old level but comprehend passages at a 7-year-old level is no better off practically than a person who reads at a 7-year-old level

overall. (Sometimes an even worse situation develops in which reading becomes a "parlor trick," separate from any meaningful activity.) The question therefore becomes how to make reading and writing meaningful, useful, and enjoyable to the adolescent with autism.

Many autistic persons have developed their own way of using their strengths and avoiding areas of difficulty by reading material such as maps, books of lists, timetables, television guides, and certain types of manuals. In these materials, the demands for comprehension are limited, but the words to be read can be quite varied. Newspapers and news magazines also fit in this category. If reading seems to be a source of pleasure for the youngster, helping him or her identify and obtain age-appropriate as well as comprehension-level-appropriate materials can be useful.

Developing a special interest in reading or writing about a topic, with a clear way of pursuing it, can be particularly exciting if there are social opportunities or activities associated with it. Thus, promoting an interest in model railroads, Trivial Pursuit, soap operas, or botany may help identify comprehensible reading material and also introduce a teenager to a population of people with similar interests. Although this strategy may appear at first glance to be exacerbating preoccupations, it is based on a recognition of individual differences in skill and interest that characterize autistic and nonautistic persons alike. Encouraging such interests in a structured way in the classroom, at home, or in a communication group is similar to the requirement in a high school class for each student to write essays and book reports on chosen topics, with the teacher's hope that an area will catch a student's fancy. For teenagers who already have such interests, finding ways that they can use their knowledge to go beyond memorization, such as volunteering in a record store or working in a special collections section of a library or even summarizing the news for family members at supper, can make the difference between a meaningless preoccupation and a meaningful interest.

Somewhere in between preoccupations and special interests that easily facilitate social interaction are activities such as word-finding games, word-oriented game shows, some computer games, making scrap books, writing simple stories, and answering offers for free brochures. If such activities are enjoyed by the youngster, then they are surely as worthwhile as reading romance novels or watching hockey games. However, their value may lie primarily in giving adolescents activities they enjoy and in which they can experience some success, rather than expanding knowledge or social opportunities.

Functional uses of language in everyday life

In the last decade, programs for severely retarded youngsters have come to focus on everyday needs almost exclusively. A paradox in many educational programs currently available is that practical aspects of communication in the community are addressed less often for higher-functioning older children and adolescents with autism than they may be for far more handicapped children. Thus, while a severely retarded child may be taught at

school to use a bus token or select groceries by matching labels, it is often left up to the family to teach a nonretarded autistic teenager what to say to a bus driver and where to sit, how to make a shopping list, or how to make and keep track of an appointment for a haircut.

Families vary enormously in the extent to which they offer their high-functioning autistic children opportunities to acquire such everyday skills. Families also differ in how structured an approach they use, if and when they try to teach these skills, and how much opportunity youngsters are given to try out and practice new behaviors, once they are mastered. Many of these skills are acquired by normally developing youngsters through modeling peers or imitating family members. Often with normally developing teenagers, the pressure comes from *them* to expand their independence. Thus, it simply may not occur to parents that their autistic youngster can and does need to learn such things and needs help to do so. For example, if no one in the family uses public transportation, parents may not realize that this is an appropriate way for their autistic teenager to travel.

In addition, teaching any particular skill may be time consuming and difficult for many reasons, particularly because the motivation for learning this skill may not be great unless it is provided externally. To expect an autistic teenager to learn to take a bus in order to go to a typing course in which he or she is not particularly interested or to make a shopping list to buy food for a well-balanced diet, may negatively bias the acquisition of that skill. For normally developing teenagers, the rewards for learning such skills include a sense of freedom and a feeling of adult social competence. These two aspects of development may not mean much yet to an autistic adolescent whose major bid for independence may be in not cleaning up his or her own room. However, extrinsic awards (e.g., taking the bus to somewhere he or she wants to go) can be coupled with new privileges to make clear the message that others value these behaviors. Altogether, specific functional objectives for communication in the community are easy to identify, clearly needed, and relatively easy to attain with planning, structured teaching, and guided practice.

• • •

In conclusion, adolescence is a time when developing communication skills may provide more specific opportunities to extend individual interests and to increase independence. New skills also can be taught that meet the specific needs of a teenager's social life. Identifying positive goals for achievements during this period is particularly important to the facilitation of reasonable, achievable objectives and treatment approaches. Deriving these goals from consideration of the desired outcome for the individual in his or her environment, rather than from specific aspects of how he or she speaks, seems most likely to result in meaningful, effective treatment and consultation.

REFERENCES

Baron-Cohen, S., Leslie, A.M., & Frith, U. (1986). Mechanical, behavioural and intentional understanding of picture stories in autistic children. *British Journal of Developmental Psychology, 4*, 113–125.

Bartak, L., & Rutter, M. (1976). Differences between mentally retarded and normally intelligent autistic children. *Journal of Autism and Childhood Schizophrenia, 6*, 109–120.

Baltaxe, C. (1977). Pragmatic deficits in the language of autistic adolescents. *Journal of Pediatric Psychology, 2*, 176–180.

Baltaxe, C.A.M., & Simmons, J.Q. (1983). Communication deficits in the adolescent and adult autistic. *Seminars in Speech and Language, 4*, 27–42.

Cantwell, D.P., Baker, L., & Rutter, M. (1978). A comparative study of infantile autism and specific developmental receptive language disorder, IV. Analysis of syntax and language function. *Journal of Child Psychology and Psychiatry, 19*, 351–363.

Cobrinik, L. (1974). Unusual reading ability in the severely disturbed: Clinical observation and a retrospective inquiry. *Journal of Autism and Childhood Schizophrenia, 41*, 163–175.

Dodge, K.A., Coie, J.D., & Brakke, N.P. (1982). Behavior patterns of socially rejected and neglected preadolescents: The roles of social approach and aggression. *Journal of Abnormal Child Psychology, 10*, 389–409.

Dorval, B., & Eckerman, C.D. (1984). Developmental trends in the quality of conversation achieved by small groups of acquainted peers. *Monographs of the Society for Research in Child Development, 49.*

Frith, U., & Snowling, M. (1983). Reading for meaning and reading for sound in autistic and dyslexic children. *British Journal of Developmental Psychology, 1*, 329–342.

Hobson, R.P. (1986). The autistic child's appraisal of expressions of emotion. *Journal of Child Psychology and Psychiatry, 27*, 321–342.

LeCouteur, A., Rutter, M., Lord, C., Rios, P., Robertson, S., Holdgrafer, M., & McLennan, J.D. (in press). Autism diagnostic interview. *Journal of Autism and Developmental Disorders.*

Lord, C. (1984). Language comprehension and cognitive disorder in autism. In L. Siegel & F. Morrison (Eds.), *Cognitive development in atypical children* (pp. 67–82). New York: Springer-Verlag.

Lord, C., & Garfin, D. (1986). Facilitating peer-directed communication in autistic children and adolescents. *Australian Journal of Human Communication Disorders, 14*, 33–49.

Lord, C., & Magill, J. (1988). Observing social behaviour in an asocial population: Methodological and clinical issues. In G. Dawson (Ed.), *Autism: New perspectives on diagnosis, nature and treatment* (pp. 46–66). New York: Guildford Press.

Lord, C., & O'Neill, P.J. (1983). Language and communication needs of adolescents with autism. In E. Schopler & G. Mesibov (Eds.), *Autism through adolescence* (pp. 57–77). New York: Plenum Press.

Lord, C., Rutter, M.L., Goode, S., Heemsbergen, J., Jordan, H., & Mawhood, L. (in press). Autism Diagnostic Observation Schedule: A standardized method of observing social and communicative behaviour in persons with autism and other severe social deficits. *Journal of Autism and Developmental Disorders.*

Lotter, V. (1974a). Factors related to outcome in autistic children. *Journal of Autism and Childhood Schizophrenia, 4*, 263–277.

Lotter, V. (1974b). Social adjustment and placement of autistic children in Middlesex: A follow-up study. *Journal of Autism and Childhood Schizophrenia, 4*, 11–32.

Magill, J. (1986). *The nature of social deficits of children with autism.* Unpublished doctoral dissertation, University of Alberta.

Magill, J., & Lord, C. (in press). An observational study of greetings of autistic, behaviour-disordered and normally developing children. *Journal of Abnormal Child Psychology.*

McGee, G.G., Krantz, P.J., & McClannahan, L.E. (1984). Conversational skills for autistic adolescents: Teaching assertiveness in naturalistic game settings. *Journal of Autism and Developmental Disorders, 14*, 319–330.

Mesibov, G.B. (1984). Social skills training with verbal autistic adolescents and adults: A program model. *Journal of Autism and Developmental Disorders, 14*, 395–404.

Mundy, P., Sigman, M., Ungerer, J., & Sherman, T. (1986). Defining the social effects of autism: The contribution of nonverbal communication measures. *Journal of Child Psychology and Psychiatry, 27*, 657–669.

Odom, S.L., & Strain, P.S. (1986). Comparison of peer-initiation and teacher antecedent interventions for promoting reciprocal social interaction of autistic preschoolers. *Journal of Applied Behavior Analysis, 19*, 59–71.

O'Neill, P.J., & Lord, C. (1982). Functional and semantic characteristics of child-directed speech of autistic children. In D. Park (Ed.), *Proceedings from the International Meetings for the National Society for Autistic Children* (pp. 79–82). Washington, DC: National Society for Autistic Children.

Prizant, B.M., & Wetherby, A.M. (1985). Intentional communicative behavior of children with autism: Theoretical and practical issues. *Australian Journal of Human Communication Disorders, 13*, 23–59.

Rumsey, J.M., Rapoport, M.D., & Sceery, W.R. (1985). Autistic children as adults: Psychiatric, social, and behavioral outcomes. *Journal of the American Academy of Child Psychiatry, 24*, 465–473.

Rutter, M. (1985). Infantile autism and other pervasive disorders. In M. Rutter & L. Hersov (Eds.), *Child and adolescent psychiatry: Modern approaches* (pp. 545–566). London: Blackwell Scientific Publications.

Rutter, M., Greenfeld, D., & Lockyer, L. (1967). A five to fifteen year follow-up study of infantile psychosis. II. Social and behavioural outcome. *British Journal of Psychiatry, 113*, 1183–1199.

Simmons, J.Q., & Baltaxe, C. (1975). Language patterns of adolescent autistics. *Journal of Autism and Childhood Schizophrenia, 5*, 333–351.

Tager-Flusberg, H. (1981). Sentence comprehension in autistic children. *Applied Psycholinguistics, 2*, 5–24.

Watson, L.K., & Lord, C. (1982). Developing a social communication curriculum for autistic students. *Topics in Language Disorders, 3*, 1–9.

Watson, L., Schaffer, B., Lord, C., & Schopler, E. (1988). *A functional approach to communication for autistic children.* New York: Irvington Press.

Williams, T. (in press). A social skills group for autistic children. *Journal of Autism and Developmental Disorders.*

Index

A

AAC. *See* Augmentative and alternative communication (AAC)
Absolute retrieval strength, 159
Abstract vocabulary, 55, 56
Abstraction, 58
Academic deficits, of secondary-school students, 174–175
Access, SSPI intervention strategies and, 121
Accountability procedures, 9
Action schema, 78
Activities, metacognitive orientation and, 179
Activities of daily living, literacy events, 6
Adolescents
  autistic, 218
    age-appropriate social relationship participation and, 221–226
    communication and, 219–220
    communication approaches, recent changes in, 220–221
    goal identification, 221–226
    IQ and, 221
    language ability and, 221
    rituals and, 222
    topic identification and, 222–224
  communication issues of, 219–220
  learning-disabled, 173–174
    academic deficits, 174–175
    characteristics, 175

    environmental demands, 175–176
    instructional interventions, 176–177
Adult-centered clinical discourse. *See* Discourse, clinical, adult-centered
Adult-child interaction
  emergent literacy and, 7–10
  in literacy events, 4–5
African-American families, 5, 9
ALL (Analysis of the Language of Learning), 18
Alliteration, 12, 19
Alphabetic systems, 140
America 2000, 116
American Sign Language (ASL), 132–133
Analysis of the Language of Learning (ALL), 18
Answering questions, on book information, 16–17
ASL (American Sign Language), 132–133
Assessment
  of emergent literacy, 17–18
  formal, of preschool print literacy, 17–18
  of metalinguistic awareness, 44
  phonological awareness and, 96–98
  of whole language program, 43–44
Attribution retraining, reading performance and, 180
Augmentative and alternative communication (AAC)
  communicative interaction and, 26–28
  as context variable, 25
  systems
    communication interaction and, 26–27
    context variables, 31
    nature of, 32

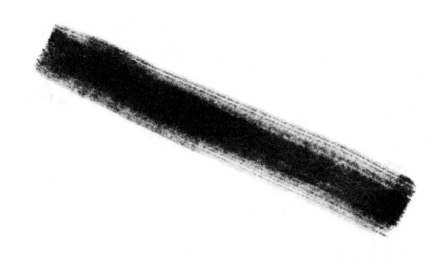

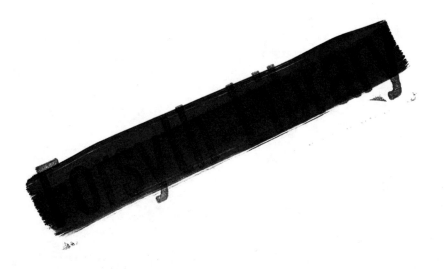